NEUROSCIENCE

A CLINICAL PERSPECTIVE

JOAN K. WERNER, P.T., Ph.D.

Director, Physical Therapy Program;
Formerly with the Department of Anatomy,
University of Wisconsin School of Medicine,
Madison, Wisconsin

ILLUSTRATIONS BY LUCY TAYLOR

W. B. SAUNDERS COMPANY

Philadelphia, London, Toronto

W. B. Saunders Company: West Washington Square
Philadelphia, PA 19105

1 St. Anne's Road
Eastbourne, East Sussex BN21 3UN, England

1 Goldthorne Avenue
Toronto, Ontario M8Z 5T9, Canada

Library of Congress Cataloging in Publication Data

Werner, Joan K

Neuroscience, a clinical perspective.

Bibliography: p.
Includes index.

1. Neuroanatomy. I. Title. [DNLM: 1. Nervous system—Anatomy and histology. 2. Nervous system—Physiology. 3. Nervous system diseases. WL100.3 W493n]

QM451.W47 611′.8 79-64779

ISBN 0-7216-9116-1

NEUROSCIENCE—A Clinical Perspective ISBN 0-7216-9116-1

Last digit is the print number: 9 8 7 6 5 4 3 2

PREFACE

This text is designed to provide a basic understanding of the nervous system for all students who are preparing for a career in the medical sciences. The major portion consists of information accumulated by the author in 12 years' experience in a variety of clinical settings and during the last seven years of teaching neuroanatomy in the Anatomy Department, University of Wisconsin Medical School–Madison.

The objective of the book is to correlate structure and function of the central and peripheral nervous systems, so that the clinician can understand abnormalities in nervous system function encountered in the clinic as well as the rationale on which treatment procedures are based. To accomplish this objective, descriptions of structures, pathways and interconnections are accompanied by numerous illustrations, and the functional implications of the morphology are discussed. Following the discussion of structure and function in each section is an application of this basic information to the clinical environment, through explanations of neurologic deficits and treatment procedures.

This is a book for the beginning neurosciences student who has some understanding of gross human anatomy. It is not intended to be a source of detailed information, which can be obtained from those textbooks designed for advanced students.

ACKNOWLEDGMENTS

I wish to thank all those who have made valuable contributions to this book: Mary Jane Meng for her help in the early stages of preparation of the manuscript and for her contribution to Chapter 14; Janet C. Lemke for her contributions to Chapter 15; T. P. Stewart for the excellent photographic work in Chapter 6; and Steven J. Phillips for his thoughtful review of and excellent suggestions for the text and illustrations. I am especially grateful to have had the opportunity to work with Lucy C. Taylor, who is responsible for the preparation of the illustrations in this text. I am most fortunate that Lucy was willing to share her incredible talent, and I thank her for her infinite patience and her persistent probing to make sure that the end product placed the emphasis of the illustrations correctly, all of which contributed to a thoroughly enjoyable relationship. I am also most grateful for the excellent cooperation and guidance in editing and preparing this text for publication given me by Marie D. Low and her editorial staff at W. B. Saunders Company.

JOAN K. WERNER, P.T., Ph.D.

CONTENTS

CHAPTER 1 • INTRODUCTION TO THE NERVOUS SYSTEM

OBJECTIVES

After reading this chapter you should: • Be able to diagram and completely label a generalized nerve cell. • Understand the functional implications of the distribution of ribonucleic acid in the nerve cell. • Understand the functions of the organelles of the nerve cell. • Be able to illustrate axons with their sheaths. • Be aware of the dangers in interpreting material stained by the various methods discussed. • Know the morphologic types of synapses that exist. • Know the sequence of events involved in impulse transmission. • Understand how the strength of the influence of the presynaptic on the postsynaptic element may vary. • Understand the function of the glial cells and know from which embryonic layers they are derived.

WHY STUDY NEUROSCIENCE?

The immediate question that arises is, why is it necessary for prospective health professionals to study and understand the nervous system? The answer is simply that one cannot understand the abnormalities that will be encountered in the nervous system without a thorough knowledge of its normal structure and function.

Throughout this book we will be searching for a basic understanding of the function of the brain, spinal cord and peripheral nervous system. In so doing, we will concentrate on the brain of man, but it is important to realize that much of our knowledge of neural organization comes from studies of subhuman primates, other mammals, and many vertebrate and invertebrate species.

We actually know relatively little about how the brain works, especially about the fundamental processes involved in speech, thought and memory. However, we do understand something of the neural mechanisms subserving various types of sensations and something about the basis of motor control, and these are the areas on which the emphasis has been put in this book.

In order to facilitate the initiation of the study of the nervous system, after examining the nerve cell, synapses and glial cells, we will start with an area with which those who have learned some gross anatomy will have some familiarity, the peripheral nervous system. Subsequently we will study the structures of the spinal cord and brain, and finally degeneration and regeneration in the nervous system, concluding with a general summary of central nervous system lesions and their evaluation. As we ascend in the central nervous system (CNS), the student will learn to understand how structures of the neuraxis are interconnected, and thus how sensory input may elicit motor responses after being processed through a number of internal neural circuits. It is this kind of understanding that is essential if we are to realize the effects that may be produced by destruction of neural structures or their interconnections, and those which we produce by sensory stimulation of our patients in the therapeutic environment.

THE NERVE CELL

Nerve cells are unique among all cells in the body because they can be depolarized and therefore are capable of propagating action potentials along their axons. Muscle cells can also be depolarized, but they do not carry information for long distances as do nerve cells. Because of this unique function of nerves, the central and peripheral nervous systems act as the primary integrating system of organisms. The CNS also determines the nature of man as distinct from other species. One of man's major advantages is the command of language, which permits the transmission of culture.

In 1891 Waldeyer formulated the neuron doctrine, which states that "the individual nerve cell is the genetic, anatomic, trophic and functional unit of the nervous system." For many years there was an active dispute between those who believed in the neuron doctrine and those who favored the syncytium theory. The latter group thought that the entire nervous system was continuous, with no membranes interposed between individual nerve cells. Relatively recently, the electron microscope and cytochemical experimentation have provided answers to many of the fine structural and functional questions regarding neurons. Information acquired by use of these experimental tools has validated all of the original tenets of the neuron doctrine, and the syncytium theory has been discarded.

The morphology of nerve cells varies greatly in different parts of the CNS (see Fig. 1–1), but it is possible to generalize and say that the vertebrate neuron consists of a cell body, also called the perikaryon, several dendrites and one axon. A specialized portion of the perikaryon which serves as the usual point of origin of the axon is called the axon hillock. The part of the axon between its origin and the site where it becomes myelinated is the initial segment of the axon. The nerve cell bodies and their processes (axons and dendrites) are surrounded by a three-layered plasma membrane similar to that of most tissue cells. The plasma membrane consists of a lipid layer approximately 30 angstroms thick, situated between two layers of protein approximately 25 angstroms thick.

Figure 1–2 shows the major features of a generalized nerve cell.

The perikaryon consists of a large, pale staining nucleus with a prominent nucleolus. The nucleus is surrounded by cytoplasm, which contains the same organelles and inclusions observed in other tissue cells, with the exception of neurofibrils, which are uniquely characteristic of nerve cells.

There are two types of nucleic acid in the cell, desoxyribonucleic acid (DNA), the location of which is restricted to the chromatin, and ribonucleic acid (RNA), which is most abundant in the perikaryon. There is also some RNA located in the dendrites, but it is absent in the axon and its hillock. The nucleic acids are contained in ribosomes, which may be loosely scattered in the cytoplasm, or in clumps called polysomes. They are also found in close association with cisternae, in which case they are called rough endoplasmic reticulum when their ultrastructure is observed, or Nissl substance when observed with the light microscope. The nucleic acids are protein producers and the implications of their distribution should be clearly understood. Since the great majority of ribosomes are located in the perikaryon, presumably most of the nerve cell proteins are produced there and are then distributed to the nerve cell processes. The proteins distribute throughout the axons by a process called axoplasmic flow, of which there is a rapid component (100 to 900 mm/day) and a slow component (1 to 4 mm/day). Distribution of proteins throughout the nerve cell is essential to maintain the integrity of the cell and to replace proteins that are continually being used by it. Because the nerve cell processes are dependent on the cell body for their supply of proteins, they will degenerate if they become separated from it.

Neurofibrils are made up of aggregations of neurofilaments (about 100 angstroms in diameter) and neurotubules (200 to 300 angstroms in diameter). They are located in all parts of all nerve cells. Their precise func-

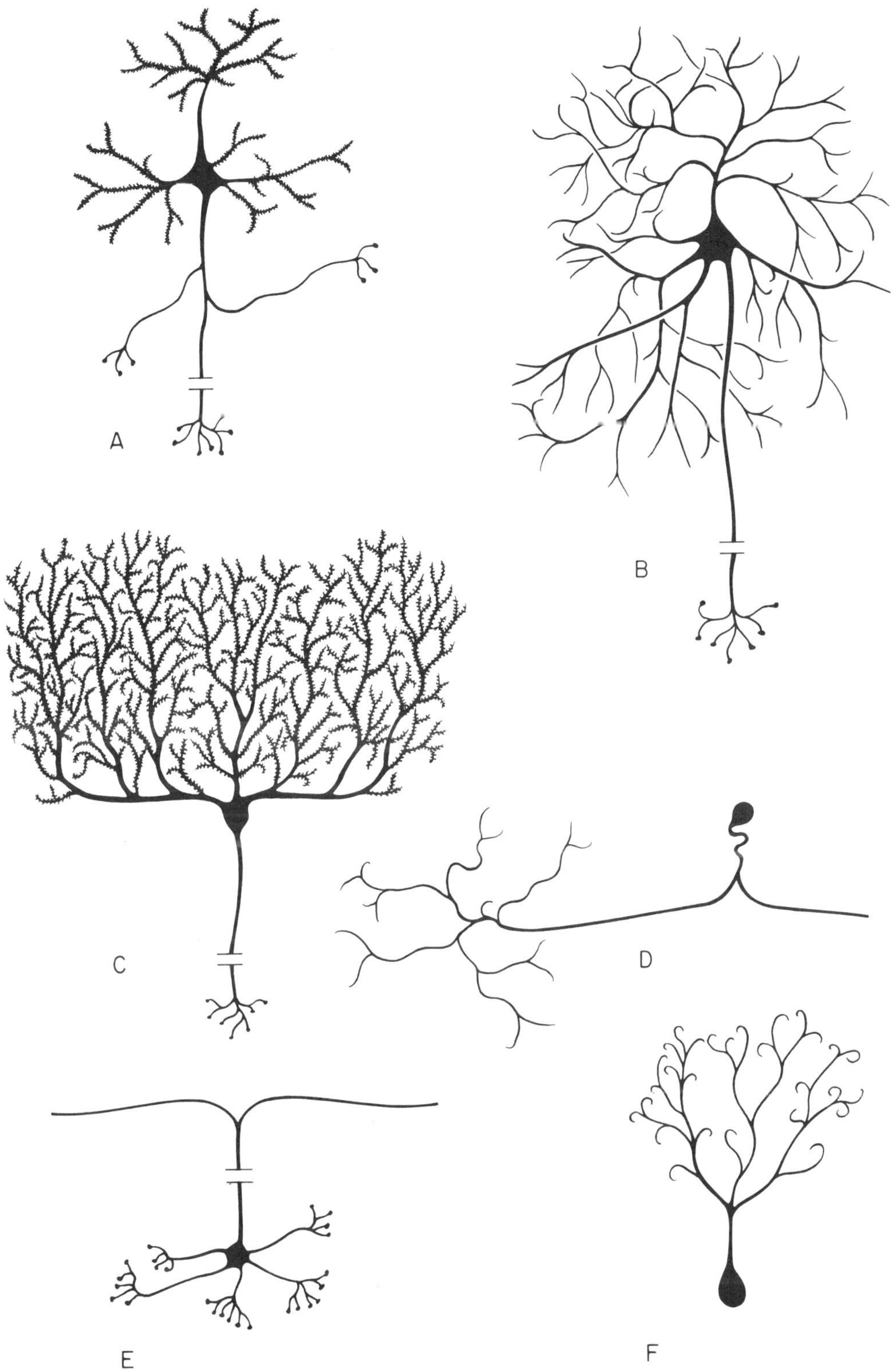

Figure 1–1. Examples of the varying morphology of different types of nerve cells. The interrupted processes indicate axons. *A,* Pyramidal cell; *B,* stellate cell; *C,* Purkinje cell; *D,* bipolar dorsal root ganglion cell; *E,* granule cell; *F,* amacrine cell.

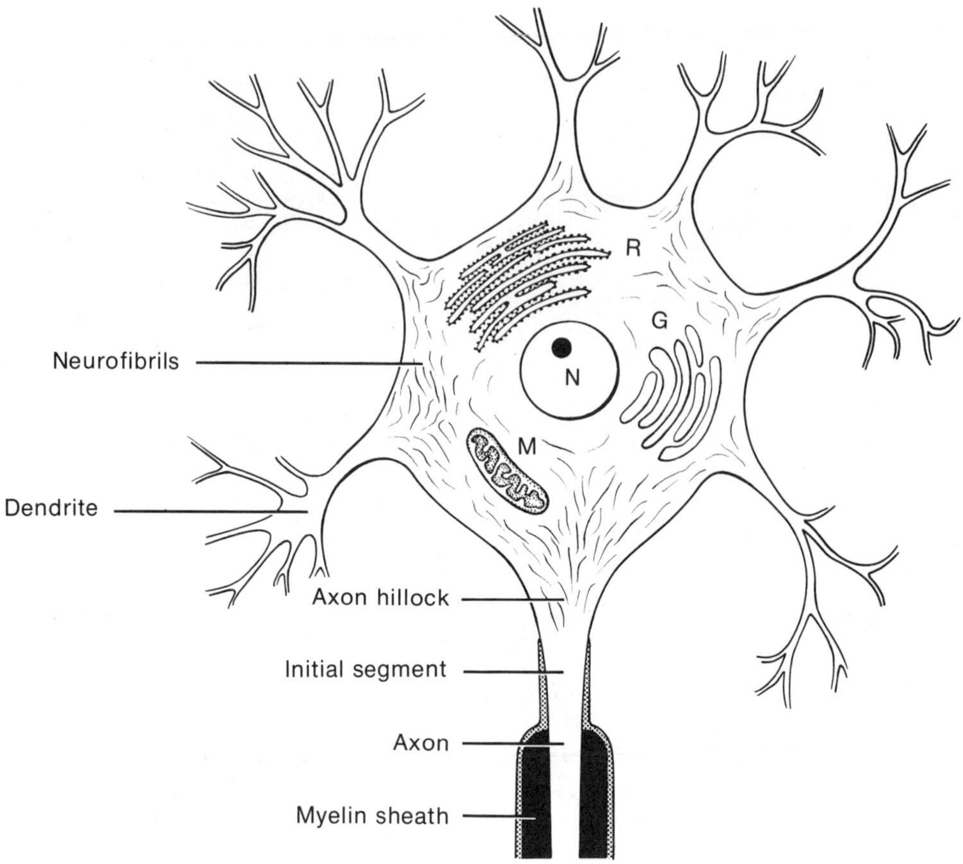

Figure 1–2. The major features of a generalized nerve cell. *R,* Rough endoplasmic reticulum; *N,* nucleus with its nucleolus; *G,* Golgi apparatus; *M,* mitochondria.

tions are unknown, but some possibilities are that they are involved in axon growth, or the transportation of essential enzyme systems through axoplasmic flow, and/or that they form synaptic vesicles. They may also contribute to the neuron's cytoskeleton.

Mitochondria are found throughout nerve cells and particularly at synapses and sensory and motor nerve terminals, i.e., wherever intense metabolic activity occurs. Their locations are consistent with what is known about their role as "mobile power plants," which supply energy for numerous chemical reactions and active transport mechanisms of the cell.

Nerve cells contain highly developed Golgi bodies which are also commonly called the Golgi apparatus. This consists of flattened vesicles called saccules which are often arranged in stacks of three to eight layers. Investigations have shown that products of the rough endoplasmic reticulum are transported to the stacks of saccules, and as these products move through the stacks they are chemically modified and packaged before being released from the cell as secretory granules or synaptic vesicles. In addition the evidence indicates that they play a role in the production and maintenance of the cell membrane.

Nerve Cell Sheaths

Nerve cell processes do not all possess the same number of outer sheaths. Dendrites usually are not myelinated; some axons are myelinated, and others are not. In the peripheral nervous system the Schwann cells, which are neural crest derivatives, produce myelin. The central nervous system contains no Schwann cells, but one of the four types of glial cells, the oligodendroglial cells, produce myelin. Myelin consists of several alternating layers of lipids and proteins which actually are successive layers of the plasma membrane of Schwann cells or oligodendroglial cells that have wrapped themselves spirally around the axons. The longitudinal dimension of this myelin wrapping is interrupted by distinct gaps in the myelin, called nodes of Ranvier. In the peripheral nervous system one Schwann cell produces the myelin between each two adjacent nodes of Ranvier.

Myelination occurs relatively late in ontogenetic development and ends sometime after birth in humans. Different fiber systems or tracts of the CNS become myelinated at different times. Myelination takes place very late in the corticospinal tracts and is not completed until close to the second year after birth. The corticospinal tracts are responsible for voluntary control of the musculature and do not function well until they become myelinated. This is why the ability to perform coordinated activities develops slowly in infants. Myelin functions as an insulator along most of the nerve fiber so that the axonal membranes are depolarized only at the nodes of Ranvier. Therefore, myelinated nerves conduct at a faster rate than do unmyelinated nerves. Multiple sclerosis is a frequently encountered disease that involves degeneration of myelin sheaths.

In addition to myelin, there are three connective tissue sheaths that surround peripheral nerve axons. Each axon, whether myelinated or not, is surrounded by collagen fibers derived from the connective tissue cells in the area. This is called the endoneurial sheath. Groups of several axons with their myelin and endoneurial sheaths are enclosed by a second connective tissue sheath, the perineurium, which presumably is derived from the pia-arachnoid (two of the connective tissue coverings of the CNS). All peripheral nerve trunks are ensheathed outwardly by a dense collagenous layer of connective tissue, the epineurium, which is derived from another of the connective tissue coverings of the brain, the dura mater. Axons that are less than 1 micron in diameter are not myelinated, but nevertheless are enveloped by a thin Schwann cell sheath and by a thin layer of endoneurium in the peripheral nervous system. Figure 1–3 illustrates the nerve cell sheaths.

Neuroanatomic Methods

Only a brief discussion of neuroanatomic methods will be included here to aid in understanding how information about the central and peripheral nervous systems has been obtained, and to provide a background for a more critical view of methods utilized in studies that may be encountered in the literature.

Probably more has been learned about the morphology of the whole single nerve cell by use of the *Golgi* method than by any other method. This involves staining with heavy metals, that is, potassium dichromate or zinc. Not all the cells in a particular area are stained, but those that are, are stained quite completely. This enables one to follow the axons for long distances in some cases, so that their patterns of terminal arborization may be observed. However, it is important to understand that this stain is used most successfully in newborn or at least very young animals, before the myelin sheaths develop. After these develop, sometimes only the unmyelinated terminal segments are shown, and an incomplete picture may result in incorrect interpretation of the material. Therefore, one should suspect cases in the literature in which this method is used in older animals.

Distribution of nerve cells in the central nervous system has been studied extensively by the *Nissl* method. This entails the use of basic aniline dyes that stain rough endoplasmic reticulum, which you will recall is located primarily in the perikaryon and the proximal segments of dendrites. This technique provides very useful information regarding the grouping of cells in the CNS. The study of cell groupings is called *cytoarchitectonics.*

The *Weigert* staining method utilizes iron hematoxylin in the central nervous system and osmium tetroxide in the peripheral nervous system. This is a myelin stain which is very useful for studying the sequence in which CNS pathways become myelinated during development, in addition to providing information about CNS tracts and connections when lesions are produced by disease or trauma. In Weigert preparations all degenerated tracts as well as nuclear aggregations remain unstained. Everything that remains myelinated is stained. The Weigert method gives only a partial picture of axon-

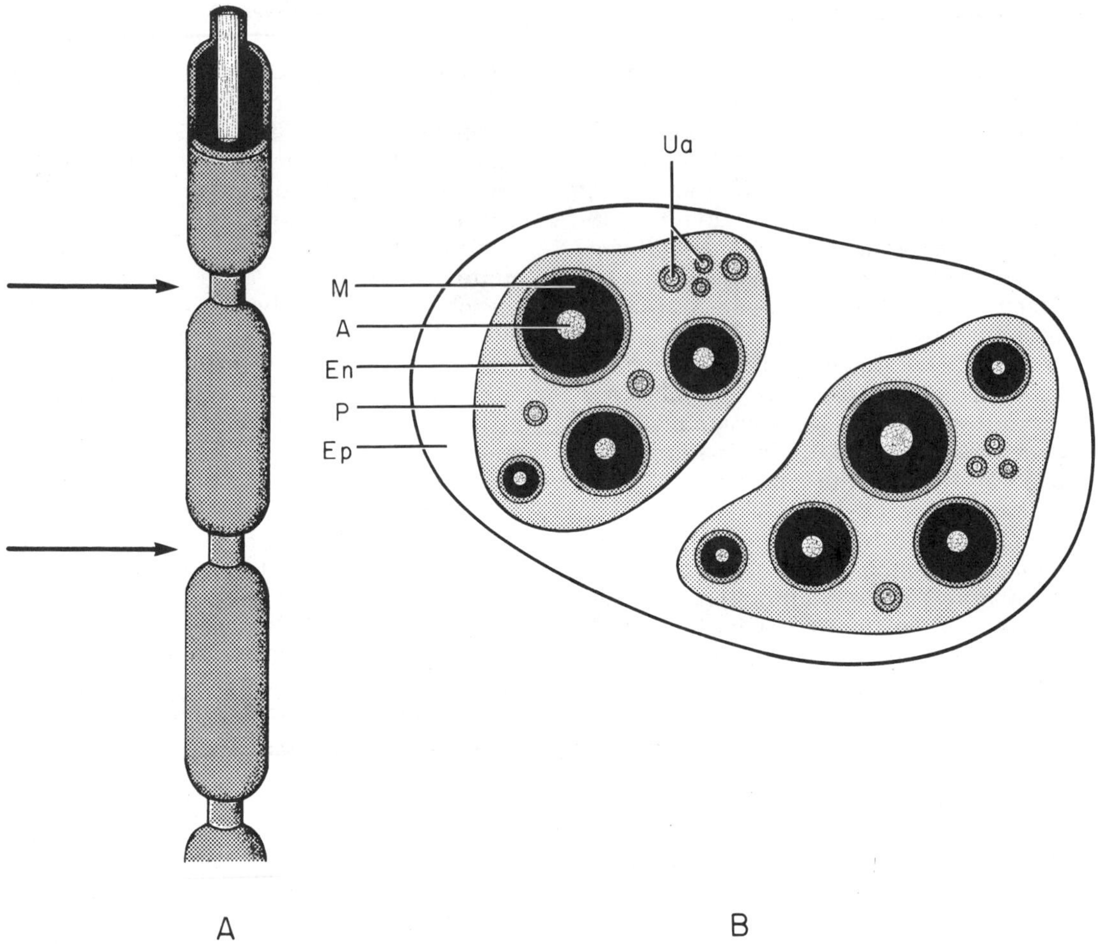

Figure 1–3. *A,* Part of the longitudinal dimension of a myelinated nerve. The arrows indicate nodes of Ranvier, which are discontinuities in the myelinated sheath.

B, A cross-section of a group of myelinated and nonmyelinated axons. Each myelinated axon is surrounded by an endoneurial sheath, as is each unmyelinated axon. In this example each group of myelinated axons and several unmyelinated axons are enclosed within a perineurial sheath, and the entire bundle of axons is surrounded by an epineurial sheath. *M,* Myelin; *A,* axon; *En,* endoneurial sheath; *P,* perineurial sheath; *Ep,* epineurial sheath; *Ua,* unmyelinated axons.

al networks, because many axons, even in the adult, are unmyelinated. Therefore, the material must be interpreted with caution. The study of the distribution of myelin is called *myeloarchitectonics.*

In order to obtain a more complete picture of neuronal networks, the axons, rather than myelin, can be stained. The best known methods for staining axons have been developed by *Cajal* and *Bielschowsky.* They both employ reduced silver nitrate, which gives preferential impregnation of the fibrillar components of the nerve cell. Therefore, these silver methods are called *neurofibrillar methods.* Since neurofibrils are located in all parts of the nerve cell, axons, cell bodies and dendrites are all stained by these methods, which have been widely used to show the distribution of axon terminals. However, one must be critical of papers written by those who use these methods for determining the *number* of synapses because many axon terminals contain no fibrillar components, and hence do not stain. Also, the finest nerve terminals may not stain.

By far the most effective tool for studying the details of synaptic morphology is the *electron microscope,* with its resolving power down to 2 to 5 angstrom units.

Two methods for tracing CNS pathways have been introduced fairly recently. They involve the use of *tritiated amino acids* and *horseradish peroxidase*. Pathways may be traced from their origins to their terminations by injecting tritiated amino acids in the vicinity of the nerve cell bodies. The amino acids are incorporated into proteins and move to the axon terminals by way of axoplasmic flow. By injection of horseradish peroxidase in the vicinity of axon terminals one can trace the pathway of the axons retrogradely toward the cell body. This peroxidase is transported toward the cell body by means of reverse axoplasmic flow.

The radioactivity in the nerve terminals that results from the administration of tritiated amino acids can be measured by scintillation counting of samples, or may be examined by autoradiography of tissue sections coated with photographic emulsion. The horseradish peroxidase can be visualized in the perikaryon by use of a histochemical reaction.

SYNAPSES

The word synapse was first used by Sir Charles Sherrington. It is derived from the Greek and the literal meaning is "to clasp." A synapse is defined as the region where some part of one nerve cell contacts the perikaryon, dendrite or axon of another nerve cell. It specifically refers to contact regions where transmission of nervous activity from one cell to another occurs. The term has also been expanded to include the neuromuscular junction, where activity of the nerve cell is transmitted to muscle.

Two types of synaptic transmission have been described: chemical and electrotonic. We have been aware of the latter synapses for only a little over a decade. At these neuro-neuronal junctions, chemical transmission is not involved. Rather, the transmission is an electrical event, with the electric current spreading bidirectionally, i.e., in either direction across the synapse. The morphology of electrotonic synapses is such that the extracellular space is almost completely obliterated by the very close apposition of the membranes of the two cells. Such a contact is called a "gap" junction. Vesicles may or may not be present as they are at chemical synapses, and there is no particular concentration of mitochondria. Electrotonic synapses are common in invertebrate species, but not at all common in mammals. The great majority of vertebrate nervous systems have the characteristics of chemical transmission. Therefore, the emphasis here will be placed on chemical synapses.

Five morphologic types of synapses have been described: axodendritic, axosomatic, axo-axonal, somatodendritic and dendrodendritic (see Fig. 1–4). The first three types are by far the most common. A typical synaptic junction in the central nervous system includes a presynaptic element, which is most often axonal, and a postsynaptic element, which is most often perikaryal or dendritic. There is usually a localized swelling of the presynaptic element at the contact site, which is called the synaptic knob. It contains numerous mitochondria and syn-

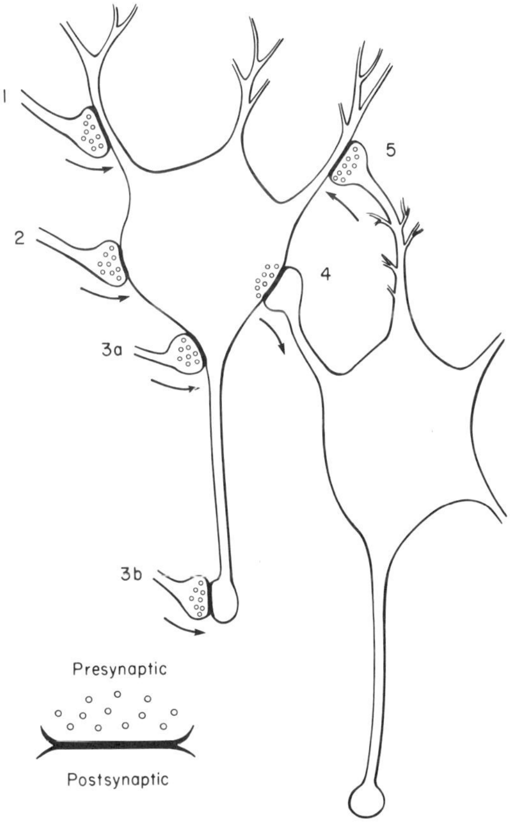

Figure 1–4. Two nerve cells that illustrate the five morphologic types of synapse. *1,* Axodendritic; *2,* axosomatic; *3a* and *3b,* two types of axo-axonal synapse; *4,* somatodendritic; *5,* dendro-dendritic. The inset below indicates that in all synapses shown in this illustration the synaptic vesicles (*small circles*) are located on the presynaptic side.

aptic vesicles which are 300 to 600 angstroms in diameter, crowded against a presynaptic thickening. The postsynaptic thickening is often somewhat wider than the presynaptic thickening. According to Katz, chemical transmission involves the release of acetylcholine or other transmitters in packets from the synaptic vesicles located in the synaptic knobs. The neurotransmitter in turn excites or inhibits the postsynaptic membrane. Impulses are transmitted only unidirectionally at chemical synapses, a process known as *dynamic polarization*.

When the amount of excitatory transmitter released by multiple presynaptic vesicles is sufficient to stimulate the postsynaptic element, "all or nothing" spikes are initiated in the postsynaptic neuron. The current flows toward the initial segment, where a spike potential is initiated, since the initial segment has a lower threshold for spike initiation than the rest of the nerve cell. The depolarization is then conducted orthodromically down the axon.

Axons may have one of two influences at the synaptic junctions: excitation or inhibition. The latter occurs when a cell becomes hyperpolarized; i.e., the membrane potential becomes more negative (moves further from the threshold for stimulation). Presumably, inhibition is produced by a different neurotransmitter from that which produces excitation. The effect of inhibition is to produce inhibitory postsynaptic potentials which prevent "all or nothing" spikes from occurring in the postsynaptic neuron.

The strength of the influence of the presynaptic cells on the postsynaptic cell may vary. There is evidence to suggest that a synapse placed close to the initial segment, where spike initiation occurs, is more effective than one placed far out on a dendrite. The number of contacts a single axon makes with a postsynaptic cell can also vary from one to many, and one postsynaptic cell may have many thousands of axons impinging upon it from different sources. In addition, one axon may terminate on several different postsynaptic elements. In general, the closer the synaptic contacts are to the initial segment and the more numerous the synaptic contacts on the postsynaptic cell, the stronger will be the influence on the postsynaptic cell by its input.

We do not know much about synaptic linkage between nerve cells in many parts of the nervous system, but we do know that synaptic junctions vary considerably in structure. A number of attempts have been made to relate structural variations to known aspects of synaptic function. Some have been successful, others have not. Some examples are:

1. Some axons contain many dense cored granular (electron opaque) vesicles. The distribution of these is associated with the distribution of catecholamines in the nervous system. Catecholamines are a specific class of neurotransmitters which include epinephrine, norepinephrine and dopamine. Therefore, granular and agranular vesicles may represent packets of different types of transmitter substances.
2. The synaptic thickenings are not the same at all synaptic junctions. Based on the appearance of synapses they have been classified as symmetric or asymmetric. E. G. Gray has called the latter *type I* synapses and the former *type II* synapses. His attempts to relate type I synapses to excitatory activity and type II synapses to inhibitory activity have been generally unsuccessful. Figure 1–5 illustrates Gray's synapses.
3. Some axon terminals contain more or less regularly shaped, spherical vesicles; others contain irregularly shaped (pleomorphic) vesicles. The evidence suggests that spherical vesicles are present in excitatory neurons, and pleomorphic vesicles in inhibitory neurons. Thus, the shape of the vesicles may give a clue to the type of transmitter contained by individual neurons. The evidence for this is not yet unequivocal, but there is no documented evidence to disprove it. In some instances round vesicles have been related to Gray's type I synapses and pleomorphic vesicles to his type II synapses, but again the evidence is not conclusive that both type I synapses and round vesicles indicate excitatory neurons and type II synapses and pleomorphic vesicles indicate inhibitory neurons.

Two types of axo-axonal synapses have been described in many parts of the nervous system. One type involves contact of one axon terminal with another (see 3b in Fig. 1–4). The postsynaptic axon terminal in turn synapses with the cell body or dendrite of another neuron. There is evidence that this type of axo-axonal synapse may account for presynaptic inhibition, as de-

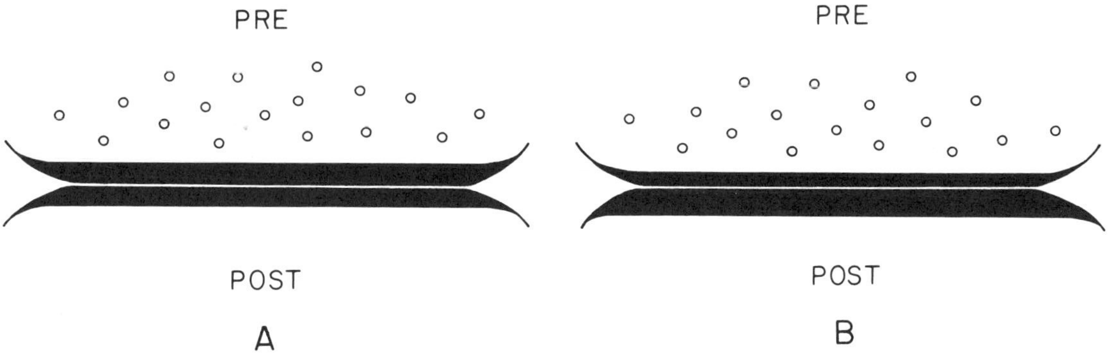

Figure 1–5. *A*, Gray's type II synapse. The thickenings on the pre- and postsynaptic sides are approximately equal. This is a symmetric type of synapse.

B, Gray's type I synapse. The thickening on the presynaptic side, which contains the round vesicles, is less than that on the postsynaptic side. This is an asymmetric type of synapse.

scribed by Eccles. The second type of axo-axonal synapse consists of a presynaptic axon terminal that synapses with the axon hillock or initial segment of the postsynaptic neuron (see 3a in Fig. 1–4). There is evidence that the influence of this type of presynaptic neuron on the postsynaptic neuron is also inhibitory.

At present, those who are studying the ultrastructure of nerve cells are able to identify different types of synaptic contacts, but very little can be said about the types of interactions that occur between them.

GLIAL CELLS

There are approximately ten times as many glial cells as there are nerve cells in the central nervous system, and they comprise about one-half of the volume of the brain. Unlike nerve cells, they are not excitable. There are four types of glial cells, the astrocytes (protoplasmic and fibrous), oligodendroglia, ependyma and microglia. The first three all originate from the embryonic ectoderm, as do the nerve cells. Microglia originate from the mesoderm and migrate into the CNS by way of the blood vessels.

Fibrous astrocytes have longer processes than protoplasmic astrocytes and are most abundant in the white matter of the nervous system, whereas protoplasmic astrocytes are most plentiful in the gray matter. Both types often have end feet on blood vessels. They play an active role in regulation of normal metabolism of neurons and in regulation of transport mechanisms between the blood and brain. They may be implicated in the blood-brain barrier.

It was mentioned previously that the oligodendroglia are the myelin producers in the CNS, both during development and during the small amount of regeneration that occurs after trauma to CNS axons.

Ependymal cells line the central canal of the spinal cord and the ventricular system of the brain. They function in secretion and absorption and may play a part in the brain–cerebrospinal fluid barrier in conjunction with the astrocytes. They are also extremely important in development because many CNS cell types are derived from them.

The microglial cells function as phagocytes. In case of disease, trauma or natural cell death, the microglia engulf and dispose of the necrotic debris.

REVIEW QUESTIONS

1. What is the neuron doctrine?
2. In what parts of the nerve cell is ribonucleic acid (RNA) located? What are the functional implications of its distribution?

3. What are the functions of a. neurofibrils? b. mitochondria? c. Golgi bodies?
4. What cell types produce myelin in the peripheral nervous system? In the central nervous system?
5. Why does the ability to perform coordinated activities develop slowly in infants?
6. Define a. cytoarchitectonics. b. myeloarchitectonics.
7. List the dangers in interpreting material stained by the a. Golgi method. b. Weigert method. c. Bielschowsky and Cajal methods.
8. What is meant by dynamic polarization?
9. According to Katz, what is involved in chemical transmission at synapses?
10. When the amount of transmitter released by the presynaptic element is sufficient to stimulate the postsynaptic element, what is the sequence of events that takes place in the postsynaptic neuron?
11. Name the four types of glial cells.
12. From what embryonic layer does each type of glial cell originate?
13. State the functions of a. astrocytes. b. oligodendroglia. c. microglia.

CHAPTER 2 • THE PERIPHERAL NERVOUS SYSTEM: DERMATOMES, BRACHIAL AND LUMBOSACRAL PLEXUSES

OBJECTIVES

After reading this chapter you should: • Understand the definitions of: a. dermatome; b. myotome. • Understand why the distribution of innervation of the trunk is uncomplicated and why the distribution of innervation in the extremities is more complicated. • Know the dermatomes that contribute to each named cutaneous nerve. • Know the distribution of each named cutaneous nerve. • Know which spinal segments contribute to the innervation of each muscle. • Know which areas of the body are innervated by posterior primary divisions and which are innervated by anterior primary divisions. • Understand how most muscles become innervated by more than one spinal segment and how one spinal segment may innervate several muscles.

DERMATOMES

The definition of a dermatome is *that cutaneous area which is supplied by a single dorsal root and its ganglia.* The distribution of dermatomes is very clear-cut in the trunk region, since each dorsal root supplies the cutaneous area that corresponds to its own segment. The cutaneous nerves supplied by these roots extend from the middle of the back to the middle of the thorax and abdomen.

In the extremities, the situation is quite different, since the segmental innervation migrates distally. Additional complicating factors are contributed by the formation of plexuses and rotation of the limbs during development. The lower extremities rotate from lateral to medial and the upper extremities from medial to lateral. Furthermore, although the available diagrams make it appear as if a single nerve root is responsible for the innervation of a clear-cut area, it should be remembered that there is a great deal of overlap in cutaneous innervation. For example, if the dorsal roots from only one spinal segment are damaged in the trunk area, there is very little, if any, deficit in sensation. A minimum of two or three adjacent spinal roots must be damaged for the patient to notice any real dificit.

Particularly important dermatomal landmarks on the trunk are:

1. T4 — at the level of the nipples.
2. T10 — at the level of the umbilicus.
3. S3 and S4 — at the level of the genitalia.

A complete representation of the derma-

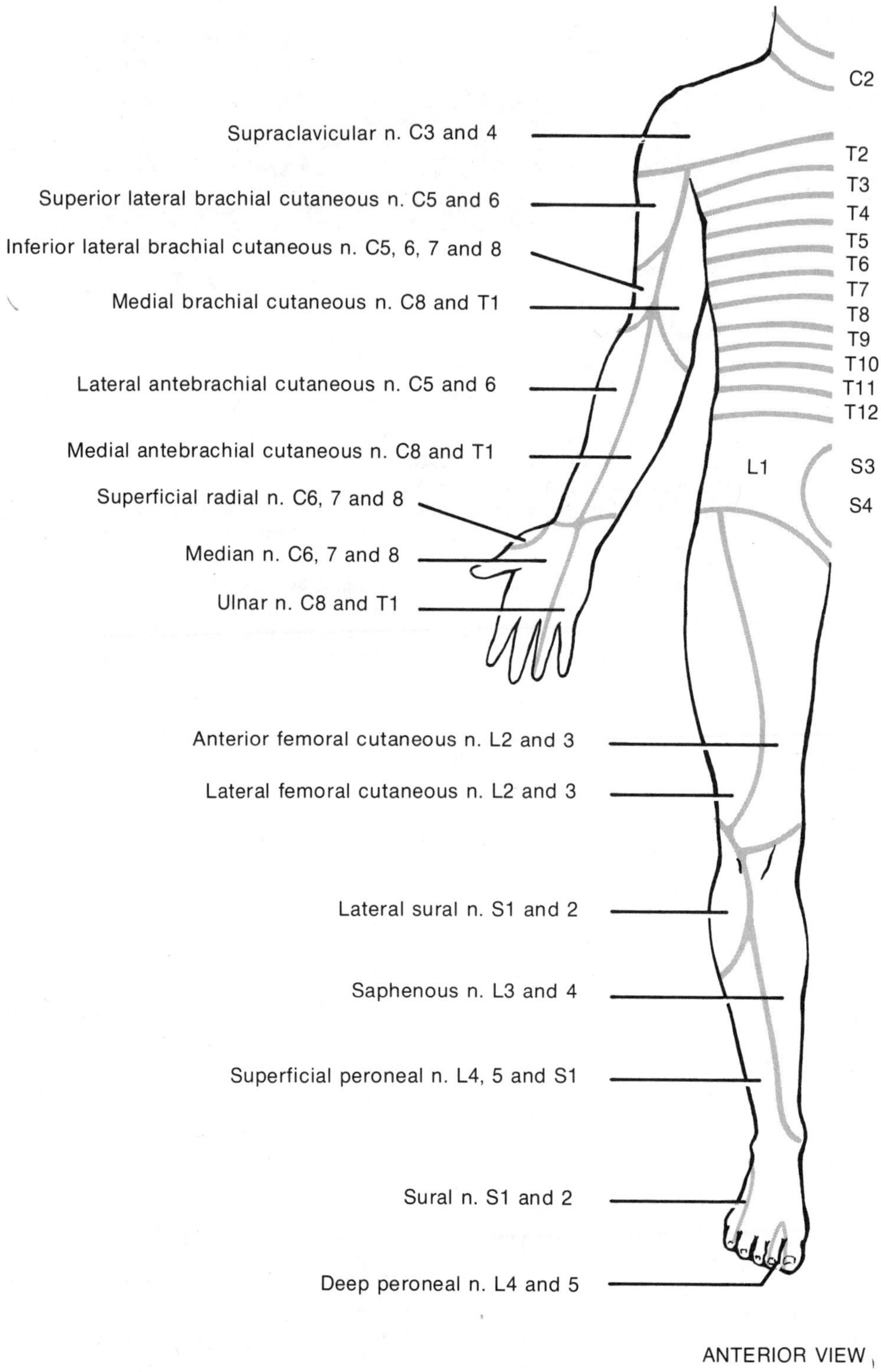

Figure 2–1. Cutaneous innervation of the trunk and extremities — anterior view.

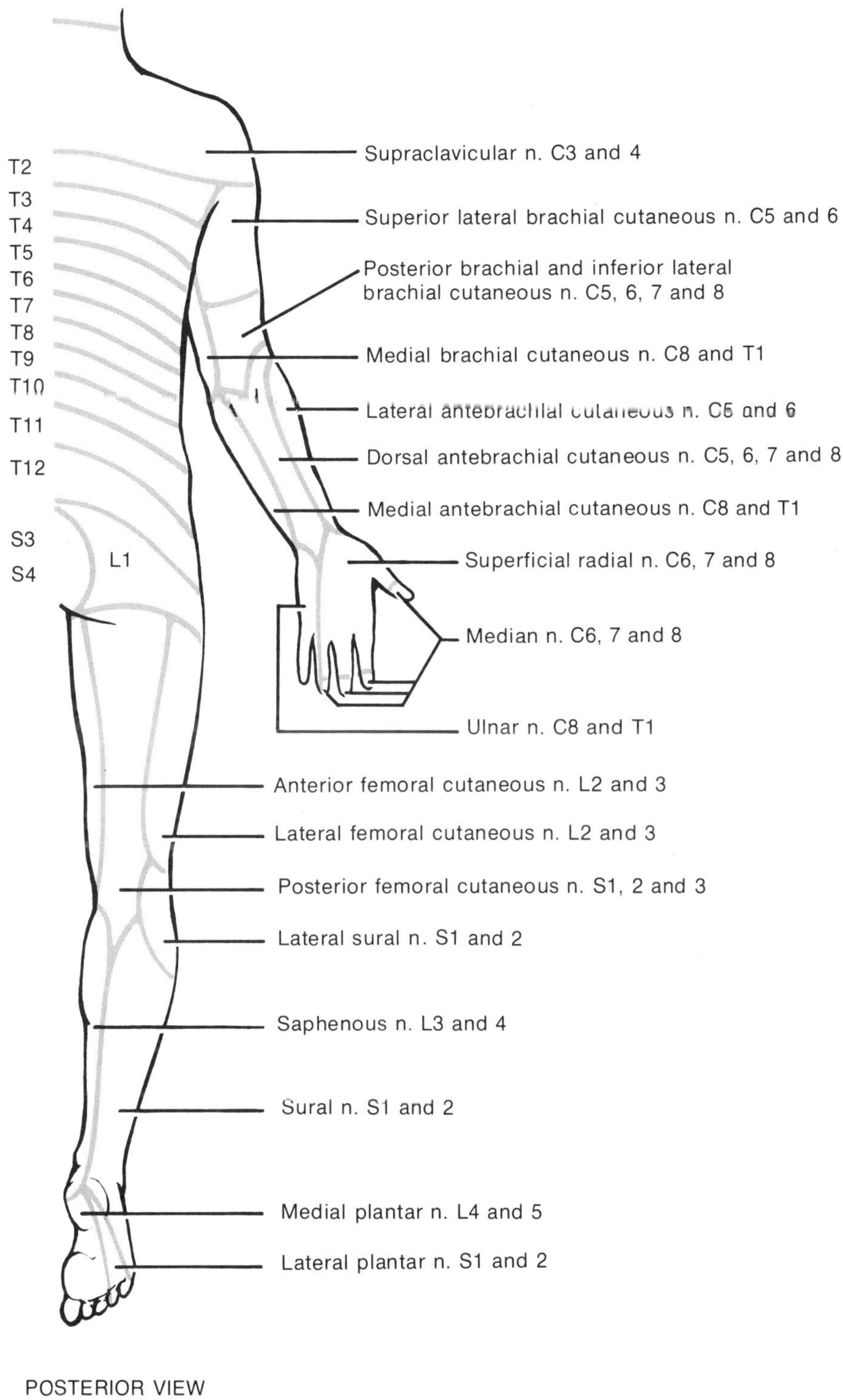

Figure 2–2. Cutaneous innervation of the trunk and extremities — posterior view.

tomes of the trunk and their contributions to the named nerves of the extremities is shown in Figures 2–1 and 2–2 and the cutaneous innervation of the head is included in Figure 2–3. Notice that in the neck and shoulder region the contribution from C4 is adjacent to that of T2 because the roots from C5 through T1 migrate down the upper extremity. In the extremities each individual dermatome is not outlined. Rather, the dermatomes that contribute to each named nerve are included. It should be understood that the more superior segments that contribute to a named nerve innervate the most proximal area which that nerve innervates, and the more inferior segmental contributions innervate the most distal area which that nerve innervates.

For those involved in patient care it is extremely important to have this type of information at hand. Some examples of how this knowledge may be applied include first, the case in which a description of the sensory deficit is available. The lesion can be localized easily. If one is asked to administer diagnostic tests to determine in which cutaneous areas sensitivity is lost or diminished, one can then make a decision concerning which spinal cord segments or dorsal roots are damaged as a result of disease or injury. Second, if a description of the lesion is available, the sensory deficit can be localized. If it is known that a lesion involves specific spinal segments or dorsal roots, the area or areas in which hypoesthesia (diminished sensation), hyperesthesia (increased sensitivity or hypersensitivity) or paresthesia (abnormal sensation) is produced can be determined. This may be very important in cases in which various forms of heat may be prescribed. It will be necessary to monitor the patient carefully for the possibility of burns if application of heat is prescribed for an hypoesthetic area. The patient may be burned seriously yet have no awareness of it. Also, a patient with a spinal cord injury may have no sensation below the level of the lesion. If he wears braces, areas where these come into contact with the skin must be checked carefully and frequently for pressures and abrasions that the patient may not feel.

THE BRACHIAL AND LUMBOSACRAL PLEXUSES

After the dorsal and ventral roots emerge from the spinal cord they join to form mixed spinal nerves that contain both sensory and motor components. These extend peripherally for only a very short distance before they divide into dorsal and ventral rami. These are also called anterior and posterior primary divisions. These rami or divisions generally are simply named for the areas which they innervate. The dorsal rami innervate the muscles and skin of the back. The ventral rami innervate the muscles and skin of the extremities and the anterolateral

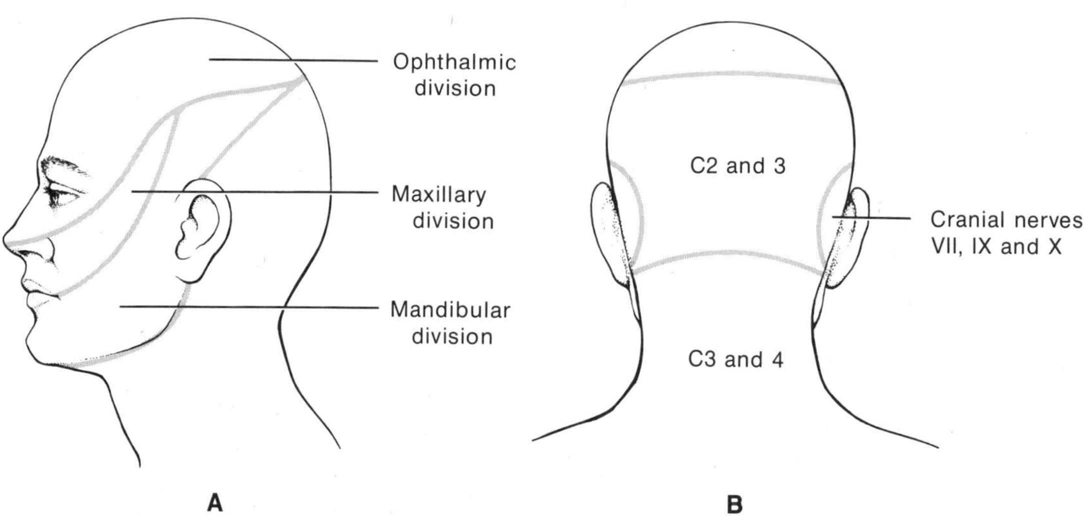

Figure 2–3. Cutaneous innervation of the head. *A,* Contributions of the three divisions of the trigeminal (Vth cranial) nerve. *B,* Contributions by the cervical plexus and the posterior auricular nerve, formed by branches of the facial (VIIth cranial), glossopharyngeal (IXth cranial) and vagus (Xth cranial) nerves.

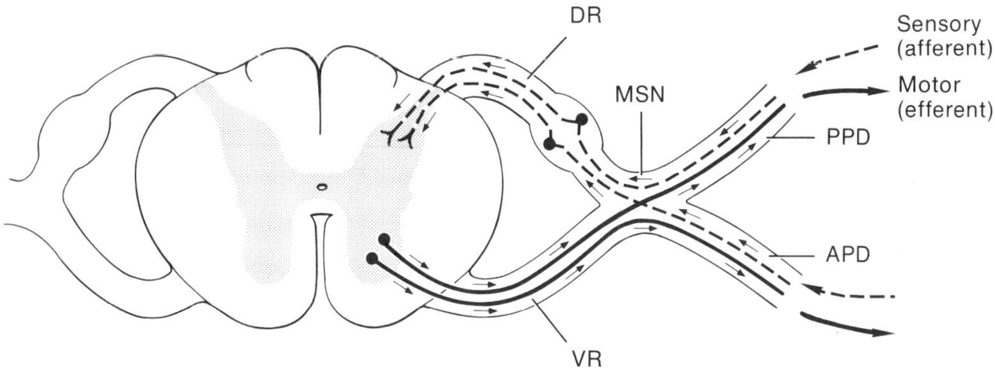

Figure 2–4. A cross-section of the spinal cord showing the distribution of motor and sensory components. *DR,* Dorsal root; *VR,* ventral root; *MSN,* mixed spinal nerve; *PPD,* posterior primary division; *APD,* anterior primary division.

body wall. Dorsal and ventral rami are often confused with dorsal and ventral roots of the spinal cord. It is important to understand the difference between the two because in the dorsal and ventral roots motor and sensory components are segregated, whereas dorsal and ventral rami each contain both sensory and motor components. These structures are illustrated in Figure 2–4.

The distribution of the posterior primary divisions is quite clear, since in general they are segmentally distributed. The distribution of the anterior primary divisions is much more difficult to understand owing to the formation of the brachial and lumbosacral plexuses, both of which are made up exclusively of anterior primary divisions. Considerable emphasis will be placed upon these two plexuses because they are extremely important clinically. As mentioned previously, there is overlap in the distribution of cutaneous innervation, and in addition there are individual variations in the segmental contributions to named peripheral nerves, muscles and cutaneous areas. For these reasons there are variations in the segmental contributions presented in different textbooks. Figures 2–5, 2–6 and Tables 2–1 and 2–2 consist of diagrammatic representations and lists of structures innervated by specific segments of the spinal cord.

It is important to learn the spinal segments that contribute to the innervation of each muscle. With this information one can determine which muscles and movements are affected when a lesion is known to have occurred at a specific level of the spinal cord, or when it is known that specific ventral roots have been damaged. Conversely, if a muscle test is administered, i.e., the strength of a patient's musculature is evaluated, one should be able to locate the level of the lesion from the information obtained regarding weakness or absence of function of each muscle. Very practically speaking, if you know the level of the lesion you will know what to expect from the patient in terms of which activities of daily living he will be capable of. For example, will it be feasible to try to teach him how to feed himself? Does he need supportive devices in order to do so? Can he ever be expected to walk after a good program of strengthening exercises with or without supportive devices? Should orthotic devices be planned for? It is extremely important to be realistic in planning short- and long-term goals for each patient. There is nothing more depressing for a patient than to have goals set for him that he is not physically capable of attaining.

As the segmental innervation of the musculature is studied it becomes obvious that most muscles are innervated by more than one spinal segment. Also one spinal segment may contribute to the innervation of more than one muscle. This leads us to the definition of a myotome, which consists of *those striated somatic muscles which are derived from a single somite.* Somites develop very early in the embryo concomitantly with the development of the neural tube. They are small masses of mesoderm which flank the neural tube and are divided into three parts — the dermatome, myotome and sclerotome. All three parts of the somites

Text continued on page 20

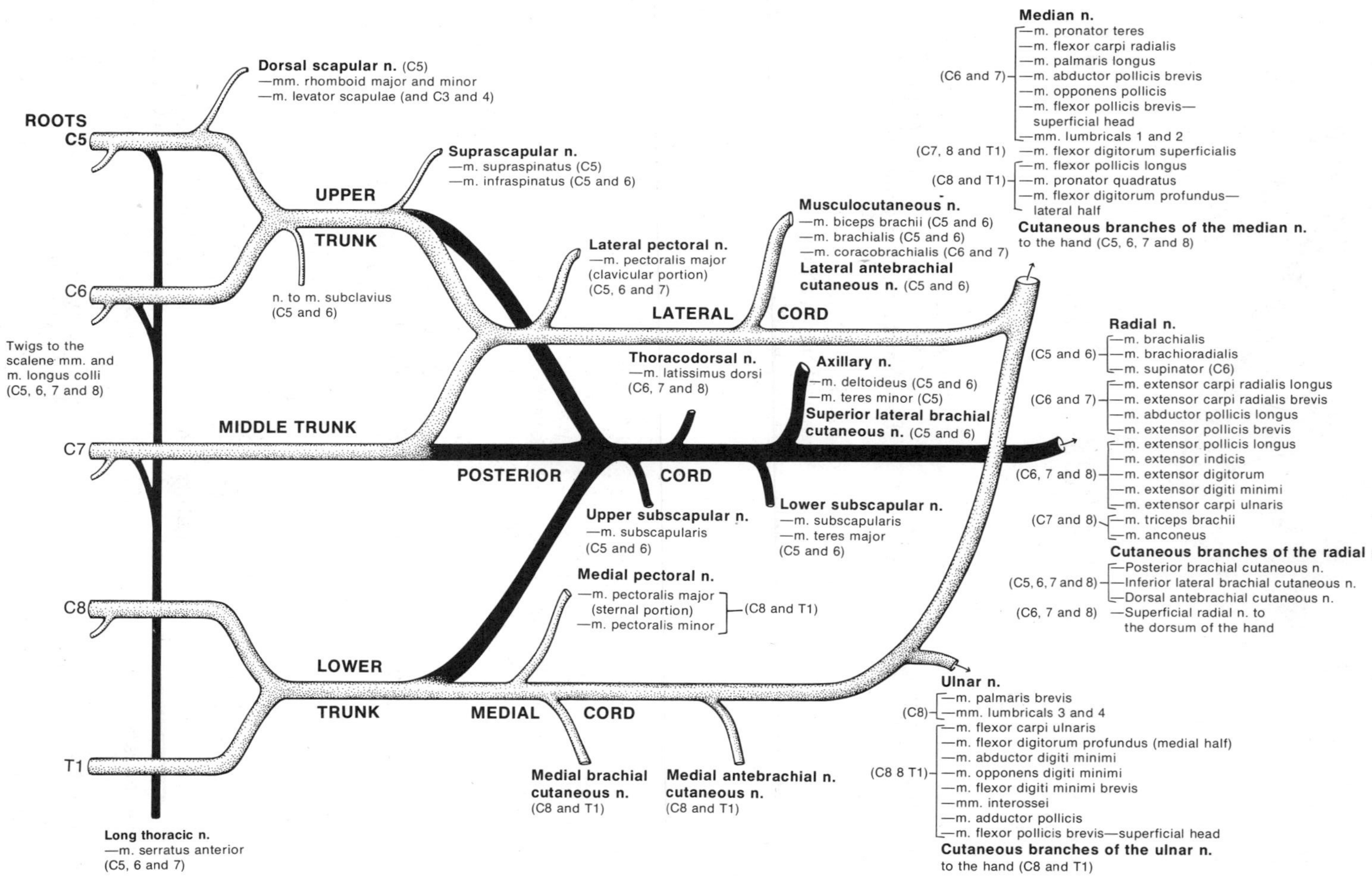

Figure 2–5. The brachial plexus.

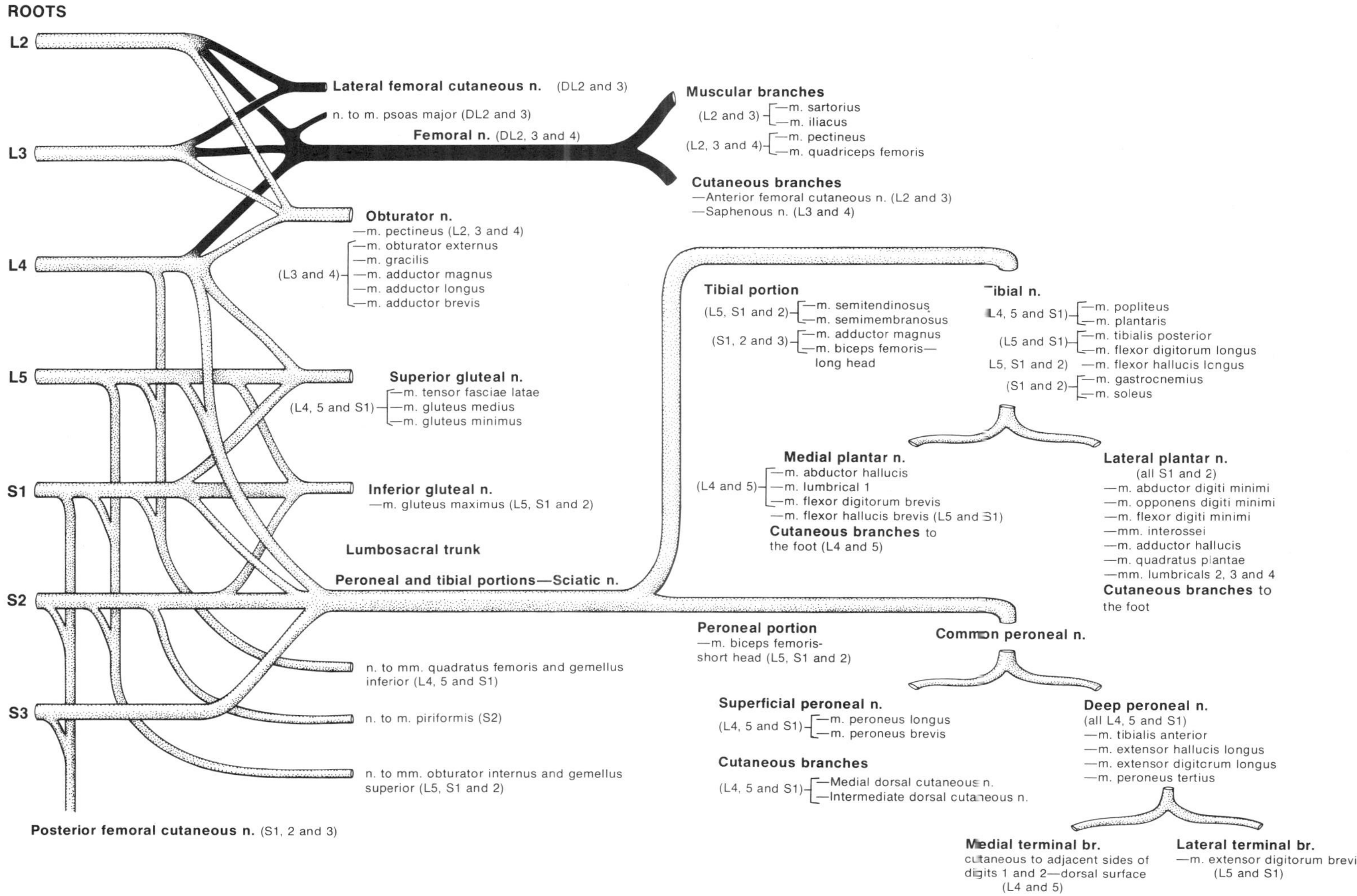

Figure 2–6. The lumbosacral plexus.

TABLE 2–1. BRACHIAL PLEXUS. SEGMENTAL INNERVATION OF INDIVIDUAL MUSCLES

C5
Rhomboid major
Rhomboid minor
Levator scapulae (+C3 and C4)
Supraspinatus
Teres minor

C5 and C6
Subclavius
Infraspinatus
Biceps brachii
Subscapularis
Teres major
Deltoideus
Brachialis
Brachioradialis

C5, C6 and C7
Serratus anterior
Pectoralis major—clavicular portion

C5, C6, C7 and C8
Scalenes
Longus colli

C6
Supinator

C6 and C7
Coracobrachialis
Extensor carpi radialis longus
Extensor carpi radialis brevis
Abductor pollicis longus
Extensor pollicis brevis
Pronator teres
Palmaris longus

C6 and C7 (continued)
Flexor carpi radialis
Abductor pollicis brevis
Opponens pollicis
Flexor pollicis brevis—superficial head
Lumbricales 1 and 2

C6, C7 and C8
Extensor pollicis longus
Extensor indicis
Extensor digitorum
Extensor digiti minimi
Extensor carpi ulnaris
Latissimus dorsi

C7 and C8
Triceps brachii
Anconeus

C7, C8 and T1
Flexor digitorum superficialis

C8
Palmaris brevis
Lumbricales 3 and 4

C8 and T1
Flexor digitorum profundus
Pronator quadratus
Flexor pollicis longus
Flexor carpi ulnaris
Opponens digiti minimi
Abductor digiti minimi
Flexor digiti minimi
Interossei
Flexor pollicis brevis—deep head
Pectoralis minor
Adductor pollicis
Pectoralis major — sternal portion

TABLE 2–1A. BRACHIAL PLEXUS. SEGMENTAL CONTRIBUTIONS TO NAMED CUTANEOUS NERVES

C5 and C6
Lateral antebrachial cutaneous nerve (branch of the musculocutaneous nerve)
Superior lateral brachial cutaneous nerve (branch of the axillary nerve)

C5, C6, C7 and C8
Branches of the Radial Nerve
- Posterior brachial cutaneous nerve
- Dorsal antebrachial cutaneous nerve
- Inferior lateral brachial cutaneous nerve

Cutaneous distribution of the median nerve to the hand

C6, C7 and C8
Cutaneous distribution of the radial nerve to the dorsal surface of the hand

C8 and T1
Medial brachial cutaneous nerve
Medial antebrachial cutaneous nerve
Cutaneous distribution of the ulnar nerve to the palmar and dorsal surfaces of the hand

TABLE 2-2. LUMBOSACRAL PLEXUS. SEGMENTAL INNERVATION OF INDIVIDUAL MUSCLES

L2 and L3
Iliacus
Sartorius
Psoas major

L2, L3 and L4
Pectineus
Quadriceps femoris

L3 and L4
Obturator externus
Gracilis
Adductor longus
Adductor brevis

L3, L4, S1, S2 and S3
Adductor magnus

L4 and L5
Abductor hallucis
Flexor digitorum brevis
Lumbrical 1

L4, L5 and S1
Gluteus medius
Gluteus minimus
Tensor fasciae latae
Quadratus femoris
Gemellus inferior
Popliteus
Plantaris
Peroneus longus
Peroneus brevis
Tibialis anterior
Extensor hallucis longus

L4, L5 and S1 (continued)
Extensor digitorum longus
Peroneus tertius
Flexor hallucis brevis

L5 and S1
Tibialis posterior
Flexor digitorum longus
Extensor digitorum brevis

L5, S1 and S2
Obturator internus
Gemellus superior
Gluteus maximus
Flexor hallucis longus
Biceps femoris—short head
Semimembranosus
Semitendinosus

S1 and S2
Gastrocnemius
Soleus
Abductor digiti minimi
Flexor digiti minimi
Quadratus plantae
Adductor hallucis
Lumbricales 2, 3 and 4
Interossei

S1, S2 and S3
Biceps femoris—long head

S2
Piriformis

TABLE 2–2A. LUMBOSACRAL PLEXUS. SEGMENTAL CONTRIBUTIONS TO NAMED CUTANEOUS NERVES

L1
Genitofemoral nerve

L2 and L3
Lateral femoral cutaneous nerve
Anterior femoral cutaneous nerve (branch of the femoral nerve)

L3 and L4
Saphenous nerve (branch of the femoral nerve)

L4 and L5
Cutaneous distribution of the medial plantar nerve to the foot.
Medial terminal branch of the deep peroneal nerve to adjacent sides of the dorsal surfaces of digits 1 and 2—foot

L4, L5 and S1
Superficial peroneal nerve
Medial dorsal cutaneous branch of the superficial peroneal nerve
Intermediate dorsal cutaneous branch of the superficial peroneal nerve

S1 and S2
Lateral sural cutaneous nerves
Sural nerve
Lateral dorsal cutaneous nerve
Cutaneous distribution of the lateral plantar nerve to the foot
Lateral calcaneal nerves

S1, S2 and S3
Posterior femoral cutaneous nerve

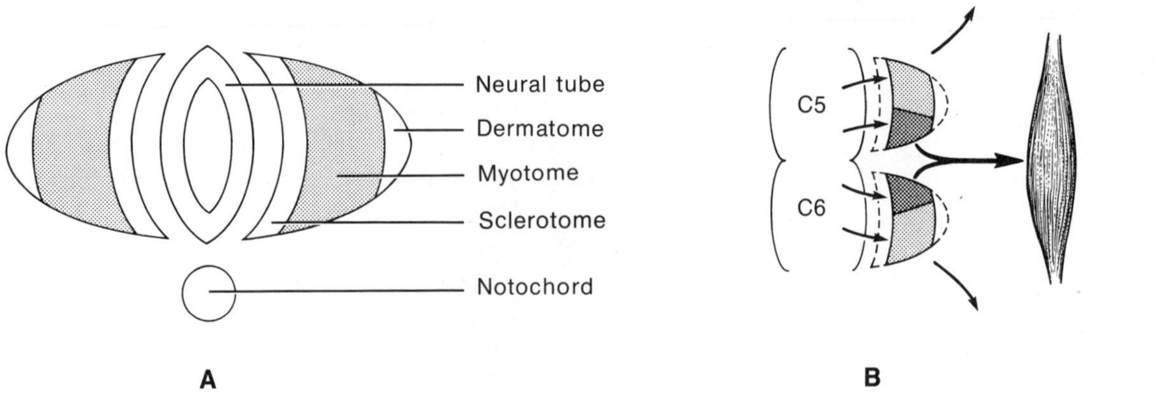

Figure 2–7. *A*, A cross-section of the neural tube with the notochord ventral to it and a pair of somites on either side of it. (This is but one of 42 to 45 somites that ultimately develop along the longitudinal dimension of the neural tube in the embryo.)

B, An example of how myotomes split to contribute to more than one muscle and how pieces of myotome fuse to form one muscle. This is a longitudinal view, showing segments C5 and C6 of the neural tube, which will develop into the spinal cord. In this example the most darkly shaded areas of the myotomes adjacent to segments C5 and C6 fuse to form m. biceps brachii, which is innervated by these segments. Notice the neural connections between the neural tube and the myotomes (*smallest arrows*). The nerves migrate peripherally with the myotomes. The more lightly shaded parts of the myotomes split away from that part which contributes to m. biceps brachii and contribute to the formation of other muscles. Thus it is seen how one muscle may become innervated by more than one spinal cord segment and how one spinal segment may innervate more than one muscle. The sclerotomes and dermatomes are indicated by the white areas enclosed by the dashed lines.

migrate. The dermatomes migrate peripherally and become subcutaneous tissue; the myotomes also migrate peripherally to contribute to the somatic musculature; and the sclerotomes migrate centrally to form the vertebral column. As the dermatomes and myotomes migrate to their final locations they are followed by innervation from the spinal cord segment adjacent to the origin of the somites from which they are derived. Thus, whenever a group of muscles share the same individual segmental innervation, they are derived, at least in part, from the same myotome. Those muscles with multiple segmental innervations are derived from several myotomes which fuse during development. It should be understood that not all of the mesoderm that contributes to the somatic musculature is of somatic origin. Much of it derives from mesoderm in the locale where the muscle develops, but the contribution of the myotomal parts of the somites explains the ultimate innervation pattern of the musculature (see Fig. 2–7).

REVIEW QUESTIONS

1. Describe in writing, discuss and demonstrate:
   a. areas in which there would be a sensory deficit with any given lesion of the spinal cord or dorsal roots, and conversely, locate the site of the lesion if an area of sensory deficit is outlined.
   b. muscles in which function will be lost or diminished when there are specific lesions of the spinal cord or ventral nerve roots, and conversely, locate the site of the lesion when specific muscles are known to have lost or diminished function.
2. What areas of the body are innervated by:
   a. ventral rami (anterior primary divisions)?
   b. dorsal rami (posterior primary divisions)?

3. What is the most peripheral structure in which there is segregration of motor and sensory components?
4. What is the definition of a dermatome? A myotome?
5. How does one muscle ultimately become innervated by more than one spinal segment? Why do some spinal segments contribute to the innervation of more than one muscle?

PERIPHERAL NERVE INJURY PROBLEMS

1. If the superficial peroneal nerve is severed at the head of the fibula: a. what muscles will be denervated or partially denervated? b. what movements will be lost or weakened? Explain. c. what might be the danger of muscle imbalance produced by this lesion? d. which cutaneous areas will be hypoesthetic? e. what spinal cord segments contribute to the severed superficial peroneal nerve?
2. If the deep peroneal nerve is severed at the head of the fibula: a. what muscles will be denervated or partially denervated? b. what movements will be lost or weakened? Explain. c. how might a patient alter his gait pattern to compensate for the muscular weakness produced by this lesion? d. which cutaneous areas will be hypoesthetic? e. what spinal cord segments contribute to the severed nerve?
3. If the median nerve is severed at the wrist: a. what muscles will be denervated or partially denervated? b. what movements will be lost or weakened? Explain. c. describe the cutaneous distribution that will be hypoesthetic. d. what spinal cord segments contribute to the part of the nerve which is severed? e. how might you detect this injury clinically, i.e., where would you expect to see atrophy or wasting of the muscles? f. what will be the functional deficits produced by such an injury?
4. If the ulnar nerve is crushed between the medial epicondyle of the humerus and the olecranon process of the ulna: a. what muscles will be denervated or partially denervated? b. what movements will be lost or weakened? Explain. c. describe the cutaneous distribution that will be hypoesthetic. d. what spinal cord segments contribute to the crushed nerve? e. do you think this injury will produce a very profound functional deficit? Why?
5. If the radial nerve is severed in the distal one-third of the arm: a. what muscles will be denervated or partially denervated? b. explain why this might be a more debilitating injury than those involving the ulnar nerve at the elbow or the median nerve at the wrist. c. what might be done to help the patient gain better function?
6. Quite commonly at birth traction results in a condition termed Erb's palsy. Most often the ventral roots of C5 and C6 are separated or "avulsed" from the spinal cord. In this situation, which muscles will be totally nonfunctional and which will be partially nonfunctional? What spinal cord segments contribute to those muscles which maintain partial function?

   What would be the effects of this injury upon movements of the: a. shoulder girdle? b. shoulder joint? c. elbow joint? d. radioulnar joints? e. wrist joint? f. joints of the digits?

   Explain your answers in terms of which muscles are nonfunctioning and which muscles are still functioning to produce the movement.

CHAPTER 3 • THE PERIPHERAL NERVOUS SYSTEM: SOMATOSENSORY RECEPTORS

OBJECTIVES

After reading this chapter you should: • Know the locations and functions of all the somatosensory receptors. • Understand how stimulation of certain receptors may be used to clinical advantage. • Understand how the gamma system functions to maintain the sensitivity of the muscle spindle at any length of the extrafusal fibers. • Understand the mechanisms underlying the tonic vibration reflex, and learn the optimum values of the parameters necessary for successful clinical application of this modality.

TYPES OF RECEPTORS

All information from the external and internal environment is transmitted to the central nervous system by way of a variety of sensory receptors located in various parts of the body. The somatosensory receptors are those which subserve the modalities of pain, temperature, touch, pressure and proprioception. Vision, hearing, taste and equilibrium, which comprise the special senses, will be dealt with in a later chapter.

The somatosensory receptors fit into three separate categories, according to location. They are:

1. Interoceptors — located within the walls of the cardiovascular system and respiratory, genitourinary and gastrointestinal tracts.

2. Exteroceptors — located immediately under the skin or external mucous membranes.

3. Proprioceptors — located in muscles, tendons and joints.

Before going into a detailed description of the structure and function of each type of receptor, some generalizations may be made. In order to react or respond to changes in the environment, receptors must possess a mechanism by which they can convert energy input into "all or nothing" spikes. In other words, if the stimulus is adequate in strength, the receptors act as transducers and the "all or nothing" spike occurs because of a change in the membrane permeability of the nerve that supplies the receptor. The change in local membrane permeability causes a localized influx of sodium into the nerve cell, followed by an efflux of potassium. This results in local depolarization, followed by a propagated action potential along the nerve that supplies the sensory receptor. In this way the information received by the receptor is conveyed via the dorsal roots into the central nervous system.

Depending on their mechanical properties, receptors may be classified as rapidly or slowly adapting. Rapidly adapting receptors do not respond after their initial response to a stimulus. Slowly adapting receptors continue to respond to an initial stimulus. All receptors fall into one of these two categories. More will be said regarding response characteristics as the individual receptors are discussed.

The receptors may also be categorized as encapsulated or unencapsulated. All of the receptors except free nerve endings and Merkel's discs are enclosed by connective tissue coverings called *capsules*.

There are five elementary qualities of conscious sensation that may be evoked by stimulation of the skin and deeper structures. Receptors that subserve touch and pressure, warmth, cold and pain are highly developed in the skin. Position sense (i.e., conscious proprioception or kinesthesia) is dependent on receptors located in all of the joints of the body. In addition, we are able to synthesize information from the tactile receptors of the skin and the joint receptors, which enables us to give a three-dimensional interpretation of objects held in our hands. This is called *stereognosis* and results from the tactile receptors providing information about the consistency of an object and the joint receptors gauging the size of an object.

There are two receptors that are responsible for subconscious proprioception. They are the Golgi tendon organ and the neuromuscular spindle, more commonly called the muscle spindle. These receptors provide us with subconscious awareness of body position, muscle tension and movement, which means that they contribute to coordinated movement on an efficient basis, since they do so without conscious effort on our part. More emphasis will be placed on the function of these two receptors than on others, not because they are more important than other receptors, but rather because an understanding of their function will make possible an easy grasp of some of the concepts on which many of the treatment procedures now being utilized clinically are based. Both Golgi tendon organs and muscle spindles are considered as muscle receptors, since the former are located in tendons and the latter, within the bellies of muscles.

ENCAPSULATED RECEPTORS

Golgi Tendon Organs

Golgi tendon organs measure approximately 1 millimeter in length and 100 microns in diameter. They consist of a few tendon fascicles, surrounded by a connective tissue capsule into which a type IB afferent nerve fiber enters. When muscle spindles are discussed, type IA afferent nerve fibers will be mentioned, and therefore the distinction between type IA and type IB nerve fibers must be made. Type I denotes the diameter of nerve fibers, so that types IA and IB fibers are the same diameter — between 12 and 20 microns. Both types of nerves are myelinated. According to Matthews, types A and B denote receptor characteristics. Type IA fibers have a very low threshold for stimulation and have the characteristics of a mechanism that lies and operates in parallel with the surrounding muscle tissues. Type IB nerve fibers have a very high threshold for stimulation and have the characteristic of a mechanism that lies and operates in series with the surrounding tendinous tissues. Actually, the nerve supply to the Golgi tendon organs only partially fulfills the requirements of type IB neurons, since they have a very low threshold for stimulation when a muscle is contracted. This fact was not known when Matthews originally classified these neurons. Type IB fibers comprise the sole innervation of Golgi tendon organs. They have no efferent nerve supply. Figure 3–1 shows the structure of a Golgi tendon organ.

Golgi tendon organs lie in series with muscle fibers in most instances, and therefore respond to both contraction and stretch of muscles. In fact, the most effective way to stimulate Golgi tendon organs is to stretch and contract a muscle concomitantly. The net effect is that the collagenous tendon fascicles are squeezed more tightly together so that the nerve endings are distorted by compression forces. If the distortion of the IB nerve ending is great enough, the threshold to produce a signal is exceeded and a propagated impulse reaches the spinal cord. Figure 3–2 illustrates a Golgi tendon organ which lies in series with the surrounding structures.

These organs have a very high threshold for stretch, requiring 90 to 100 grams of

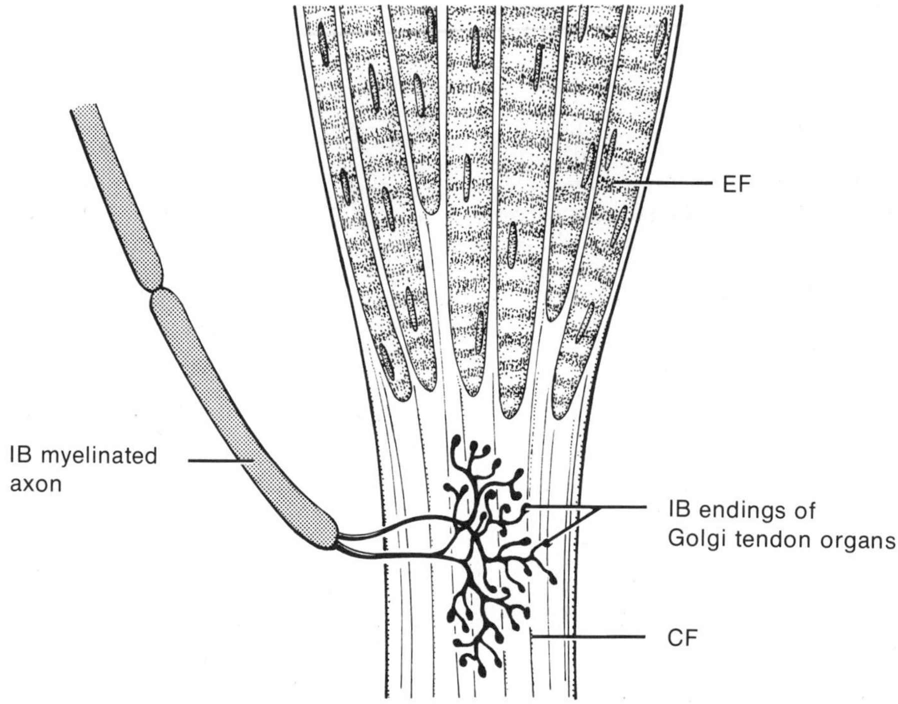

Figure 3–1. IB endings of Golgi tendon organs embedded within the collagenous tendon fascicles (*CF*) of an extrafusal muscle (*EF*).

stretch for stimulation to occur. However, they have a very low threshold for contraction. As little as 0.1 gram of contraction is sufficient to stimulate them. When the stimulus is great enough to evoke a response, the nerves that supply the muscle in which the stimulated Golgi tendon organs are located and its synergists are inhibited, and the activity in the nerves that supply the antagonists (muscles which do the opposing movement) is enhanced on the ipsilateral side. On the contralateral side the opposite effects are produced. These are reflex responses that occur by way of disynaptic contacts within the gray matter of the spinal cord. That is, there is one internuncial neuron between the IB sensory neuron and the alpha motor neuron, which is the efferent component of the reflex arc. The response is a rather diffuse one, involving not only the muscles at one particular joint, but also those muscles which control adjacent joints. For example, if a population of Golgi tendon organs is stimulated in the quadriceps femoris muscle as illustrated in Figure 3–3, there is not only inhibition of the nerves to the knee joint extensors and enhancement of activity in the nerves to the knee joint flexors, but in addition the nerves to the physiologic extensors (plantar flexors) at the talotibial joint are inhibited and those to the physiologic flexors (dorsiflexors) are excited. Because the muscle in which the stimulated Golgi tendon organs are located is always inhibited, the response is termed *autogenic inhibition.*

Clinically, Golgi tendon organs are responsible for the *clasped knife reflex.* This is not found normally but is seen in patients with upper motor neuron lesions (lesions of descending pathways of the central nervous system) that display some degree of hypertonic (increased muscle tone) resistance to passively imposed movements. The reflex is elicited by attempting to passively move a muscle in which hypertonicity or spasticity resists the movement; suddenly the muscle relaxes so that the extremity is moved easily through the available range of motion. The sudden relaxation is the clasped knife reflex. A specific example is a case in which a spinal cord-damaged patient has spasticity in the extensors of the lower extremities. As one attempts to flex the patient's hip and knee joints concomitantly, resistance to the imposed flexion is met; then suddenly the

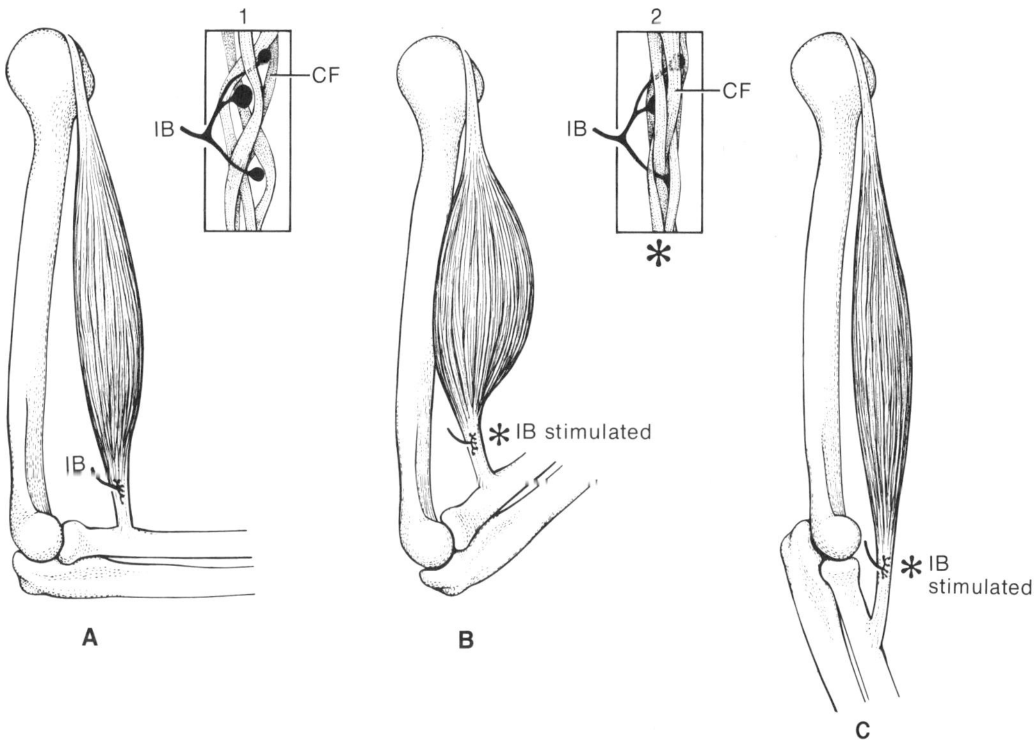

Figure 3–2. The IB endings of a Golgi tendon organ are shown in *A, B,* and *C.* Inset 1 shows that when a muscle is in a relaxed state (*A*) the collagenous tendon fascicles (*CF*) of that muscle are on slack and somewhat separated so that there is no compression (i.e., no stimulation) of the IB endings. Inset 2 shows what occurs when the muscle contracts (*B*) or is elongated (*C*). The collagenous tendon fascicles are compressed together, which squeezes the IB endings, thus stimulating them.

resistance "melts away" and the two joints can be taken into flexion easily, much as an open jackknife may be closed.

Golgi tendon organs function normally as a protective mechanism in situations in which a muscle is elongated slightly beyond its physiologic limits. A muscle tear may be prevented by the relaxation of the muscle provided by the reflex activity of the Golgi tendon organs. Also, the very low threshold of these receptors to muscle contraction enables them to function as feedback control mechanisms for fine control of movement through their connections with the cerebellum.

The central connections of Golgi tendon organs are those reflex connections at the spinal cord level that have just been discussed, as well as projections to the ipsilateral cerebellum by way of the dorsal and ventral spinocerebellar tracts, and some to the contralateral cerebellum by way of the ventral spinocerebellar tracts.

For those familiar with the Proprioceptive Neuromuscular Facilitation rehabilitation techniques, the Golgi tendon organs presumably are responsible for the increases in range of motion produced by means of the "contract–relax" method. This involves elongation of a muscle or muscle group through the comfortable range combined with resistance to an isometric contraction of the muscles in which the increase in range is desired. For example, if a patient has been in a cast for six weeks with the elbow joint flexed to 90 degrees for immobilization of a fractured humerus, he will have decreased range of motion in both the elbow joint flexors and extensors. To gain range in the elbow joint flexors, the patient actively *extends* the elbow joint as far as possible. Resistance is then given on the anterior aspect of the wrist joint as the patient attempts to move into elbow joint *flexion*. Movement is not allowed. The contraction should be isometric. This is repeated a

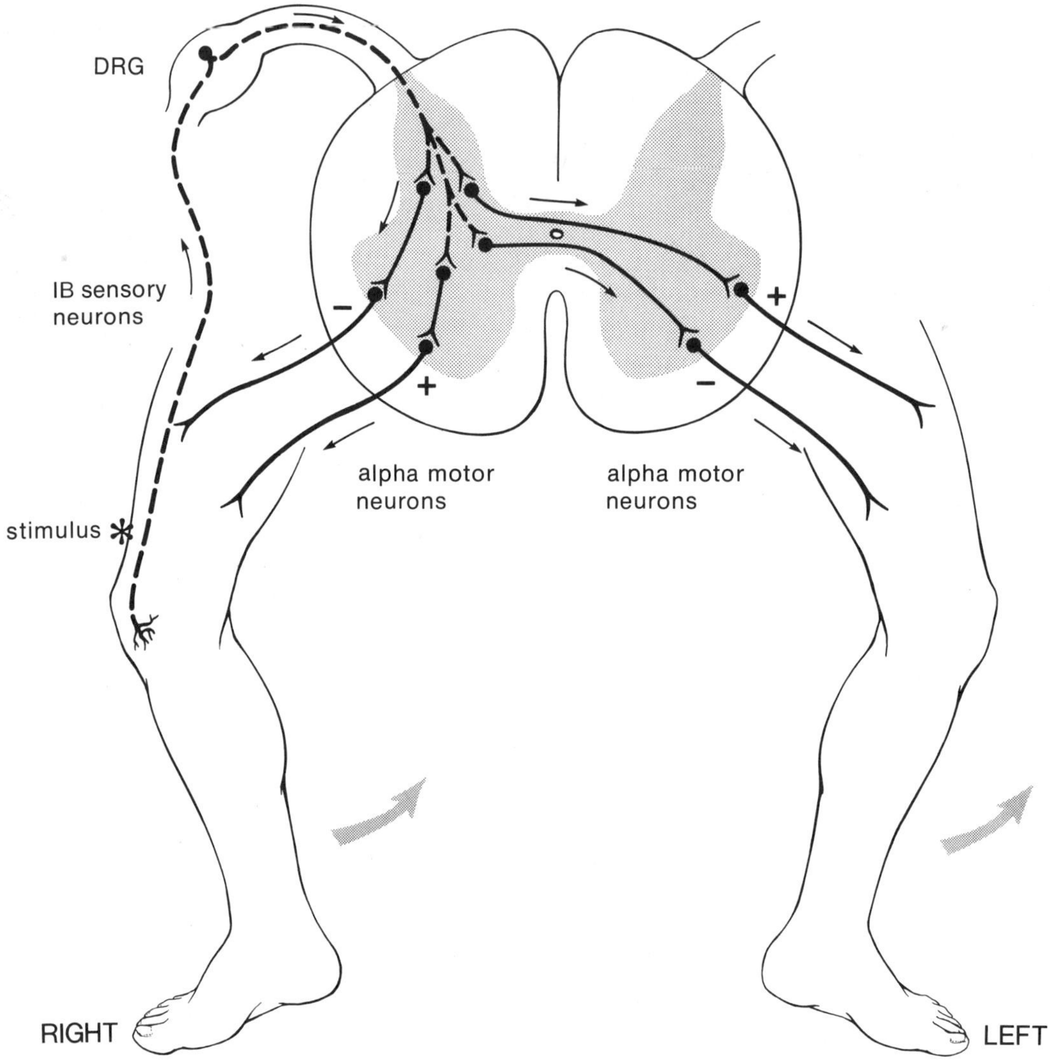

Figure 3–3. Reflex activity initiated by stimulation (*) of Golgi tendon organs in the right quadriceps femoris muscle. The impulses produced by the stimulation travel to the spinal cord via IB sensory neurons. These synapse with interneurons, which in turn synapse with alpha motor neurons. The latter project back to the musculature as shown. The net direction of leg movement due to the enhancement of activity in the knee joint flexors on the ipsilateral side and of knee joint extensors on the contralateral side is shown by the large gray arrows. Knee joint extension is inhibited on the ipsilateral side and knee joint flexion is inhibited on the contralateral side. The muscle in which the stimulated Golgi tendon organs are located is inhibited. This is called *autogenic inhibition.* + = enhancement of activity; − = inhibition of activity.

few times, after which the patient again actively extends the elbow joint as far as possible. He will probably be able to move a few degrees further into extension than on his initial attempt. To gain range in the elbow joint extensors, the patient actively *flexes* the elbow joint as far as possible. Resistance is given on the posterior aspect of the wrist joint as the patient attempts to move into elbow joint *extension.* Again, movement is not allowed. Repeat a few times and then have the patient actively *flex* the elbow as far as possible.

Both of these examples involve contraction of the muscle in its elongated state, which is the optimum combination for inhibiting the nerves that supply the muscle in which the stimulated Golgi tendon organs are located. The inhibited nerves produce relaxation in the muscle.

Muscle Spindles

Muscle spindles are located within muscle, and monitor both the amount of change in length and the rate of change in length of muscles. In man, the dimensions vary somewhat, but some are as large as over 1 centimeter in length and 100 to 200 microns in diameter. Spindles consist of very small muscle fibers which are classified into two types, nuclear bag and nuclear chain fibers. The classifications are based on morphologic differences. The major differences at the light microscopic level are that nuclear bag fibers (1) are longer and larger in diameter than nuclear chain fibers and (2) have an aggregation of many nuclei clumped together at the equatorial zone, whereas nuclear chain fibers contain a single row of nuclei in the equatorial zone. Nuclear chain and nuclear bag fibers are called collectively *intrafusal* muscle fibers, as opposed to the large *extrafusal* muscle fibers that produce joint movement. Intrafusal fibers contain contractile sarcomeres identical to those of extrafusal fibers in their polar regions, but are practically devoid of contractile proteins in the equatorial region where the nuclei are located. Although intrafusal fibers have contractile polar regions, the fibers are far too small to produce any joint movement when they contract.

The number of intrafusal fibers per muscle spindle varies from spindle to spindle and from species to species. For example, adult rat spindles quite consistently contain two nuclear bag and two nuclear chain fibers, whereas human spindles generally contain three or four nuclear bag fibers and anywhere from four to 11 nuclear chain fibers. The intrafusal fibers are enclosed within a connective tissue capsule which is derived from the perineural epithelium (one of the nerve cell sheaths) of the nerves that supply them. The number of muscle spindles in different muscles is variable, but in general muscles subserving fine coordination contain the largest number, those subserving gross movements contain the least and postural muscles contain an intermediate number. Figure 3–4 is a diagrammatic representation of the morphology of nuclear bag and nuclear chain fibers.

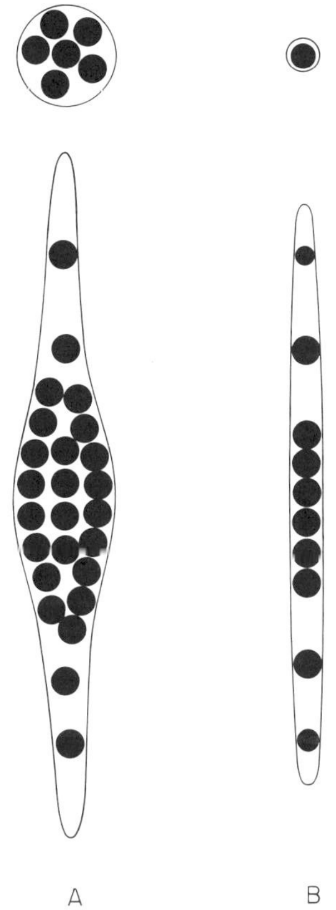

Figure 3–4. The morphology of nuclear bag (*A*) and nuclear chain (*B*) fibers. The upper figures in *A* and *B* show cross-sections of the nuclear bag and nuclear chain fibers at the midequatorial zone, and the lower figures show the longitudinal shape of the intrafusal fibers and the distribution of nuclei within these.

In contrast to Golgi tendon organs, muscle spindles are innervated by motor nerves as well as sensory nerves. The sensory innervation, which consists of type IA and type II afferent fibers, will be considered first. As mentioned earlier, type IA nerve fibers measure from 12 to 20 microns in diameter and have a very low threshold to stimulation. In fact, they respond to as little as 2 to 3 grams of stretch, in contrast to the 90 grams of stretch required to stimulate Golgi tendon organs. Muscle spindles are attached in parallel with extrafusal fibers so that contraction of those fibers does not stimulate them, but *elongation of extrafusal fibers does stimulate them.* Contraction of extrafusal fibers causes spindle firing to cease. This is what is meant by possessing the characteristics of a mechanism which is located in parallel with surrounding muscle structures — one of the requirements of Type IA nerve fibers (see Fig. 3–5).

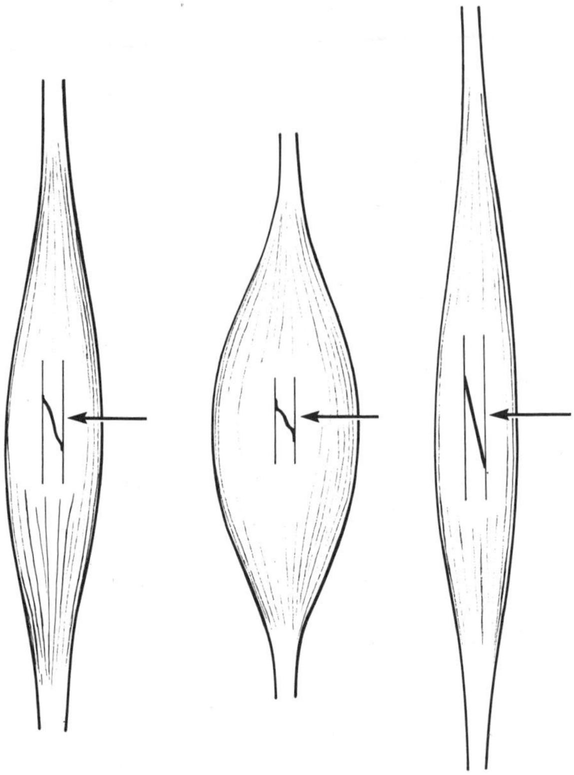

Figure 3–5. The arrows in *A, B,* and *C* indicate the same muscle spindle with the extrafusal muscle within which it is located at resting length (*A*), contracted (*B*), and elongated (*C*). The ends of the muscle spindle are attached to two adjacent extrafusal fibers (*two vertical lines*) in this example. Therefore, when the muscle as a whole shortens or contracts, the spindle is put on slack and its sensory innervation is not stimulated. When the muscle is elongated, the longitudinal dimension of the spindle increases so that the sensory nerve endings that terminate upon it are distorted and thus stimulated. Note that the spindle is not located exactly parallel with the surrounding structures, but it responds in the same manner as a mechanism that lies in parallel.

Each muscle spindle is innervated by one IA sensory nerve fiber which branches and terminates as primary (annulospiral) endings. These supply the equatorial zones of all intrafusal fibers, both nuclear bag and nuclear chain fibers. Type II sensory nerve fibers measure 8 to 12 microns in diameter and have a slightly higher threshold than type IA fibers. They require 19 to 20 grams of stretch for stimulation to occur. Each spindle is innervated by zero to 5 type II fibers. They terminate as secondary (flower spray) endings in the juxtaequatorial regions of both nuclear bag and nuclear chain fibers, but they are distributed primarily to nuclear chain fibers. Those secondary endings which terminate upon nuclear chain fibers do so in a spiral type of arrangement, and those which terminate upon nuclear bag fibers do so in a flower spray type of configuration, which reflects the older terminology for them (see Fig. 3–6).

The response elicited by stimulation of the primary endings of muscle spindles is the opposite of autogenic inhibition, which is produced by stimulation of Golgi tendon organs. The muscle in which the stimulated muscle spindles are located contracts and the nerves to the antagonistic muscles are inhibited. On the contralateral side, the opposite effects are produced. The example illustrated in Figure 3–7 involves stimulation of spindles which are located in the knee joint extensors. In this case the extensors contract and the flexors are inhibited on the ipsilateral side. On the contralateral side the extensors are inhibited and activity in the flexors is enhanced. If the stimulated spindles are located in flexors, the flexors will contract, with concomitant relaxation of extensors on the ipsilateral side; on the contralateral side the extensor activity will be enhanced and flexor activity inhibited in the corresponding muscles. Note that the connections of the IA fibers with alpha motor neurons that innervate the muscle in which the stimulated spindles are located (homonomous alpha motor neurons) are

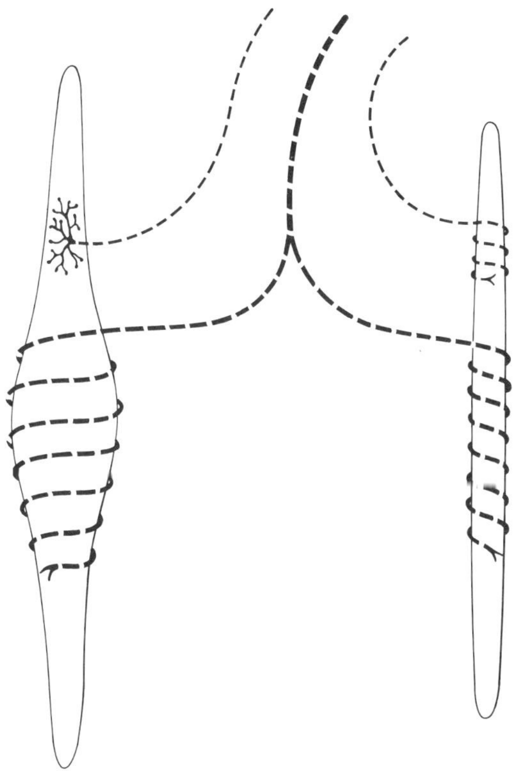

Figure 3–6. A nuclear bag fiber (*A*) and a nuclear chain fiber (*B*) innervated by primary (*heavy dash*) and secondary (*thinner dash*) sensory nerve endings.

monosynaptic within the spinal cord. This means that the response to stimulation occurs very rapidly. The connections of the IA fibers with all of the alpha motor neurons that innervate other muscles (heteronomous alpha motor neurons) are polysynaptic. The response elicited by stimulation of the primary endings is more localized than that elicited by stimulation of Golgi tendon organs; i.e., it is limited to muscles controlling the joint or joints upon which the stimulated muscle acts. The response is the well-known *stretch* or *myotatic reflex*.

The response of the secondary endings to stimulation is a little more difficult to understand. If the muscle in which the stimulated secondary endings of the muscle spindles are located is an extensor, activity in that muscle and its synergists will be inhibited and the flexors will be concomitantly facilitated. Conversely, on the contralateral side activity of the extensors will be facilitated and activity in the flexors will be inhibited. If the muscle in which the stimulated secondary endings are located is a flexor, the flexors on the ipsilateral side will again be facilitated and the extensors will be inhibited, and again, the effect on the contralateral side is facilitation of extensors and inhibition of flexors. Because the response on the ipsilateral side is always facilitation of flexors and inhibition of extensors, no matter in what muscles the stimulated secondary endings are located, these responses are called *flexor reflexes*. In addition, the response on the contralateral side consistently is facilitation of extension, regardless of where the stimulated secondary endings are located. This is called the *crossed extension reflex*. An example of reflex activity produced by stimulation of secondary endings is illustrated in Figure 3–8. Some recent investigations have provided some suggestion that stimulation of secondary endings does not always enhance flexion. However, until further research is completed in this area, this author prefers the above description of function.

Consideration of the sensory innervation of the muscle spindle only clarifies the means by which the spindle functions on a reflex level. However, the spindle does much more than this. It contributes to the production of smooth, controlled, coordinated movement, and to understand how this is accomplished the motor innervation of intrafusal fibers must be considered.

According to Barker, who has studied the ultrastructure of spindle innervation, there are three types of motor nerves which terminate on intrafusal fibers. The designation of types of motor nerves is based on differences in diameter and on the morphology of their terminals. They are called *trail ends* and *P1* and *P2 plates*. The details will not be considered here, but it is important to know the terminology in order to recognize them as gamma or fusimotor innervation when encountering them in the literature. In general, their diameters vary from 3 to 7 microns. Barker's work shows that the nerve fibers that terminate as P2 plates are the largest, and those that terminate as trail ends are the smallest.

The fusimotor or gamma motor neurons innervate the polar, contractile regions of the intrafusal fibers. Impulses transmitted to the contractile regions of the intrafusal fibers via gamma motor neurons produce

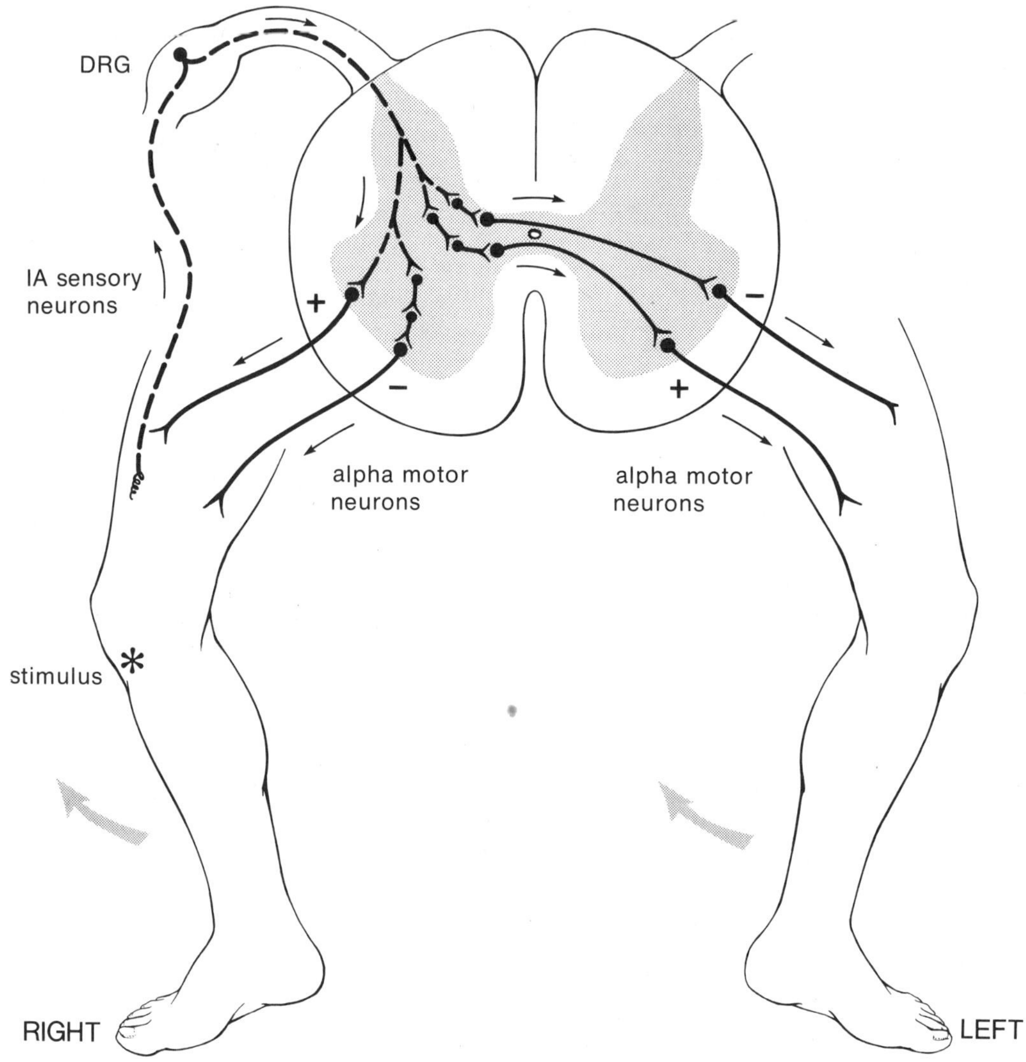

Figure 3–7. Reflex activity elicited by stimulation (∗) of the primary endings of the right quadriceps femoris muscle. The impulses produced by the stimulation travel to the spinal cord via IA sensory neurons. The synapses with homonomous motor neurons are direct (monosynaptic), and all other connections with alpha motor neurons are indirect (polysynaptic). The alpha motor neurons project back to the musculature as shown. The large gray arrows indicate enhancement of activity in the knee joint extensors on the ipsilateral side and of knee joint flexors on the contralateral side. Knee joint flexion is inhibited on the ipsilateral side and knee joint extension is inhibited on the contralateral side. The muscle in which the stimulated primary endings are located is always stimulated. This is the *stretch reflex*, which is also called the *myotatic reflex*. + = enhancement of activity; − = inhibition of activity.

contraction of the intrafusal muscle fibers, just as impulses transmitted to extrafusal fibers via alpha motor neurons produce muscle contraction and joint movement. When the polar regions of the intrafusal fibers contract they shorten, and since they have fixed attachments to the endomysium of adjacent extrafusal fibers at both ends, the shortening of the polar regions results in lengthening of the longitudinal dimension of the equatorial zone (see Fig. 3–9). This has the same effect as stretching extrafusal muscle fibers and stimulates the primary endings to depolarize and send propagated impulses to the spinal cord. From that point on the response is the same as illustrated for the myotatic reflex.

There is no evidence that gamma motor

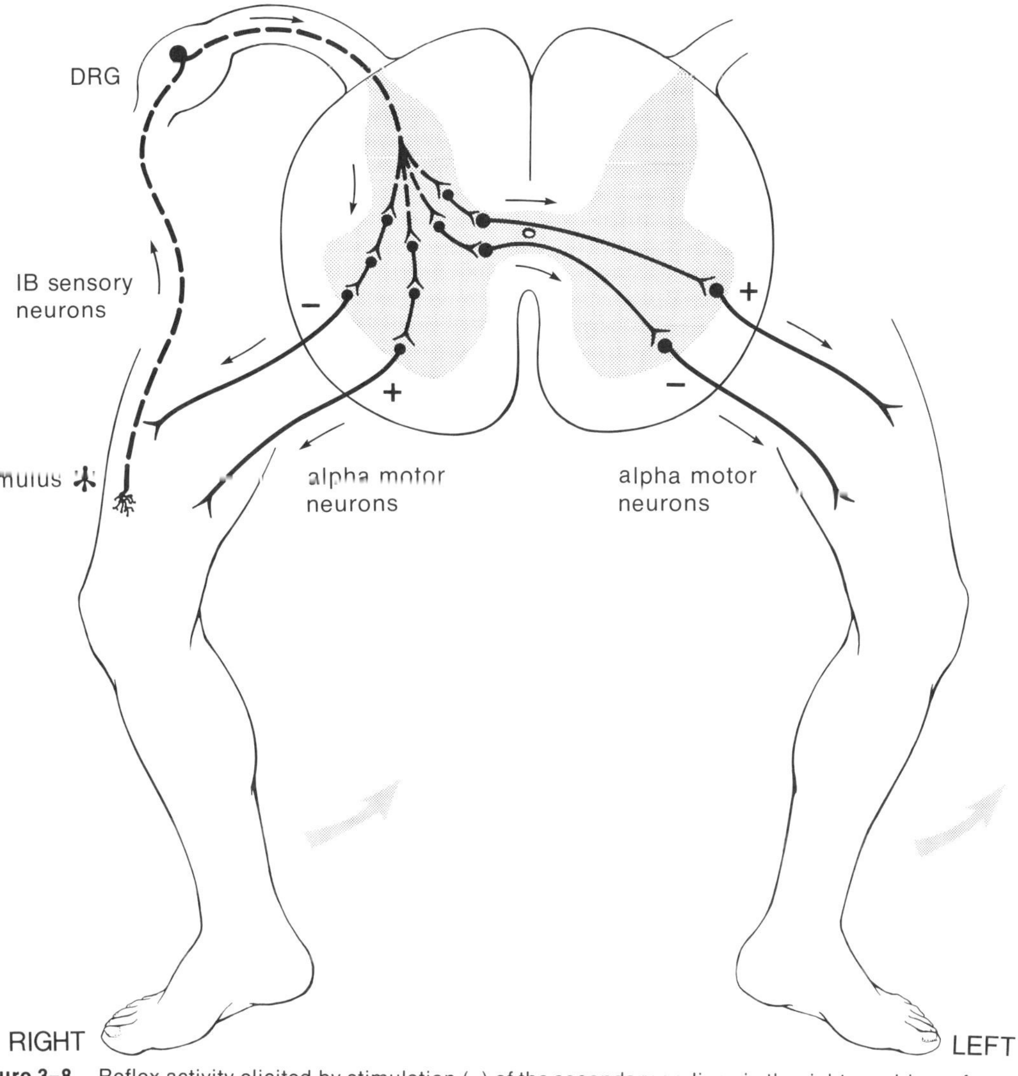

Figure 3–8. Reflex activity elicited by stimulation (∗) of the secondary endings in the right quadriceps femoris muscle. The impulses produced by the stimulation travel to the spinal cord via type II sensory neurons. All synapses with alpha motor neurons are indirect (polysynaptic). The alpha motor neurons project back to the musculature as shown. The large gray arrows indicate enhancement of activity in the knee joint flexors on the ipsilateral side and of knee joint extensors on the contralateral side. Knee joint extension is inhibited on the ipsilateral side and knee joint flexion is inhibited on the contralateral side. No matter what muscle the stimulated secondary endings are located in, the response of the ipsilateral side is enhancement of flexion. These responses are called *flexor reflexes.* + = enhancement of activity; − = inhibition of activity.

neurons are ever directly contacted by IA sensory neurons, but they are contacted by axons from a number of different sources, which either excite or inhibit them. The descending pathways that influence gamma motor neuron activity arise from brain stem structures. They are the reticular formation (reticulospinal tract), the red nucleus (rubrospinal tract) and perhaps the lateral vestibular nucleus (vestibulospinal tract). The reticular formation is a rather ill-defined region located deep within the brain stem, extending through the medulla, pons and midbrain. The red nucleus is a large oval nucleus located in the midbrain and caudal diencephalon. The lateral vestibular nucleus is one of four vestibular nuclei that lie inferior to the floor of the fourth ventricle.

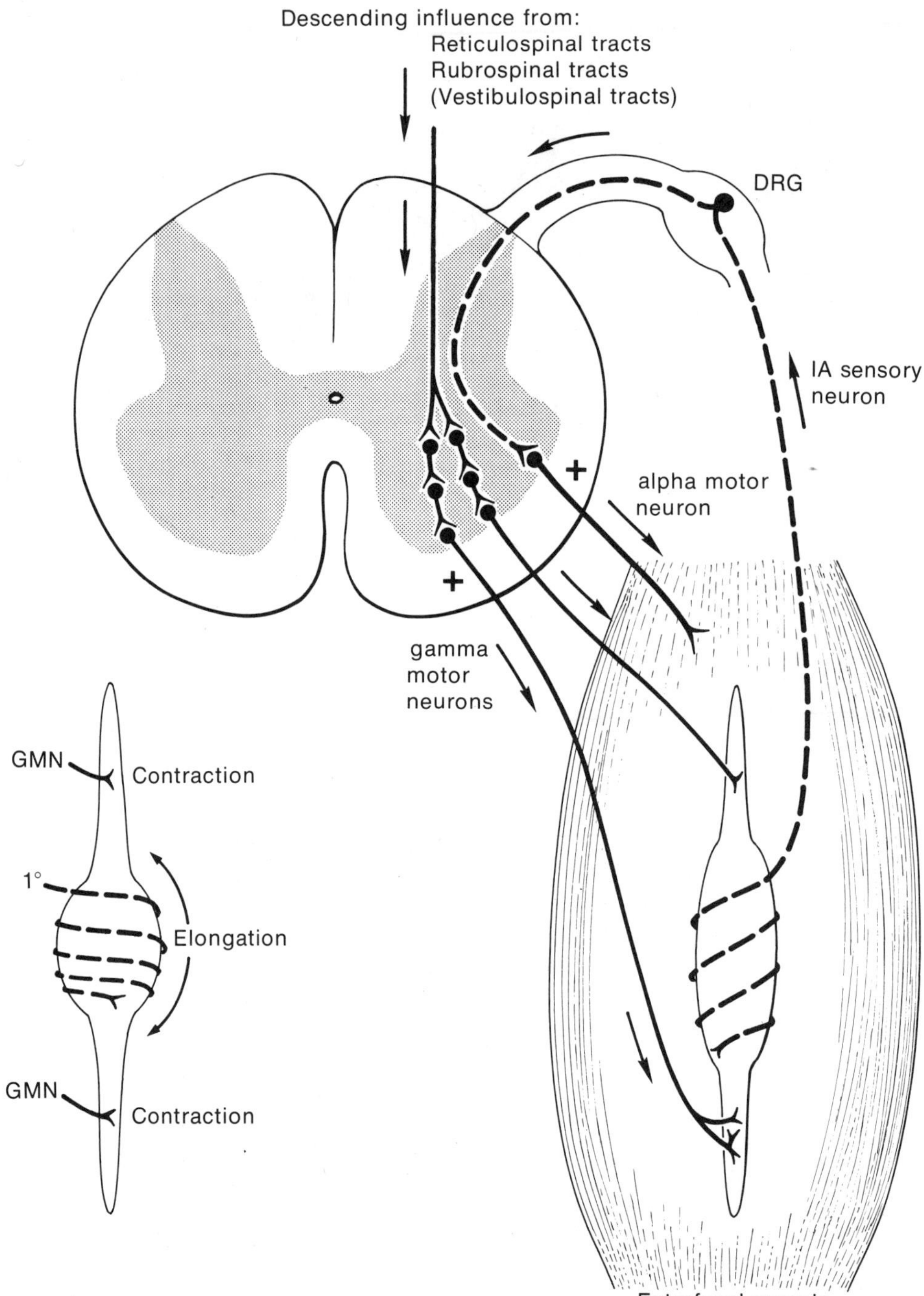

Figure 3–9. The response when gamma motor neurons are excited. On the right descending excitatory influences are shown. They synapse with gamma motor neurons which terminate in the polar regions of intrafusal fibers. The gamma motor neurons cause the polar regions of the intrafusal fibers to contract, which results in elongation of the equatorial region. This elongation produces distortion of the primary endings, which results in a propagated impulse back to the spinal cord by way of IA sensory neurons. The IA sensory neurons make monosynaptic contacts with alpha motor neurons, which in turn project back to the extrafusal muscle in which the stimulated muscle spindles are located and cause it to contract. On the left, the inset shows the intrafusal fiber in a relaxed state and indicates where contraction and elongation will occur when stimulated by gamma motor neurons. *GMN* = gamma motor neuron; 1° = primary ending.

There is no reliable evidence that axons of the corticospinal tracts make synaptic contacts with gamma motor neurons. The latter are also influenced by local afferents that originate in the skin and subcutaneous tissues. The pathways involving local afferents function on the spinal cord reflex level and provide the framework for some of the therapeutic procedures commonly utilized in the clinic (Margaret Rood). These treatment procedures involve brushing and icing of the skin in an attempt to enhance or inhibit gamma motor neuron activity, according to the needs of the patient.

Figure 3–9 illustrates the response when gamma motor neurons are excited by only supraspinal influences. It does not show the results when local afferent neurons are stimulated, nor does it illustrate the effects of inhibition of gamma motor neurons. In that case, if the gamma motor neurons are inhibited, the polar regions of the intrafusal fibers relax so that the extrafusal muscle may elongate to a certain extent without distorting the equatorial regions. Thus, no impulses will be propagated along the IA sensory fibers and no reflex activity will occur.

Owing to this "biasing" activity of the gamma motor neurons, the sensitivity of intrafusal fibers to stretch is continually adjusted so that IA sensory fibers can be activated when the muscle is contracted as well as when it is stretched. Inhibition of gamma motor neurons makes it possible to elongate an extrafusal muscle without eliciting the stretch reflex, thus allowing smooth movements to take place. The intrafusal muscle fibers are always aligned in length to extrafusal muscle fibers in normal individuals, and therefore they help provide for coordinated movement. This appears to be quite an efficient system, since it all occurs independently of conscious thought. The system is actually a subconscious monitor, gauging the length of neighboring extrafusal fibers.

It was mentioned earlier that muscle spindles monitor both change in length and the rate of change in length. What components of the spindle are responsible for each? The change in length is monitored by both primary and secondary endings. This is called the *static* component of spindle function. The rate of change in length is monitored by the primary endings alone. This is called the *dynamic* component of spindle function.

The central connections of the spindle afferent neurons are those that have been discussed at the spinal cord level as well as long ascending projections to supraspinal levels. Both type IA and type II fibers send impulses to the ipsilateral cerebellum via the dorsal and ventral spinocerebellar tracts and to the contralateral cerebellum by way of the ventral spinocerebellar tract. Some impulses also reach the cerebral cortex via the dorsal column (medial lemniscal) system. There is no good evidence that these impulses reach consciousness, but rather that they probably function in the integration of movement.

The Tonic Vibration Reflex (TVR)

In connection with muscle spindles, it is important to include some discussion about vibration, since at present it is a popular technique used clinically for enhancing muscle function, and this exemplifies one way in which spindles can be stimulated for therapeutic benefit.

The motor responses elicited by vibration are (1) active contraction of the vibrated muscle (called the tonic vibration reflex or TVR) and (2) depression of excitability of motor neurons which innervate the antagonistic muscles by means of reciprocal innervation. The latency of the response of the TVR is very short; in fact it is identical to that of the stretch reflex, and the tension in the muscle progressively increases over the first 20 to 25 seconds of stimulation. A plateau is then reached so that further stimulation does not produce greater magnitudes of tension. It is important to realize that the maximum amount of tension developed by the TVR is never more than a small fraction of that developed during a maximum voluntary effort. This is because only a small percentage of the motor neuron pool can be activated reflexly by vibrating a muscle.

It is known that the TVR is a reflex mechanism since it cannot be elicited in a denervated muscle, nor in a deafferented muscle. However, the TVR is not just a simple segmental spinal reflex, as shown by the following evidence:

1. Spinal transection abolishes the TVR permanently. Therefore, higher neural centers must play an important role in supporting the TVR.

2. Barbiturates depress the TVR without altering tendon reflexes. Since barbiturates preferentially depress small reticular neurons and interneurons, the reticular formation must be involved with the TVR.

The TVR survives cerebellectomy in decerebrate animals. Therefore, the cerebellum and the cerebral cortex are not involved in control of the TVR.

The major factors that influence the TVR are the following:

1. The initial length of the muscle — "the longer the initial length of the muscle (within reason), the stronger the isometric TVR." (Bishop, 1974, 1975)
2. Application of the stimulus — if two stimuli are applied simultaneously to antagonistic muscles, neither muscle will contract.
3. Central nervous system excitability —
   a. cooling an individual increases the magnitude of the TVR;
   b. changing the position of the head with respect to the body alters the TVR by means of the tonic neck and tonic labyrinthine reflexes.
4. Caloric stimulation of the labyrinths, which activates vestibular reflexes and increases the TVR on the ipsilateral side.
5. Parameters of the vibratory stimulus —
   a. an increase in the amplitude of the stimulus up to 150 microns increases the strength of the TVR. Further increases in the stimulus do not further augment the response. The increase in the magnitude of the TVR is produced by recruitment of more receptors, which activates a larger fraction of the motor neuron pool;
   b. a major determinant of the strength of the TVR is the frequency of stimulation. The most commonly used frequency of stimulation is 100 to 300 Hz.

The components of the TVR consist of the primary endings of muscle spindles; i.e., the afferent pathway of the TVR and the monosynaptic myotatic reflex is identical. In addition, the reticulospinal system interacts to enhance the TVR in a way that is not fully understood.

Joint Receptors

The joint receptors are responsible for kinesthesia or conscious proprioception. They function as absolute detectors of movement and position, and respond to even the slightest change of angle between two bony segments. Four types of joint receptors have been described. They are the Ruffini end organs, Golgi-Mazzoni corpuscles, Golgi type endings and free nerve endings. All of these, with the exception of free nerve endings, are subserved by type II neurons, which are myelinated and from 8 to 12 microns in diameter.

Ruffini end organs, which are associated with joints, are located exclusively in fibrous joint capsules. They are oval-shaped with a thin connective tissue capsule. A myelinated nerve enters each Ruffini end organ, after which the axon loses its myelin and arborizes freely within the capsule (see Fig. 3–10). This type of ending responds strongly when the joint is moved. These are slowly adapting stretch receptors which monitor the direction and speed of movement.

The largest of the joint receptors resemble Golgi tendon organs and are called *Golgi type endings.* These are located primarily in joint ligaments. Their response characteristics are almost identical to Ruffini end organs; i.e., they are slowly adapting, but they have a somewhat higher threshold to stimulation than the latter. Golgi type endings monitor the position of the bony segments that contribute to a joint.

Golgi-Mazzoni corpuscles closely resemble pacinian corpuscles, but are smaller (see Fig. 3–11). They are very sparsely distributed and are located in the loose pericapsular

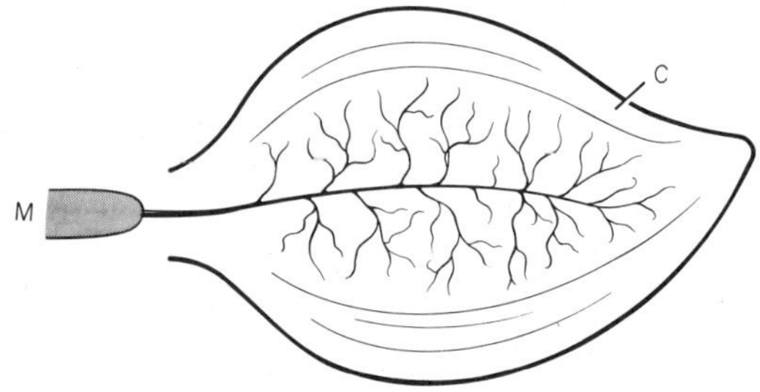

Figure 3–10. A Ruffini end organ. *M* = myelinated axon which loses its myelin and arborizes extensively after entering the capsule (*C*).

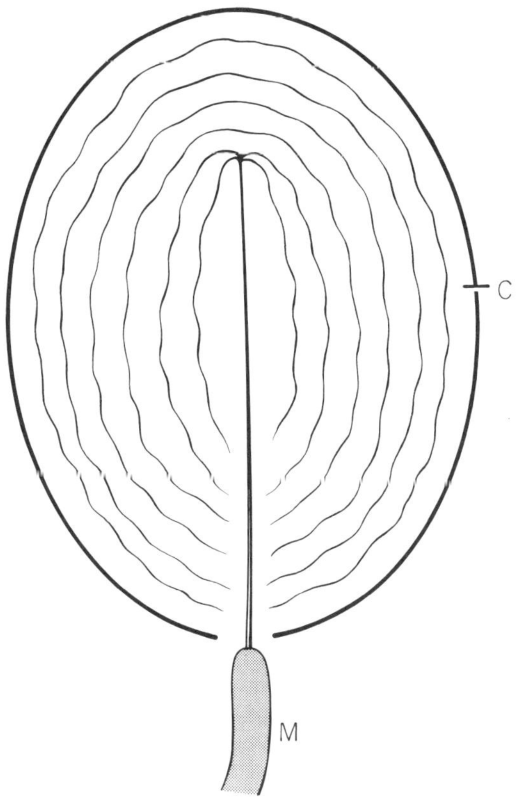

Figure 3–11. A Golgi-Mazzoni corpuscle. These resemble pacinian corpuscles but are smaller. The capsule (*C*) consists of several laminations, and the receptor is innervated by a single myelinated axon (*M*) which loses its myelin as it enters the capsule.

tissues. Whereas Ruffini end organs and Golgi type endings are slowly adapting, Golgi-Mazzoni corpuscles are very rapidly adapting. Presumably, they monitor the rate of rapid joint movements.

Plexuses of fine, unmyelinated *free nerve endings* of less than 1 micron in diameter are found in profusion in fibrous joint capsules, ligaments, synovial membranes and fat pads related to joints, but they do not function as monitors of joint movement. Rather, they are the pain receptors of the joints.

The nerves that terminate in joint structures may join either cutaneous nerves or nerves that innervate the musculature en route to the central nervous system. Recollection of Hilton's law (which states that a joint is innervated by the nerves that supply the muscles that move or cross that joint) will aid in identifying which joints are supplied by specific named nerves and spinal segments.

The joint receptors subserve an extremely important function. In normal individuals they provide conscious awareness of the positions of the limbs at all times. Loss of their function deprives one of this kinesthetic sense so that visual cues are necessary to determine the relationships of the parts of the body to each other. One of the most striking examples of a disease that destroys the joint receptors is rheumatoid arthritis. A patient with this disease may be so severely involved as to have very little kinesthetic sense, and thus may have great difficulty with balance if he is deprived of visual cues.

Cutaneous Receptors

Meissner's Corpuscles

Meissner's corpuscles are located in the dermal papillae, primarily in glabrous skin, which is most abundant on the volar surfaces of the fingers, toes, hands and feet. They are oblong, encapsulated structures innervated by one to four myelinated type II, and perhaps some type III, afferent neurons. After the nerves enter the capsule they immediately lose their myelin sheaths and spiral into a very tangled configuration (see Fig. 3–12). These receptors are responsible for monitoring two-point discrimination.

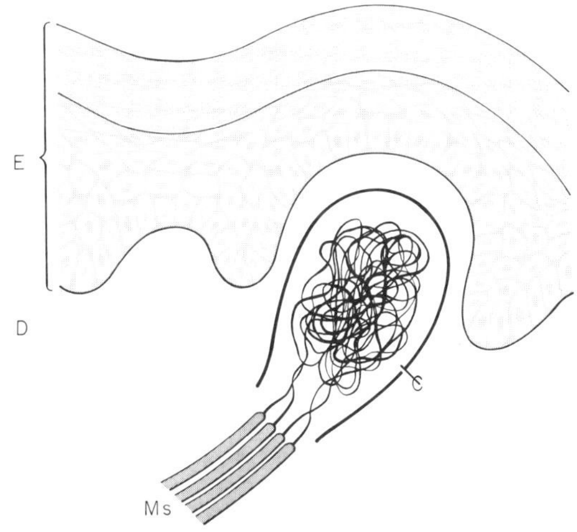

Figure 3–12. A Meissner's corpuscle located deep to the epidermis (*E*) in a dermal (*D*) papilla. In this illustration four myelinated nerves (*Ms*) enter the capsule (*C*). They lose their myelin as they enter the capsule and spiral into a very tangled configuration.

Pacinian Corpuscles

Pacinian corpuscles are the largest and most widely distributed of the encapsulated receptors. They have a very well-defined morphology, consisting of many concentric layers of connective tissue that resemble the layers of an onion and are innervated by one large myelinated nerve fiber. The nerve loses its myelin just after entering the capsule, and courses straight up the center of the corpuscle. Figure 3–11 illustrates the morphology of a Golgi-Mazzoni corpuscle, which is identical to a pacinian corpuscle, only smaller. Pacinian corpuscles are so large (3 to 4 mm in length) that they can be seen without the aid of a microscope in the mesentery of cats. They are located in the mesentery of mammals, the dermis, subcutaneous and intramuscular connective tissue, periosteum, ligaments and occasionally in muscle. These are very rapidly adapting mechanoreceptors that are often located near blood vessels. They are thought to signal changes in local blood supply and to monitor vibration and deep pressure. Although pacinian corpuscles monitor vibration, the evidence presented thus far indicates that they are not responsible for the tonic vibration reflex.

Golgi-Mazzoni Corpuscles

Golgi-Mazzoni corpuscles are present in the subcutaneous tissue of the fingers and on the surfaces of tendons, as well as in the fibrous capsules of joints. They are very similar to pacinian corpuscles, but smaller. Their functions are also similar to those of pacinian corpuscles, i.e., they monitor deep pressure and vibration and are supplied by type II, and perhaps some type III, sensory neurons.

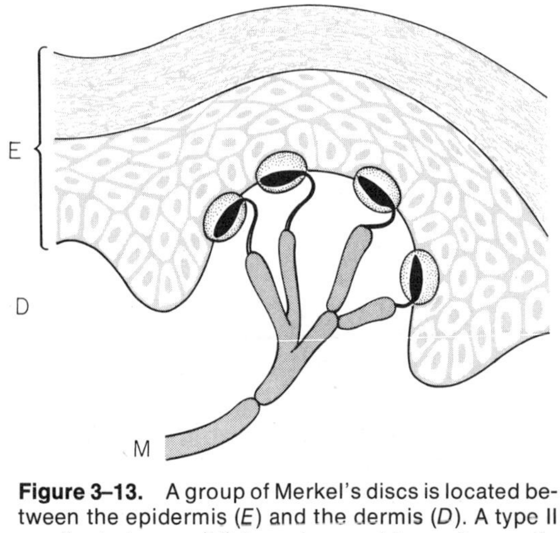

Figure 3–13. A group of Merkel's discs is located between the epidermis (*E*) and the dermis (*D*). A type II myelinated axon (*M*) branches and loses its myelin just before innervating the discs.

Ruffini Endings

Ruffini endings along with Golgi-Mazzoni corpuscles were mentioned earlier in the discussion related to joint receptors. They are also located in the deep connective tissue and in fascial sheaths. Their morphology is the same as that shown in Figure 3–10. They convey impulses when stimulated by deep pressure.

Krause End Bulbs

Krause end bulbs are present in the dermis all over the body. They consist of a round connective tissue capsule and are innervated by small, myelinated type III afferent nerve fibers. After entry into the capsule, the nerve loses its myelin sheath and immediately forms a tangled arborization within the capsule. The morphology is very similar to that of the Meissner's corpuscle illustrated in Figure 3–12 except that Krause end bulbs are round instead of oblong. There is some ground for belief that Krause end bulbs respond to cooling, but many regard this evidence as tenuous.

UNENCAPSULATED RECEPTORS

Merkel's Discs

Merkel's discs are produced by branching nerve fibers (primarily type II myelinated sensory fibers) which branch in the dermis and induce some of the cells in the deeper layers of the epidermis to differentiate into neurofibrillar discs (see Fig. 3–13). One nerve may branch to produce many such discs. They are located primarily in glabrous skin on the volar surfaces of the fingers, on the lips and external genitalia. They are believed to be touch receptors that respond to deformation of the skin.

Free Nerve Endings

Free nerve endings are the most widely distributed nerve endings in the body. Some of them are myelinated, but most are unmyelinated. If myelinated they lose their myelin as they approach their receptive surfaces. Most free nerve endings innervate the dermis of the skin; they do not reach the surface of the skin. They are also found in mucous membranes, muscle, deep fascia, connective tissue of visceral organs, joints, the cornea (where they terminate right on the surface) and around the bases of hair follicles. Those that terminate around the bases of hair follicles are sensitive to movements of the hairs. Free nerve endings monitor sensations of pain, temperature and diffuse touch. The best evidence for their function is that the cornea contains only free nerve endings, yet is sensitive to all three modalities, touch, pain and temperature.

For many years there has been controversy among neurophysiologists concerning how the quality of a stimulus is transmitted from receptors to the central nervous system; i.e., how does the CNS interpret a stimulus or differentiate between stimuli such as pain, cold, touch, etc.? There are two classic theories which attempt to explain how this might occur: the *fiber specific theory* and the *pattern specific theory*. The interpretation of those who favor the former is that there are morphologically different receptors for each quality of sensation. The theory is also based partially on the fact that there is some correlation between sensations mediated and the diameters of the first order neurons that mediate them. Proponents of the pattern specific theory believe that one morphologic type of receptor can respond to different kinds of stimuli. They believe that the interpretation of the quality of the stimulus is dependent on the pattern of impulse transmission in the axons, assuming that the pattern is different for each type of stimulus. For example, pain might be represented by an impulse pattern that looks like:

//// //// //// ////

whereas diffuse touch might be represented by:

///////////////////////////

There are several instances in which one can see evidence for the fiber specific theory, i.e., for morphologically specific receptors that convey precise qualities of sensory information to the CNS. Examples include Meissner's corpuscles, Golgi tendon organs, muscle spindles, etc. In other cases there is evidence for the pattern specific theory, particularly related to free nerve endings, which convey a variety of sensory modalities to the CNS. Therefore, it must be concluded that the evidence is equivocal.

REVIEW QUESTIONS

1. Which modalities would be lost if there was an isolated lesion in a nerve supplying a muscle? From which specific somatosensory receptors would the afferent nerves be interrupted?
2. Which modalities would be lost if there was an isolated lesion in a cutaneous nerve that supplies the skin? Associate the specific types of receptors responsible for each modality lost.
3. What is meant by slowly and rapidly adapting receptors? Can you think, in general, how you might utilize this information when attempting to evoke a therapeutic response from a patient?
4. Explain and demonstrate how you might go about stimulating the Golgi tendon organs in a variety of muscles. Show in a detailed diagram the responses you would expect. In your diagram and accompanying your demonstration, specify the muscle in which the stimulated GTO is located. Can you think of a clinical situation in which this procedure might be of therapeutic value?

5. What are considered to be the normal functions of the Golgi tendon organ?
6. Explain, using diagrams, the reflex activity evoked upon stimulation of:
   a. primary spindle receptors.
   b. secondary spindle receptors.
7. Explain how the gamma system operates to maintain the sensitivity of muscle spindles so that they respond when extrafusal muscle fibers change their length.
8. If you stimulate the skin, is it possible to evoke a response from one specific type of receptor?
9. Name the joint receptors. Indicate their locations, specific functions and mechanical characteristics.
10. Discuss the two classic theories that attempt to explain how the quality of a stimulus is transmitted to the central nervous system. What is the evidence for each?
11. What are the motor responses elicited by vibration of a muscle?
12. What are the major factors that influence the TVR?
13. What is the optimum amplitude to elicit the TVR? Optimum frequency?
14. Name the components of the TVR.

CHAPTER 4 • ASCENDING AND DESCENDING SYSTEMS OF THE SPINAL CORD

OBJECTIVES

After reading this chapter you should: • Be familiar with Rexed's laminar arrangement of the spinal cord. This is very important to an understanding of the literature pertaining to the spinal cord. • Know the anatomy and components of the ascending and descending tracts of the spinal cord well enough to determine the consequences of lesions of the major tracts at any level of the spinal cord (i.e., in terms of sensory modalities lost on the ipsilateral and contralateral sides of the body in addition to motor losses). • Be able to locate the level of the spinal cord lesion and the side of the lesion, and know which major tracts are involved when presented with the symptoms resulting from trauma. • Be familiar with the somatotopic organization of the ascending and descending systems. • Know the difference between upper and lower motor neuron lesions.

ORGANIZATION OF THE SPINAL CORD

Before the ascending and descending systems are discussed, it is necessary to know something about the organization of the spinal cord. It consists of an ependymal layer, which provides the lining for the central canal; a mantle layer, which is equivalent to the spinal gray matter; and a marginal layer, which consists of white matter (see Fig. 4–1).

The spinal gray varies considerably in shape and size at different segmental levels. The ventral and dorsal horns are especially well-developed at the segmental levels that contribute to the brachial and lumbosacral plexuses, because the extremities require more motor innervation and send more sensory information to the spinal cord than do the neck and trunk. In the thoracic region, the intermediolateral horns are well-developed, since this is the region in which the preganglionic cells of the sympathetic nervous system are located. In high cervical regions both the dorsal and ventral horns are somewhat attenuated. Figure 4–2 illustrates the structure of the gray matter at different levels of the spinal cord.

Sensory fibers that enter the dorsal roots synapse directly or indirectly with local spinal motor neurons for reflex mechanism activity, and they also project to higher centers of the nervous system through a variety of ascending pathways.

The motor neurons, which are located in the ventral horns, may receive synaptic contacts directly or indirectly from nerve fibers

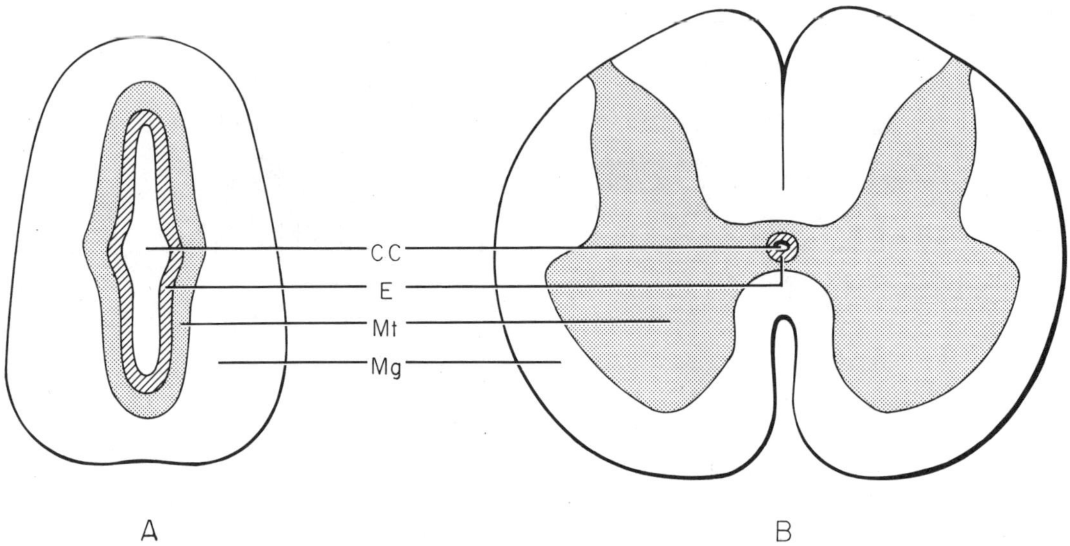

Figure 4–1. *A,* The developing spinal cord. *B,* The mature spinal cord. *CC,* Central canal. *E,* Ependymal layer. *Mt,* Mantle layer, which is the presumptive spinal gray. *Mg,* Marginal layer, which is the presumptive white matter.

that enter the dorsal roots via mono- or polysynaptic connections, as well as contacts from adjacent regions of the spinal cord, and also receive long descending fibers from the cerebral cortex and brain stem. Thus, a single alpha motor neuron may receive many thousands of synapses from a variety of sources.

The spinal gray contains several more or less distinct neuronal regions, based on differences in nerve cell size and distribution. Rexed has numbered these areas, and this classification, known as *Rexed's laminae,* is widely used. It is necessary to understand the organization of the spinal cord in order to pinpoint the sites of the terminations of afferent fibers discussed in the literature. The distribution of the laminae varies somewhat at different segmental levels of the spinal cord, but a typical cross-section at the level of T1 is shown in Figure 4–3.

Nerve fibers that convey impulses from pain and temperature receptors enter the spinal cord by way of Lissauer's tract, where they may ascend or descend for variable distances giving off branches that enter the dorsal horn.

Lamina 1 is a very thin layer that caps the dorsal horn. Lamina 2 is also called *substantia gelatinosa* because in unfixed material it has a clear, jellylike appearance. In the ventromedial part of the dorsal horn, in lamina 6, there is a column of very large cells, called *Clarke's column* or *nucleus dorsalis.* This nucleus extends from segmental levels C8 to L3 and is an important synaptic way-station for systems mediating subconscious proprioception. Note that lamina 9 consists of groups of cells that are surrounded by lamina 7. Lamina 9 contains both alpha and gamma motor neurons as well as numerous interneurons.

In general, the cell bodies of motor neurons that supply the muscles of the trunk (axial musculature) are located in the ventromedial portion of the ventral horn, and in the cervical and lumbar regions the cell bodies of motor neurons that supply the muscles of the extremities are located in the ventrolateral portion of the ventral horns (see Figure 4–4). The locations of the latter explain why the ventral horns are so prominent at cervical and lumbar levels.

Ascending Systems

Information from exteroceptors, interoceptors and proprioceptors enters the spinal cord by way of the dorsal roots. The cell bodies of these first order neurons in the somatic afferent pathways are located in the dorsal root ganglia. The major dorsal root afferent systems may be divided roughly

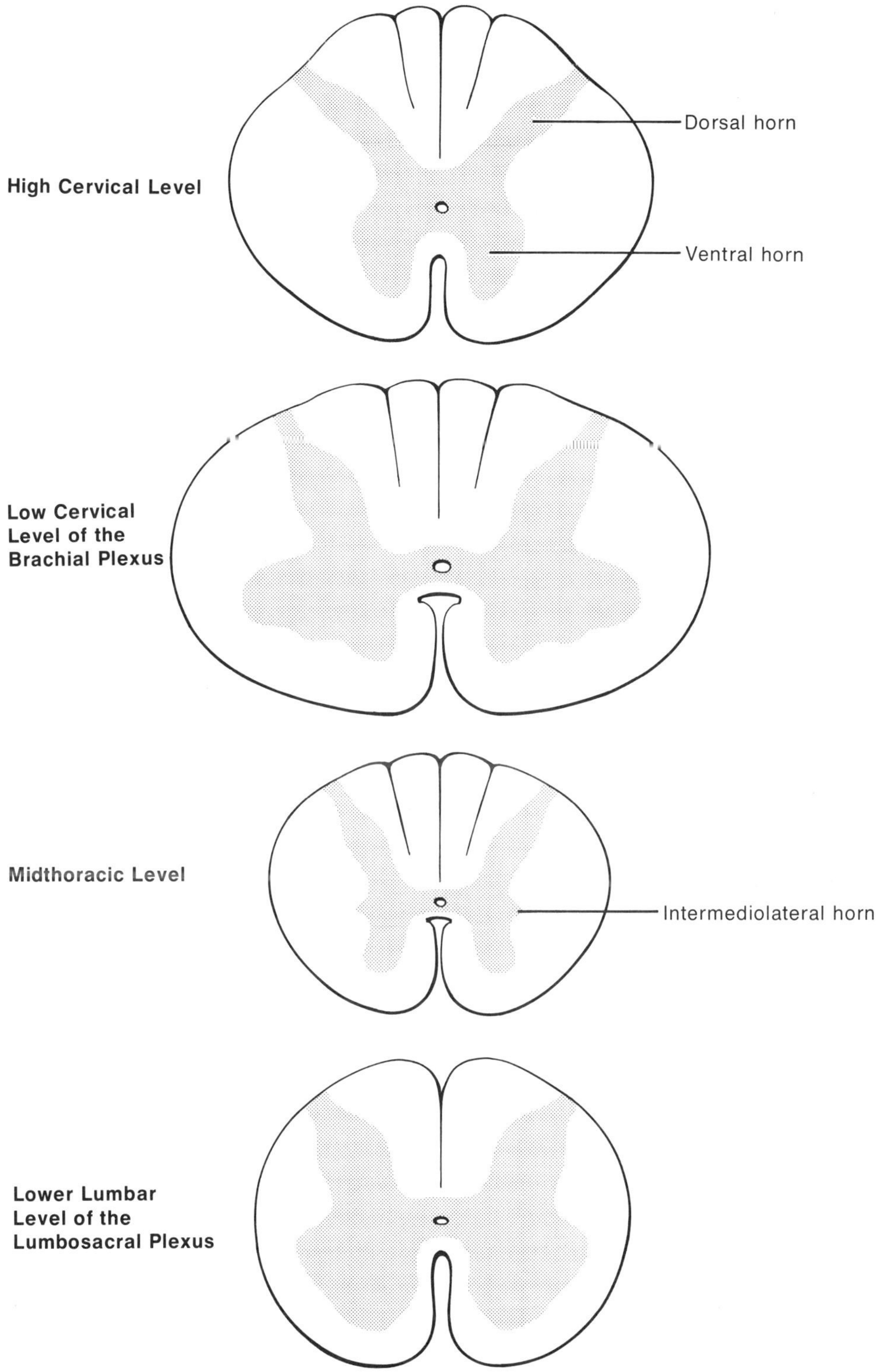

Figure 4–2. Cross-sections of the spinal cord at different levels to show variations in the shape of the spinal gray. The dorsal and ventral horns of gray matter are especially well developed at the levels that correspond with the emergence of the brachial and lumbosacral plexuses because of the large motor and sensory representation of the upper and lower extremities. The intermediolateral horn is present primarily in the thoracic region where the cell bodies of preganglionic sympathetic neurons are located. The white matter gradually increases from caudal to rostral as more ascending sensory neurons collect and descending neurons terminate.

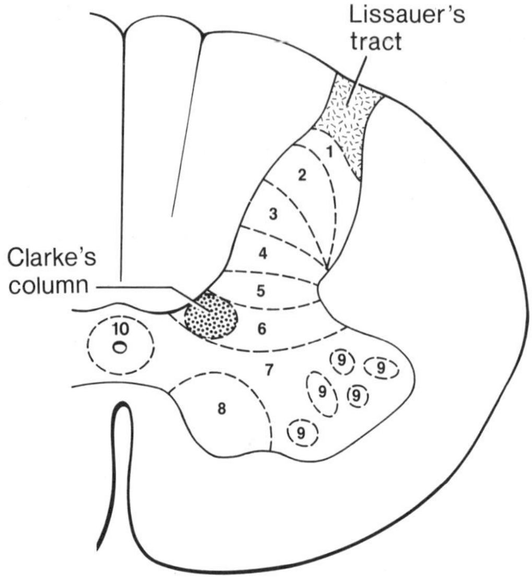

Figure 4–3. A cross-section of the spinal cord at the first thoracic level showing Rexed's laminar distribution.

into large fiber systems, which contain myelinated axons greater than 6 microns in diameter, and small fiber systems, which include myelinated and unmyelinated axons less than 6 microns in diameter.

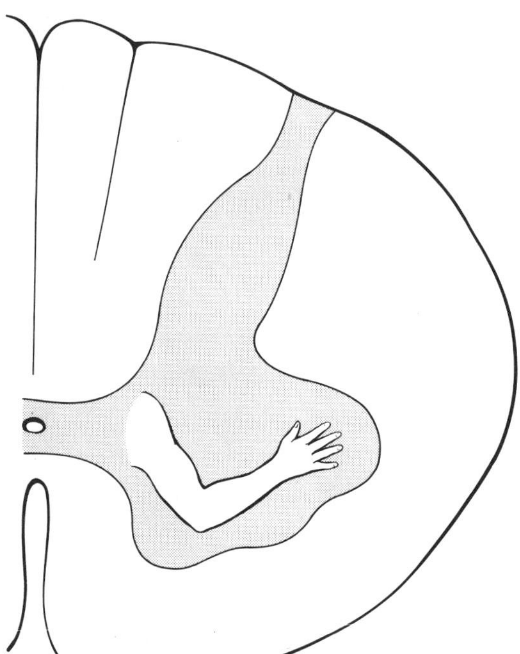

Figure 4–4. A cross-section of the spinal cord at the level of the brachial plexus illustrating the representation of the upper extremity. The motor neurons that supply the muscles of the trunk and proximal extremities are located in the ventromedial portion of the ventral horn, and those that supply the distal parts of the extremities are located in the ventrolateral portion of the ventral horn.

In general, the neurons comprising the large fiber systems enter the dorsal horn of the spinal cord more medially than do those of the small fiber systems. After entering the spinal cord the neurons may: (1) ascend to higher centers; (2) participate in monosynaptic reflex arcs; or (3) participate in polysynaptic reflex arcs. It is possible for one nerve fiber to branch and make all three of these types of connections.

Large Fiber Systems

The large fiber systems include the:
1. dorsal column (medial lemniscal) system.
2. dorsal spinocerebellar system.
3. ventral spinocerebellar system.

THE DORSAL COLUMN (MEDIAL LEMNISCAL) PATHWAY

The dorsal column system contains nerve fibers that convey impulses from receptors which subserve:
1. two-point discrimination (Meissner's corpuscles).
2. pressure (pacinian corpuscles, Golgi-Mazzoni end organs).
3. vibration (pacinian corpuscles).
4. kinesthesia (joint receptors — Ruffini end organs, Golgi type endings and Golgi-Mazzoni end organs).
5. stereognosis (joint receptors, Meissner's corpuscles and other cutaneous receptors).

There is evidence that this system also contains some IA fibers from muscle spindles. Therefore, it is composed of large axons that carry information to the central nervous system from both cutaneous and deep structures. It is a very rapidly conducting system because the axons are large and myelinated and because they synapse very few times en route to the cerebral cortex.

After the first order neurons enter the medial portion of the dorsal root, they enter either the *fasciculus gracilis* or *fasciculus cuneatus* on the ipsilateral side. See Figure 4–5 for the entire route of this system. Those fibers that enter the spinal cord from the lower extremities and lower thoracic region ascend in the fasciculus gracilis; those that enter from the upper thoracic region and upper extremities ascend in the fasciculus cuneatus. As the axons ascend they give off

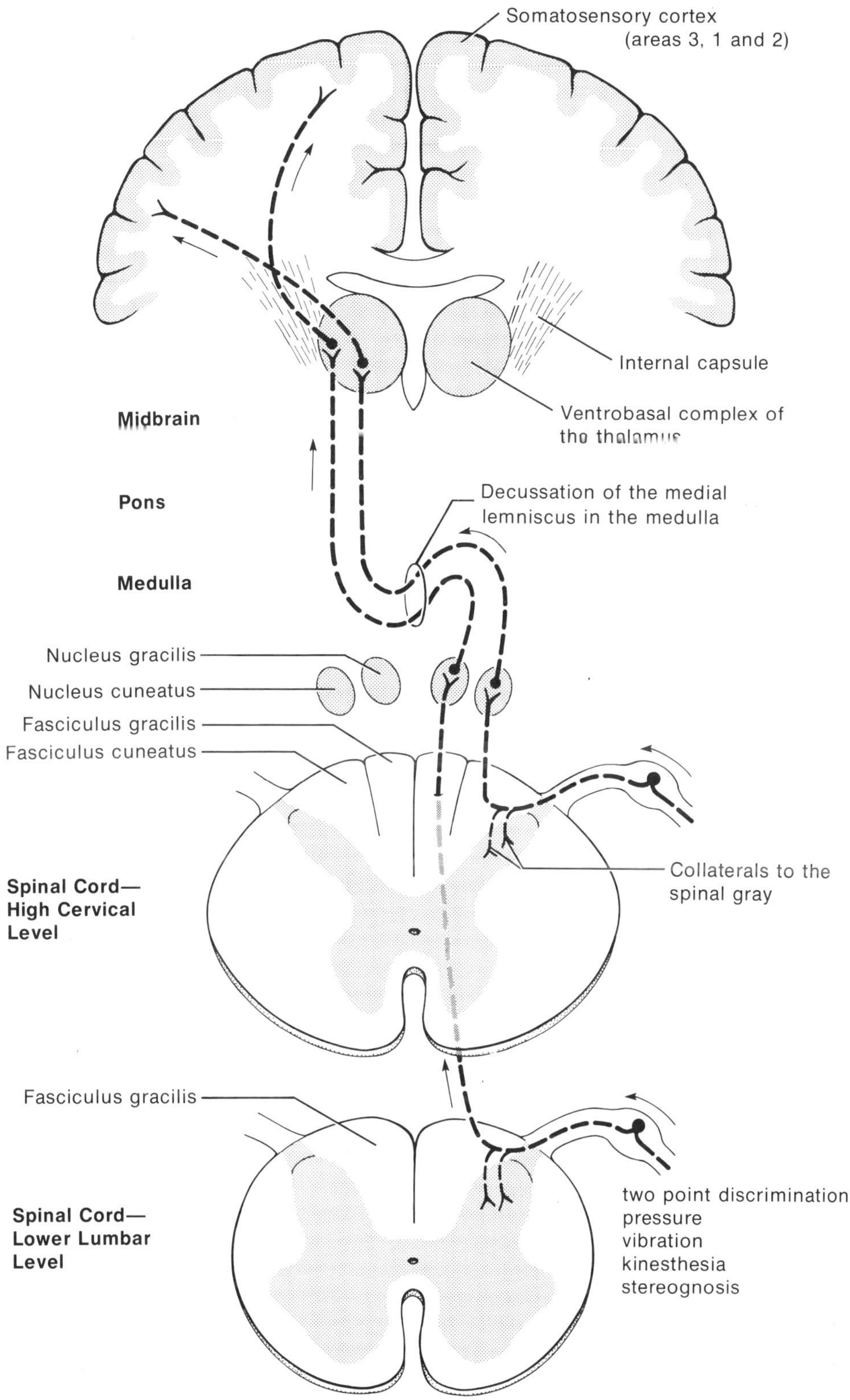

Figure 4–5. The dorsal column (medial lemniscal) system. Note that the neurons that originate in lumbar regions ascend in the fasciculus gracilis, and those that originate in upper thoracic and cervical regions ascend in the fasciculus cuneatus.

numerous collaterals to the spinal gray. This system also gives off descending collaterals. These collaterals either make reflex connections at the spinal cord level or end on neurons that give rise to secondary ascending fibers to the cerebral cortex.

En route to the cerebral cortex the dorsal column fibers synapse with the second order neurons in either the *nucleus gracilis* or *nucleus cuneatus*. These are called the *dorsal column nuclei* and are located in the posterior portion of the medulla (see Figs. 6–4 and 6–5). As the second order neurons continue to ascend, they cross to the contralateral side in the *decussation of the medial lemniscus* (see Fig. 6–4). They continue rostrally through the pons and midbrain to the thalamus. Here they synapse in what is called the *ventrobasal complex*. These are thalamic nuclei in which the great ascending pathways relay en route to the cerebral cortex. The third order neurons then ascend through the *posterior limb of the internal capsule* (a large mass made up of fibers going to and from the cerebral cortex) to terminate in areas 3, 1 and 2 of the somatosensory cortex. The latter is located in the postcentral gyrus of the cerebral cortex, as shown in Figure 4–6. Rostral to the nuclei gracilis and cuneatus no collaterals are given off. The only projection is to the ventrobasal complex of the thalamus.

The dorsal column system is organized somatotopically throughout, i.e., there is an organized central representation of the somatic periphery. In the fasciculus gracilis, sacral regions are represented posteriorly, lumbar regions in an intermediate position and low thoracic regions anteriorly; in the fasciculus cuneatus upper thoracic regions are represented posteriorly and cervical regions anteriorly. As the fibers cross in the decussation of the medial lemniscus, the somatic representation is like that of a headless man, i.e., cervical fibers are located posteriorly and sacral fibers anteriorly. Rostral to the decussation, the headless man lies down, so that cervical regions are represented medially and sacral regions laterally. Here, representation of the head is added on by the trigeminal complex. This entire representation is maintained up to the level of the thalamus; after this the fibers cross so that the sacral regions are represented most medially and the head is represented laterally in the cerebral cortex. Figure 4–7 illustrates the somatotopic organization of the dorsal column system at the levels discussed.

The fibers of this system are highly specific for temporal and spatial discrimination. The modality specificity is as precise for second as for first order neurons, which implies that single dorsal column nuclei cells receive their peripheral presynaptic

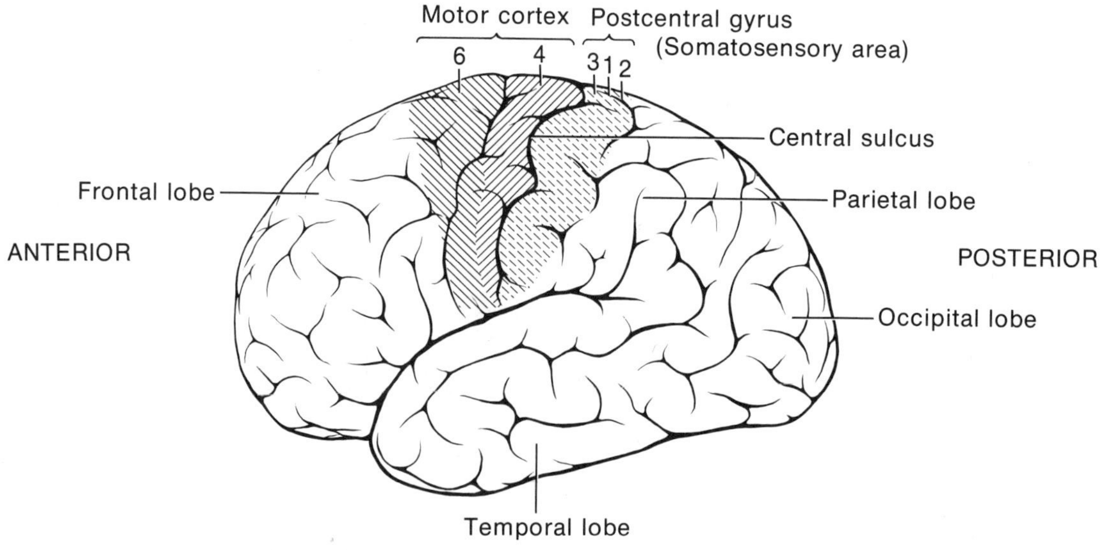

Figure 4–6. A lateral view of the cerebral cortex showing the primary motor and somatosensory areas.

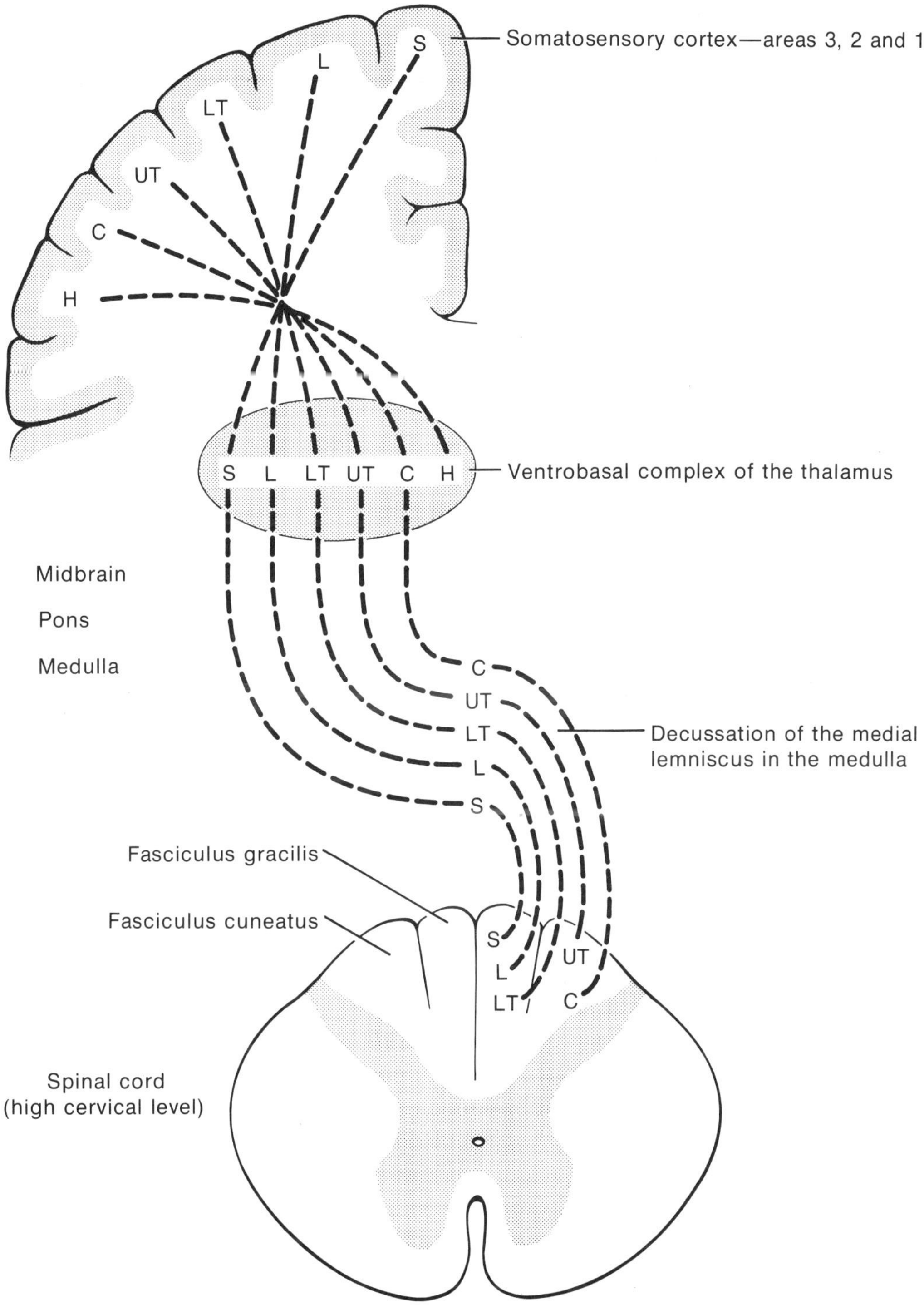

Figure 4–7. The somatotopic organization in the dorsal column (medial lemniscal) system. *S*, Sacral representation. *L*, Lumbar representation. *LT*, Lower thoracic representation. *UT*, Upper thoracic representation. *C*, Cervical representation. *H*, Head representation (added on by the trigeminal nerve complex).

input only from first order neurons that subserve a single modality type.

Lesions of the dorsal columns produce loss of:

1. two-point discrimination.
2. kinesthesia.
3. vibration sense.
4. pressure sense.
5. stereognosis.

These losses all occur on the ipsilateral side, i.e., on the same side on which the lesion occurs if it is below the decussation of the medial lemniscus. If the lesion is above the level of the medial lemniscus, where this system crosses, the losses will occur on the contralateral side of the body.

Tabes dorsalis, which may arise as a consequence of syphilis, presents initial symptoms of difficulty with balance. This is because the large dorsal root ganglion cells are damaged first so that the dorsal column system is affected. As a result, there is a paucity of information transmitted to the central nervous system from the joint receptors that are responsible for detecting the positions of the extremities.

DORSAL SPINOCEREBELLAR TRACT

Large, myelinated fibers, derived predominantly from muscle and some fibers from skin, ascend via the dorsal spinocerebellar tracts to the cerebellum. This system mediates subconscious proprioception which originates in muscle spindles and Golgi tendon organs. The primary constituents are types IA, IB and II nerve fibers.

After the first order neurons enter the medial side of the posterior horn of the spinal cord, they immediately proceed to Clarke's column (nucleus dorsalis), where they synapse with second order neurons. These then course laterally across the spinal gray to the dorsal spinocerebellar tract on the side ipsilateral to their original entry into the spinal cord. They then ascend without any further intervening synapses to the ipsilateral side of the cerebellum by way of the inferior cerebellar peduncles (see Fig. 4–8), which connect the medulla and cerebellum (see Fig. 6–6).

Since Clarke's column extends only from segmental levels C8 to L3, types IA, IB and II axons that enter the spinal cord inferior to the level of L3 ascend to that level via the fasciculus gracilis. They then enter Clarke's column. Those axons that enter the spinal cord superior to the level of C8 either descend for a short distance to enter Clarke's column or they enter the accessory cuneate nucleus (see Fig. 6–5). This nucleus may be thought of as the upper extremity homologue of Clarke's column, since the first and second order neurons synapse there and then proceed through the inferior cerebellar peduncles to the ipsilateral cerebellum, as do those fibers that enter Clarke's column directly.

The dorsal spinocerebellar tracts are also somatotopically organized, with sacral segments roughly represented posteriorly, thoracic segments anteriorly and lumbar segments in an intermediate position. In the cerebellum this system exists in both the anterior and posterior lobes. In the anterior lobe the lower extremities are represented rostrally, the face caudally and the upper extremities in an intermediate position. In the posterior lobe the lower extremities are represented caudally, the head rostrally, and the upper extremities again in the intermediate position.

This is a very rapidly conducting system, since there is only one synapse involved en route to the cerebellum and because the axons are very large in diameter and myelinated.

Pure lesions of the dorsal spinocerebellar tracts essentially are never seen in man. They are usually combined with lesions that also involve other tracts. When pure lesions of this tract are produced in experimental animals, disorders of movement occur on the ipsilateral side consisting of hypotonia (decreased muscle tone) and ataxia (loss of coordination). Position sense remains intact since it is mediated by the dorsal column system.

VENTRAL SPINOCEREBELLAR TRACT

The ventral spinocerebellar tracts convey information from the same types of receptors as do the dorsal spinocerebellar tracts. However, there is a greater concentration of type II axons from secondary endings than type IA axons from primary endings of muscle spindles. These tracts also contain some very small axons from the skin.

In contrast to the first two ascending systems that have been discussed, the ventral spinocerebellar system is a *crossed* system (see Fig. 4–9). After entering the dorsal horn, the first order neurons synapse with

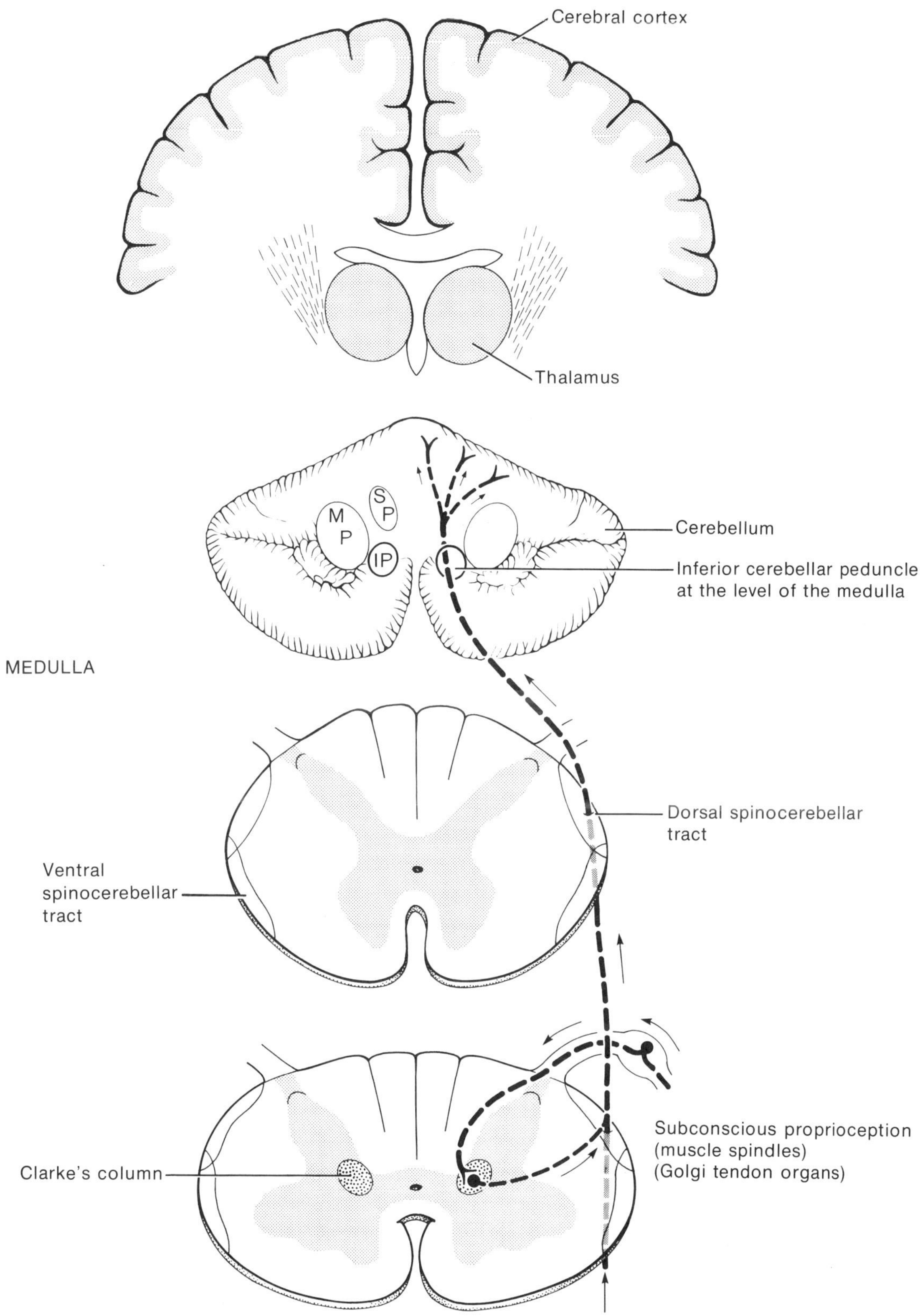

Figure 4–8. The dorsal spinocerebellar system. Note that the primary afferent neurons synapse in Clarke's column, after which the secondary neurons ascend in the dorsal spinocerebellar tracts, which enter the cerebellum by way of the inferior cerebellar peduncles. *SP*, Superior cerebellar peduncle. *MP*, Middle cerebellar peduncle. *IP*, Inferior cerebellar peduncle.

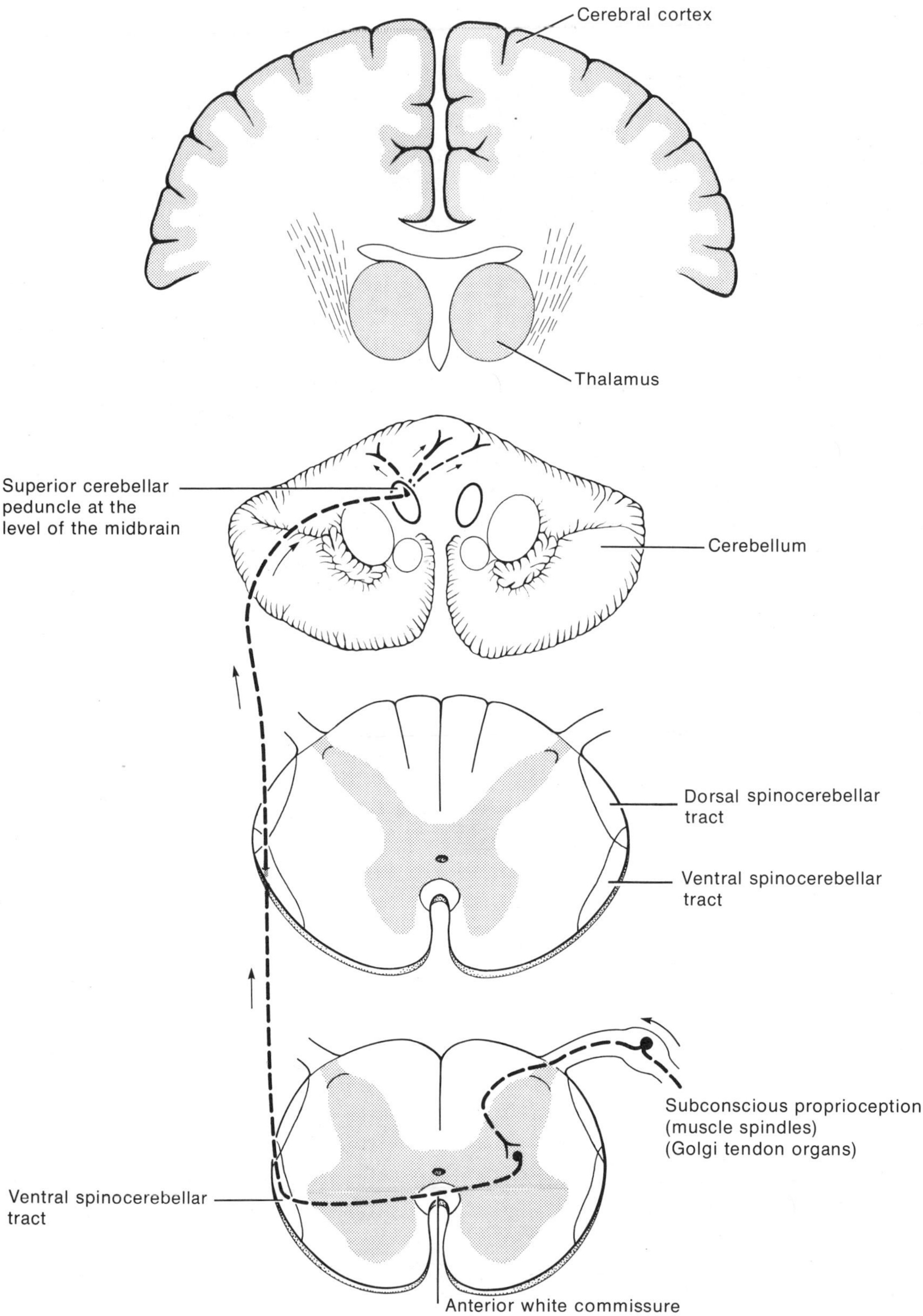

Figure 4–9. The ventral spinocerebellar system. Note that this system enters the cerebellum by way of the *superior* cerebellar peduncles. After entering the cerebellum, most fibers terminate ipsilateral to the side of their entry into the spinal cord; a few fibers remain on the contralateral side.

the second order neurons in the dorsal horn. The second order neuron then crosses to the contralateral ventral spinocerebellar tract via the anterior white commissure of the spinal cord. Without further synapses the fibers ascend and enter the cerebellum by way of the superior cerebellar peduncles. These latter connect the midbrain and the cerebellum and may be seen in Figure 6–7. Some of the fibers then recross to the side of the cerebellum that is ipsilateral to the side on which the nerve fibers initially entered the spinal cord, and some remain on the contralateral side. Therefore, the ventral spinocerebellar system is represented bilaterally in the cerebellum.

Presumably, the fibers of the ventral spinocerebellar system convey information concerning movement and posture of entire limbs rather than about changes of tension in individual muscles. Both the posterior and ventral spinocerebellar tracts project primarily to the anterior lobes of the cerebellum, but also send a few projections to the posterior lobe.

The effects of lesions of the ventral spinocerebellar tracts have not been properly determined because invariably other tracts are involved concomitantly in the lesion.

Small Fiber Systems

The small fiber systems are the:

1. anterolateral (AL) or spinothalamic system.
2. spinotectal system.
3. spino-olivary system.
4. spinovestibular system.
5. spinoreticular system.

The small fiber system axons enter more laterally in the dorsal horns of the spinal cord and the smallest of them are collected in Lissauer's tract. Most small fibers synapse with dorsal horn neurons within one or two segments of their level of entry. There is no evidence that these fine fibers go directly into the ventral horns as do some of the larger fibers. Fibers from the skin terminate further dorsally in the dorsal horn than those from the musculature.

ANTEROLATERAL (SPINOTHALAMIC) SYSTEM

Some of the textbooks separate the spinothalamic system into anterior and lateral tracts, but recent investigations have shown that there is no anatomic or physiologic basis for doing so. Therefore, in this discussion they will be treated as one system which will be referred to as the anterolateral system. This overlaps the anterior part of the ventral spinocerebellar system and is intermixed with neurons from the spinotectal and spino-olivary tracts.

The anterolateral tracts contain fibers that mediate:

1. pain.
2. visceral pain.
3. crudely localized touch.
4. temperature.

Therefore, it contains small diameter fibers, primarily types III and C fibers, many of which are unmyelinated. Because the axons are small in diameter and the pathway is a multisynaptic one, the AL is a relatively slow conducting system (Fig. 4–10).

The first order neurons enter the lateral portion of the dorsal horn, after which there are one or several synapses involving interneurons, before the fibers cross to the contralateral side of the spinal cord via the anterior commissure of the spinal cord. As these anterolateral neuron fibers cross the spinal cord they usually ascend for a distance of about two spinal segments from their level of entry. For example, if the axons enter the spinal cord at the fourth lumbar level, subsequent fibers will ascend to the second lumbar level by the time they have crossed to the contralateral side. These axons ascend in the anterolateral tracts on the contralateral side to the brain stem (medulla, pons and midbrain), where they give off numerous collaterals to the reticular formation. They continue to ascend to the ventrobasal complex of the thalamus. There they synapse with the last neurons in the system, which then terminate in areas 3, 1 and 2 of the somatosensory cerebral cortex.

Although the vast majority of AL axons cross to the contralateral side of the spinal cord close to their level of entry, a small percentage of axons do not cross and ascend in the ipsilateral AL tract. These axons reach the cerebral cortex by the same route as those that cross. The existence of these uncrossed fibers explains why there is sometimes return of pain after surgical tractotomy of the

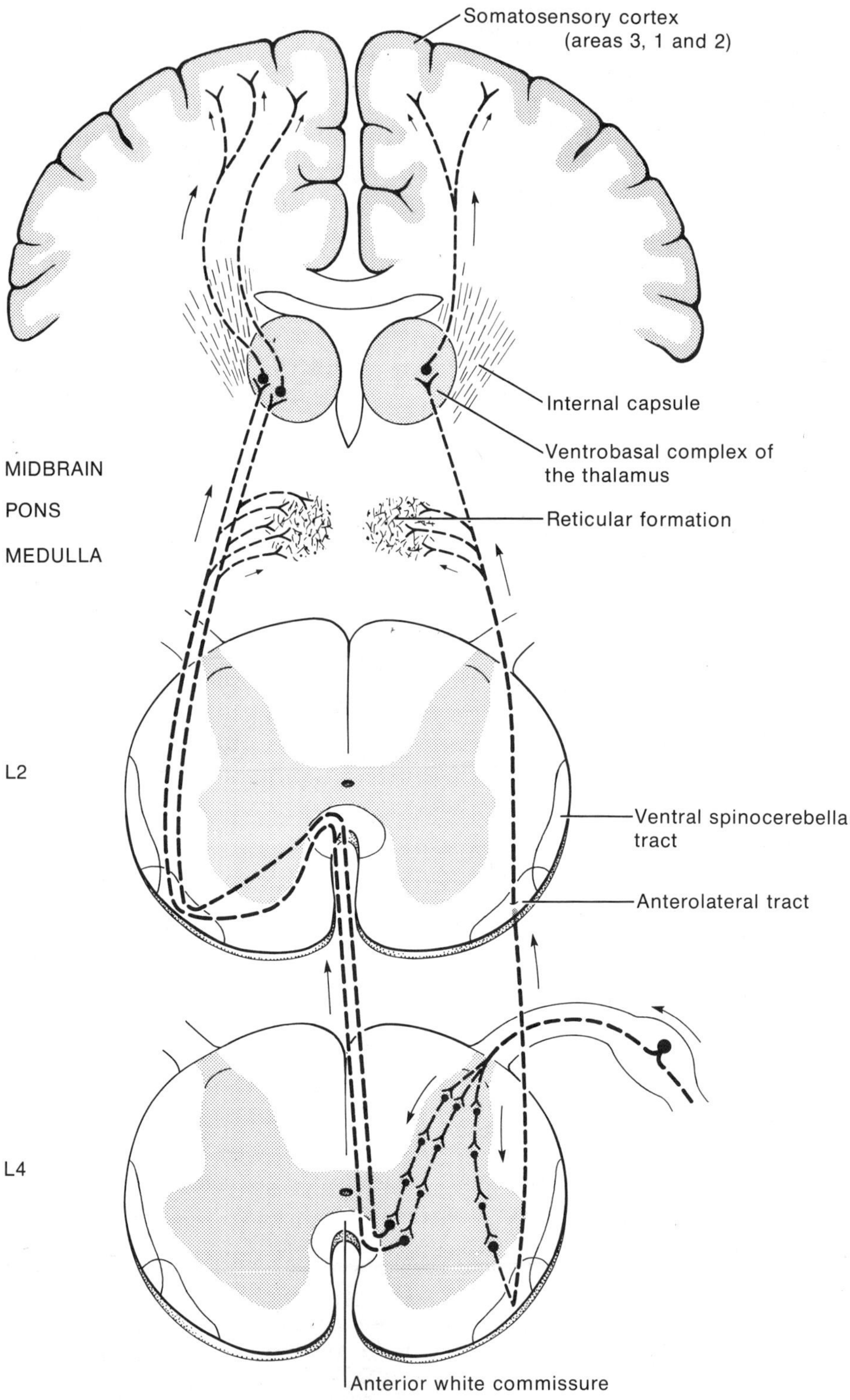

Figure 4–10. The anterolateral system. The great majority of neurons in this system cross to the contralateral side at or near their level of entry into the spinal cord. A few remain uncrossed.

anterolateral tract for relief of intractable pain.

The somatotopic organization of the AL system is not as precise as it is in the dorsal column or spinocerebellar systems because there is more overlap in this system. Although this overlapping does exist there is still a generalized representation of sacral regions in the dorsal part of the tract and cervical regions in the ventral part of the tract. The somatotopy is maintained throughout the system, as it is in the dorsal column system (see Fig. 4–7). The fibers of the AL system synapse in an area posterior to those of the dorsal column system in the ventrobasal nucleus of the thalamus. Anterolateral fibers, like dorsal column fibers, are redirected en route from the thalamus to the cerebral cortex, so that the final cortical representation is the same as that of the dorsal column system. The head is represented most laterally and the sacral region most medially. A pictorial sensory representation of the body in the cerebral cortex of man is called an *homunculus*.

A great dichotomy exists in the two great afferent systems which carry information that reaches the cerebral cortex. The *dorsal column system* has a high degree of somatic representation and of specificity for certain receptor organs (joint receptors, Meissner's corpuscles, pacinian corpuscles). In addition it is a phylogenetically new system. These qualifications fulfill the requirements of an *epicritic* type of sensibility, which means it has a high degree of specificity and that it is phylogenetically advanced. It is also a much more rapidly conducting system than the AL system because it contains fewer synapses and is composed of myelinated fibers that are large in diameter. The *anterolateral system* has a less well-defined somatotopic organization, is more diffusely distributed in the central nervous system (primarily owing to the numerous collaterals it sends to the reticular formation) and is not specific for certain receptor organs. It conveys information from receptors that subserve a variety of sensibilities, primarily via free nerve endings and type C fibers. This system is much older phylogenetically than the dorsal column system. The AL system fulfills the requirments of a *protopathic* type of sensibility. It is a much more slowly conducting system than the dorsal column system because of its many synapses and axons that are for the most part unmyelinated and small in diameter.

SPINOTECTAL TRACT

Evidence indicates that the spinotectal tract arises only from cervical levels. The axons associated with this tract enter the lateral portion of the dorsal horns and cross to the contralateral side of the spinal cord close to their level of entry, after synapsing one or several times. This tract ascends in close association with the anterolateral system, but terminates in the superior colliculus, which is located in the midbrain and is a reflex center for coordination between the visual system and movements of the neck (see Fig. 6–12). Evidence suggests that it may be part of a multisynaptic pathway that transmits nociceptive impulses as well as constituting the afferent limb of reflexes associated with coordination of head and eye movements.

SPINO-OLIVARY TRACT

Information concerning the spino-olivary tract is sparse. The evidence indicates that it originates at all levels of the spinal cord, and as it ascends it follows the spinotectal tract in conjunction with the anterolateral system. At the level of the medulla more than one-half of the fibers cross to the contralateral side, and both crossed and uncrossed fibers terminate in the inferior olive. The function of this system is unclear, although it is known that the inferior olive sends very heavy crossed projections to the cerebellum. It has been suggested that the spino-olivary system comprises a component of a spinocerebellar pathway similar to the posterior spinocerebellar system.

SPINOVESTIBULAR SYSTEM

The spinovestibular system originates from spinal levels as far inferior as the lumbar segments; it ascends ipsilaterally and also overlaps the anterolateral and ventral spinocerebellar systems. It terminates primarily in the lateral vestibular (Deiter's) nucleus and functions in the control of postural reflex mechanisms.

SPINORETICULAR SYSTEM

Spinoreticular fibers originate from all levels of the spinal cord and project diffusely to the reticular formation. The fibers ascend in the lateral part of the anterior funiculus of the spinal cord and are both crossed and uncrossed. Those fibers that project to the pontine reticular formation terminate bilaterally, and the great majority of those that project to the medullary reticular formation are uncrossed. The spinoreticular system is polysynaptic and, by way of the projections from the reticular formation to the cerebral cortex, its function is to maintain a state of alertness. In addition, some of the fibers of this system project to the lateral reticular nucleus of the medulla, which in turn projects to the cerebellum. Therefore, another function of this system may be to relay impulses from the cutaneous receptors to the cerebellum.

The dorsal column and AL systems are the only ascending systems in which symptoms of lesions are clear-cut. This is not to be interpreted to mean that damage to other systems is not important, but since the other ascending systems overlap to such a great extent, specific lesions of the individual tracts probably do not occur and cannot be clearly diagnosed.

Some clinical conditions that result from spinal cord damage are interesting and provide good examples of why it is important to learn the anatomy of the spinal cord pathways. One such condition is called the *Brown-Séquard syndrome.* This involves a complete spinal cord hemisection, i.e., either the right or left half of the spinal cord is completely destroyed. In this case all of the modalities conveyed in the dorsal column system (two-point discrimination, pressure, vibration, kinesthesia and stereognosis) are lost on the ipsilateral side, and all of those modalities conveyed in the anterolateral system (pain, temperature, crude touch and visceral pain) are lost on the contralateral side. The loss of pain, temperature, crude touch and visceral pain are experienced approximately two segments inferior to the level of the lesion, since these fibers ascend for a distance of one or two spinal segments as they cross to the contralateral side. There is also loss of voluntary control on the ipsilateral side owing to interruption of the descending corticospinal tracts (see Fig. 4–11).

Another instructive example of a spinal cord lesion is called *syringomyelia.* This disease involves progressive degeneration of the spinal cord, beginning with enlargement of the central canal. The degeneration proceeds in an anterior direction first so that the anterior commissure is destroyed. Later in the course of the disease the gray matter may also degenerate. Because the anterolateral system crosses in the anterior commissure, pain, temperature, crude touch and visceral pain may be lost in bands instead of at all levels of the body below the level of the lesion (see Fig. 4–12).

Friedreich's ataxia is an hereditary disease characterized by degeneration of the dorsal column system, the spinocerebellar tracts and the spino-olivary tracts. Destruction of these tracts produces the marked ataxia characteristic of people with this disease. The disease may be accompanied by damaged peripheral nerves, resulting in areflexia (loss of reflexes).

Descending Systems

The descending systems of the spinal cord originate from supraspinal levels of the central nervous system and influence the activity of the spinal neurons in a variety of ways, depending on their site of origin.

CORTICOSPINAL (PYRAMIDAL) TRACTS

The corticospinal tracts are also called pyramidal tracts because as they descend they course through the medullary pyramids. All other descending pathways are referred to as extrapyramidal because they do not course through the pyramids.

It was once thought that the corticospinal tracts functioned only in motor activities. Although their origin is exclusively from the cerebral cortex, there is now evidence that these projections of the cortex modulate and influence the ascending sensory systems as well as motor activity.

Most of the axons that contribute to the corticospinal tracts are myelinated and measure less than 6 microns in diameter. There are some very large myelinated fibers greater than 12 microns in diameter, but

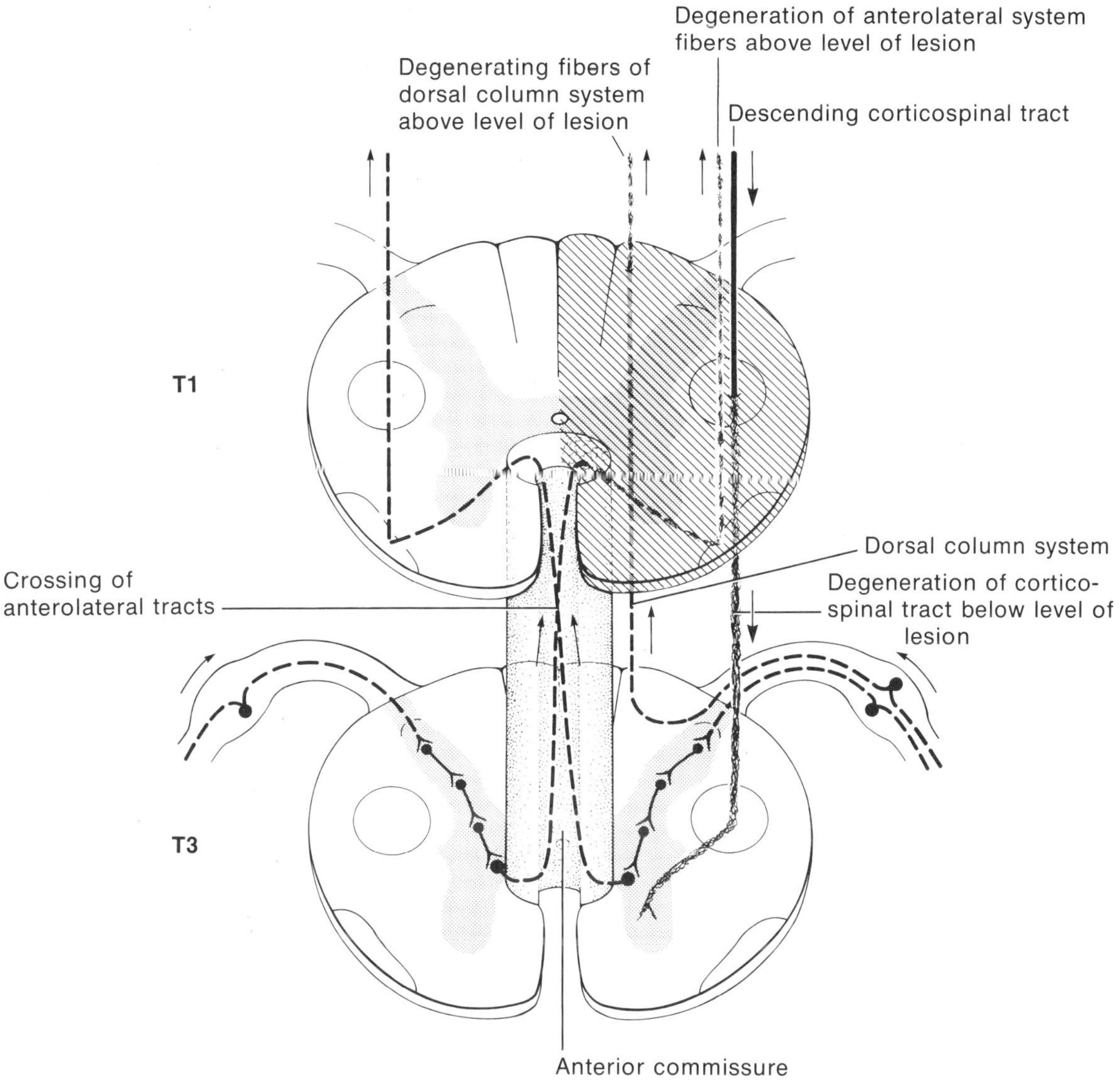

Figure 4–11. Brown-Séquard syndrome. In this example the right half of the spinal cord has been severed at the level of T1 (*indicated by the lined area*). The modalities conveyed in the anterolateral system will be lost on the contralateral side approximately two segments below the level of the lesion. The dorsal column system is interrupted at the level of the lesion on the ipsilateral side, and there will be no voluntary control of structures below the level of the lesion on the ipsilateral side owing to interruption of the corticospinal tract. The wavy lined portions of the tracts indicate degenerated neurons. The parts of the neurons that are cut off from the nerve cell bodies of origin degenerate.

these probably comprise less than one-fourth of the total number of fibers in the corticospinal system.

The specific sites of origin of the corticospinal tracts are from the *motor* (precentral) *cortex*, which accounts for about 55 per cent of the fibers, and the *sensory* (postcentral) *cortex*, which provides about 35 per cent of the fibers; the remainder have their cell bodies in other areas of the *parietal*, *temporal* and *occipital cortices* (see Fig. 4–6).

From their cells of origin the axons descend through the *corona radiata* (a massive area of white matter just deep to the cerebral cortex), the posterior limb of the internal capsule, the cerebral peduncles (see Figs. 6–11, 6–12 and 6–13, the pons and the medulla. In the decussation of the medullary pyramids (see Fig. 6–4) 80 to 95 per cent of

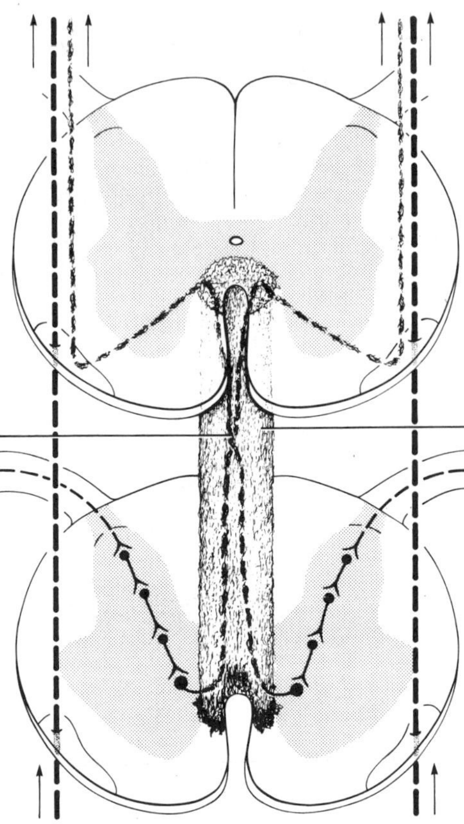

Figure 4–12. Syringomyelia. Those neurons of the anterolateral system that cross through the anterior commissure at the level or levels of the lesion will be destroyed so that they cannot convey impulses to higher centers. Those neurons that have originated at lower levels of the spinal cord have crossed to the contralateral side inferior to the level of the lesion. Therefore, they are not damaged and continue to convey impulses to higher centers. Thus, a band of loss of pain, temperature, crude touch and visceral pain occurs in those areas subserved by the anterolateral fibers that cross at the level of the lesion.

the fibers *cross* and descend in the lateral corticospinal tracts. The remaining fibers descend on the ipsilateral side in the ventral corticospinal tracts. However, essentially all fibers of the corticospinal tracts are crossed, since those fibers that do not decussate in the medullary pyramids cross at their levels of termination in the spinal cord (see Fig. 4–13). They terminate throughout the central gray at all levels of the spinal cord. Those fibers that originate in the motor cortex terminate in the base of the dorsal horn and throughout the ventral horn. Fibers that originate in the sensory cortex terminate in the dorsal horn and in the dorsal column nuclei. These are the projections which modulate activity in the ascending sensory systems by inhibiting ascending impulses that normally are destined for the cerebral cortex. It has been shown by extensive physiologic investigation that the modification of incoming sensory information at various levels along the sensory pathways is by presynaptic inhibition, which functions as a filtering mechanism so that the brain is not bombarded with excessive information.

In primates there are monosynaptic connections between large corticospinal neurons and alpha motor neurons that supply the distal musculature of the extremities. There is evidence that the large neurons, which are greater than 12 microns in diameter, originate from huge cells, called *Betz cells*, which are located in motor cortical area number 4 (see Fig. 4–6). Motor neurons which supply the axial and proximal limb musculature appear to receive polysynaptic corticospinal connections by

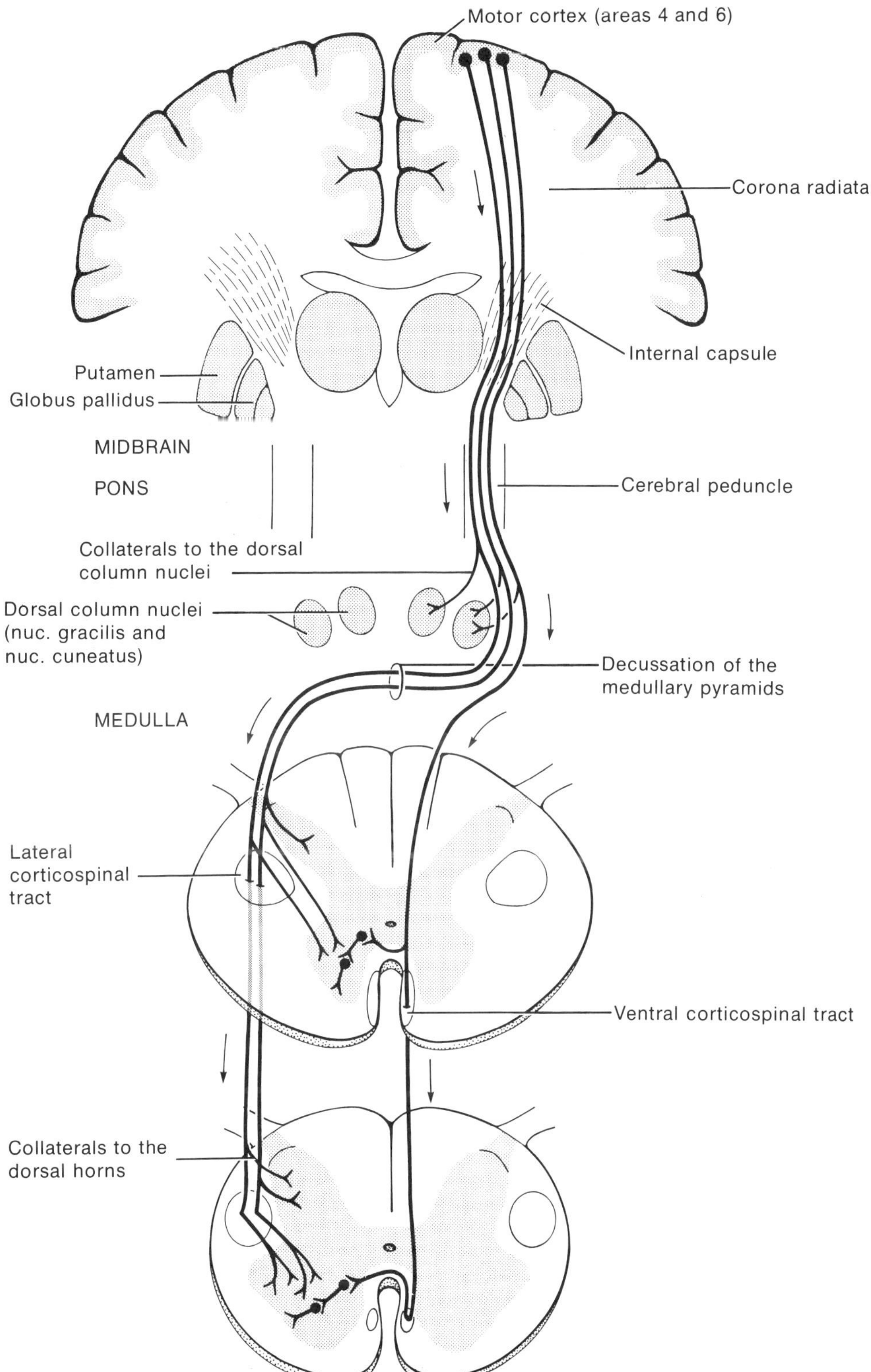

Figure 4–13. The corticospinal tracts. In this illustration only those neurons that originate in the motor cortex are included.

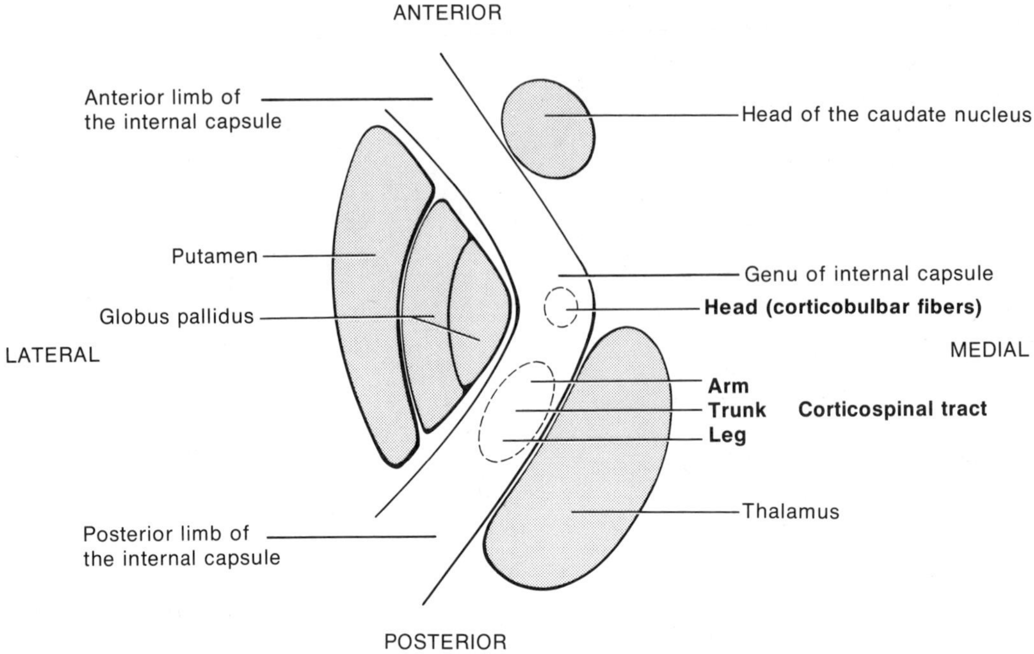

Figure 4–14. The somatotopic organization of the corticobulbar and corticospinal systems in the posterior limb of the internal capsule.

way of spinal cord interneurons. Thus, those motor neurons which innervate the muscles responsible for fine coordination are under direct rapid control by the cerebral cortex. Postural muscles and muscles that subserve gross movements are less directly and more slowly controlled by the cortex. There is no evidence to suggest that corticospinal fibers project to gamma motor neurons, which thus are not voluntarily controlled.

The corticospinal system has a high degree of somatotopic organization in the posterior limb of the internal capsule (see Fig. 4–14). Here, the face is represented anteriorly and the arm, trunk and lower extremity areas are located successively more posteriorly. Elsewhere, the somatotopic organization is not as well defined as the dorsal column and anterolateral systems, but roughly, in the lateral corticospinal tracts, cervical fibers are located more medially and sacral fibers more laterally.

Figure 4–14 shows the location of the human corticospinal tract within the internal capsule that has been accepted for many years. However, Englander et al (1975) have added to an accumulating body of evidence that the corticospinal tracts are located more posteriorly in the internal capsule, in the third quarter of the posterior limb.

RUBROSPINAL TRACTS

The rubrospinal tracts originate in the red nuclei of the mesencephalon (midbrain), *cross* immediately and descend in the lateral funiculi of the spinal cord, where they partially overlap the corticospinal tracts. The fibers terminate by making connections with alpha and gamma motor neurons at all levels of the spinal cord. Neurons of the rubrospinal tracts *do not make monosynaptic connections with gamma motor neurons,* but there is now evidence that they make monosynaptic as well as polysynaptic connections with alpha motor neurons (see Fig. 4–15).

The rubrospinal system functions to increase tone in contralateral flexor muscles and to decrease tone in the ipsilateral extensors through the described connections. There is also some evidence to suggest that this pathway may take over some of the function of the corticospinal tracts if they are damaged. This is possible because there are heavy projections from diffuse areas of the cerebral cortex to the red nucleus, which

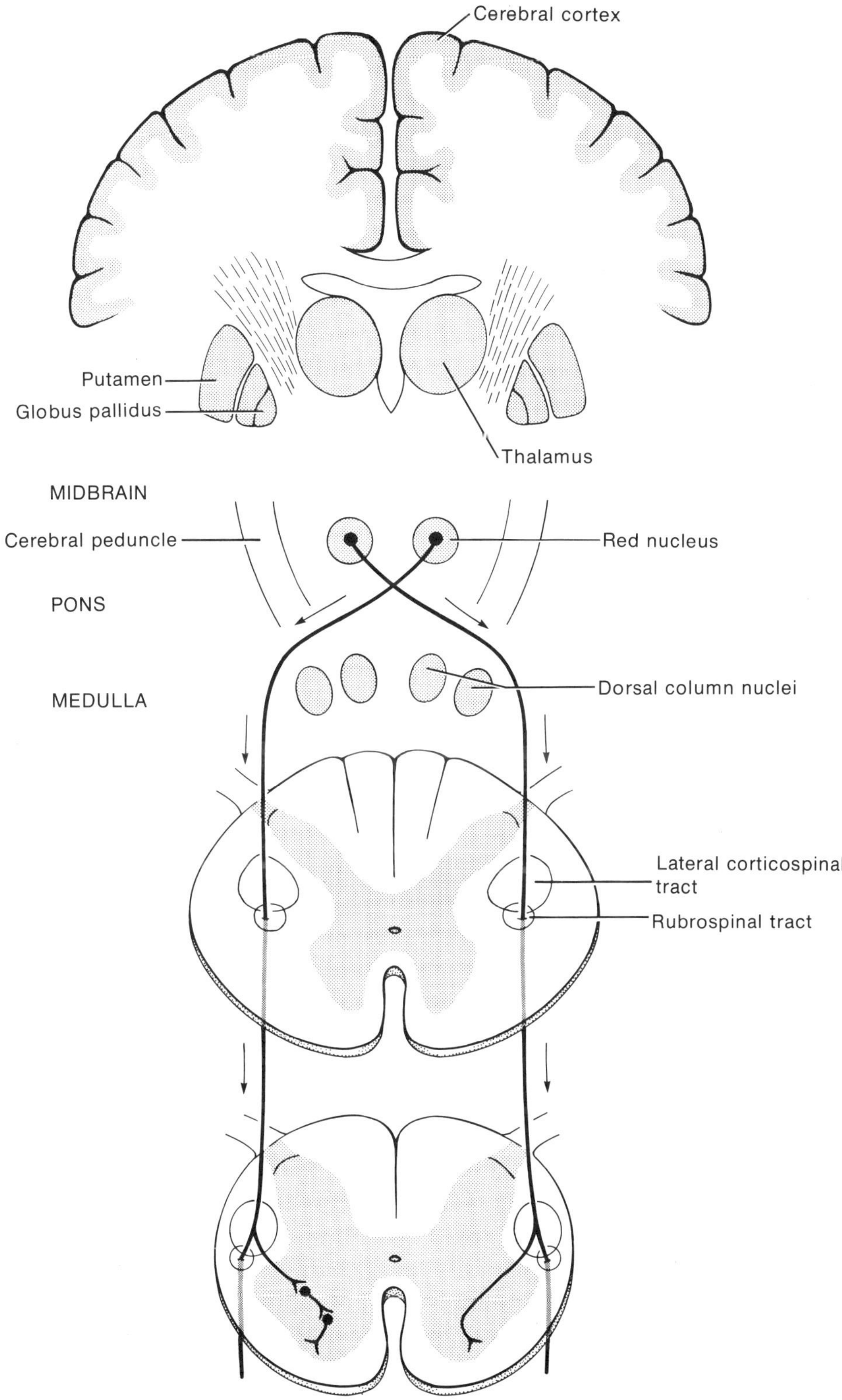

Figure 4–15. The rubrospinal tracts. In this illustration, a neuron with monosynaptic connections is shown on one side and a neuron with polysynaptic connections on the other. It should be understood that both types of connections are present on both sides.

completes a corticorubrospinal system that closely parallels the corticospinal system. This will be dealt with in more detail later, but it should be understood that the corticorubrospinal system, which is primarily polysynaptic, is much slower than the monosynaptic corticospinal system which subserves the distal musculature, and the control is not as direct. Therefore, the fast, coordinated movements cannot be controlled by the corticorubrospinal linkage.

The somatotopic organization of the rubrospinal system is similar to that of the lateral corticospinal system, i.e., fibers from cervical regions are located medially and fibers from the sacral regions are located laterally in the spinal cord. The fibers that project to the red nucleus from the cerebral cortex are located posterior to those of the corticospinal tracts as they descend in the internal capsule.

VESTIBULOSPINAL TRACTS

The vestibulospinal tracts have their cells of origin primarily in the lateral vestibular (Deiter's) nucleus, which is one of four vestibular nuclei located in the floor of the fourth ventricle. This is an uncrossed system, which descends in the anterior funiculus of the spinal cord to all levels, but the projections to the lumbar and cervical levels are most pronounced. This is a very important projection system which is involved with postural reflexes. The fibers project both directly and via interneurons to *alpha* motor neurons and perhaps to *gamma* motor neurons in the ventral horns, where they enhance spinal reflex activity by increasing extensor tone in the upper and lower extremities. See Figure 4–16 for the route taken by this system.

The lateral vestibular nucleus receives fibers from the labyrinths by way of the vestibular division of the eighth cranial nerve, and from the cerebellum. This system is responsible for the *tonic labyrinthine reflexes,* in which changing the position of the head in space changes the amount of extensor tone in different muscle groups. In a decerebrate animal with labyrinths intact, extensor tone in all the extremities is maximal when the animal is supine with the angle of the mouth 45 degrees above the horizontal, and minimal when the animal is prone with the mouth 45 degrees below the horizontal. However, Tokizani et al. have shown that in healthy human adults total extensor tone is maximal in the vertical head-down position, and minimal in the vertical head-up position. This system is also responsible for the *labyrinthine righting reactions,* in which the muscles of the neck respond to keep the head in its normal upright position regardless of the position of the body, through stimulation from the labyrinths. If an animal or individual is in the lying position, the head can be manipulated to elicit the appropriate reflexes to cause him to rise to his feet. *The tonic neck reflexes* are demonstrated best in the absence of the labyrinths. They may be either symmetric or asymmetric. If the head is passively ventroflexed, extension of the upper extremities is inhibited and extension of the lower extremities is facilitated. If the head is passively extended, extension of the upper extremities is facilitated and the lower extremities flex. These are symmetric tonic neck reflexes. Asymmetric tonic neck reflexes may be elicited by turning the head to one side. In this case, on the side to which the head is turned, extensor tone in both upper and lower extremities increases while it is diminished on the opposite side. The same response may be elicited by cervical intervertebral joint abduction. These reflexes originate in the proprioceptors of the neck, and the responses last as long as the head is retained in the new position. In normal animals, in which both tonic neck and labyrinthine reflexes are intact, the two types of reflexes show an algebraic summation. In abnormal people these exaggerated reflexes may be disadvantageous, but proper positioning to elicit these responses may also be of therapeutic value in some instances.

RETICULOSPINAL TRACTS

The reticulospinal tracts originate in the pontine and medullary reticular formations. Most of the fibers remain uncrossed as they descend, but a small percentage do cross as they descend to the spinal cord. Therefore, the distribution of these tracts to the spinal cord is *bilateral*. The fibers descend in the anterior and anterolateral funiculus to terminate upon both *alpha* and *gamma motor neurons* at all levels of the spinal cord. The connections with both alpha and gamma

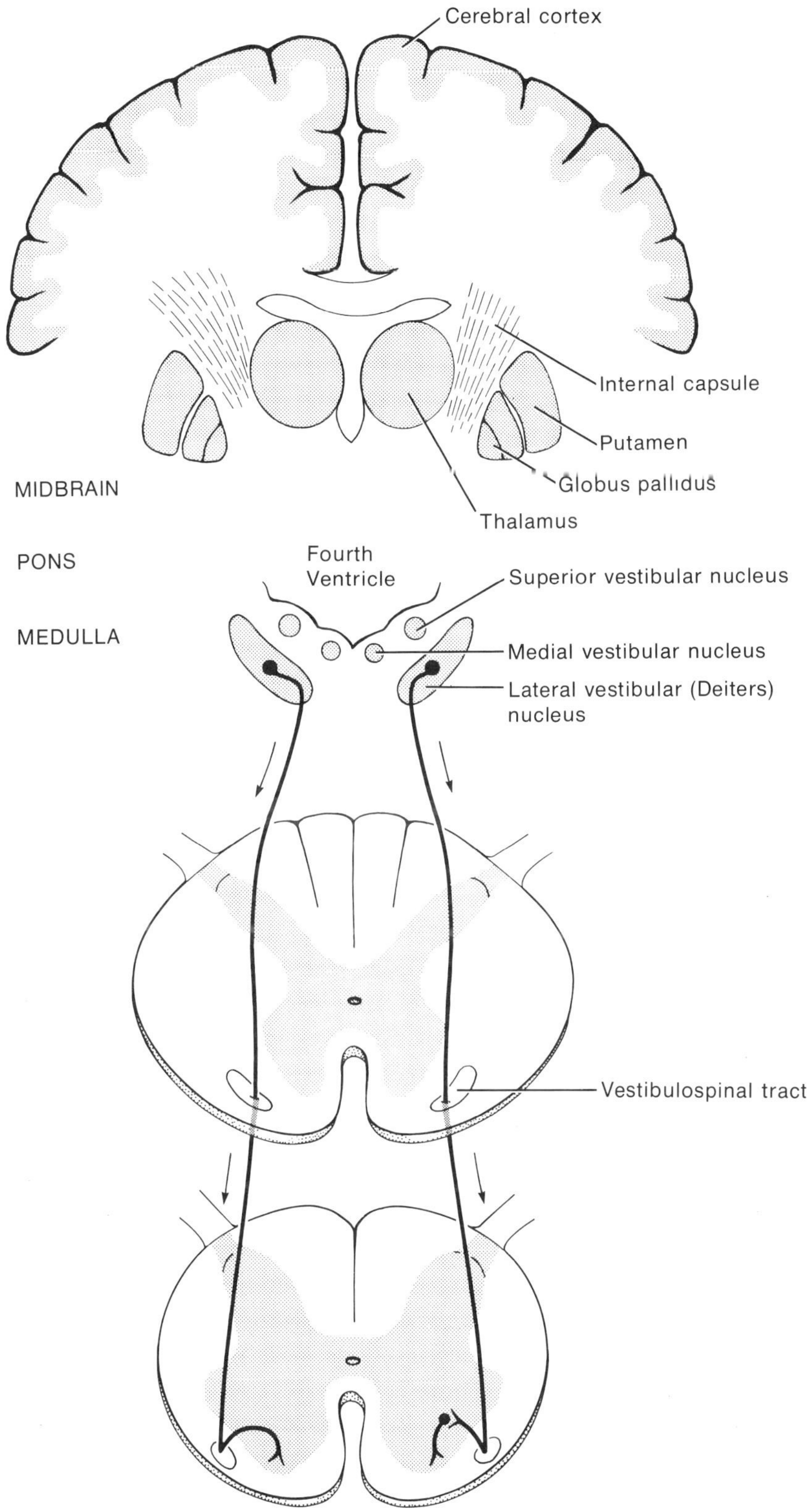

Figure 4–16. The vestibulospinal tracts. The inferior vestibular nucleus is not in the plane of this section. In this illustration, a neuron with monosynaptic connections is shown on one side and a neuron with polysynaptic connections on the other. It should be understood that both types of connections exist on both sides.

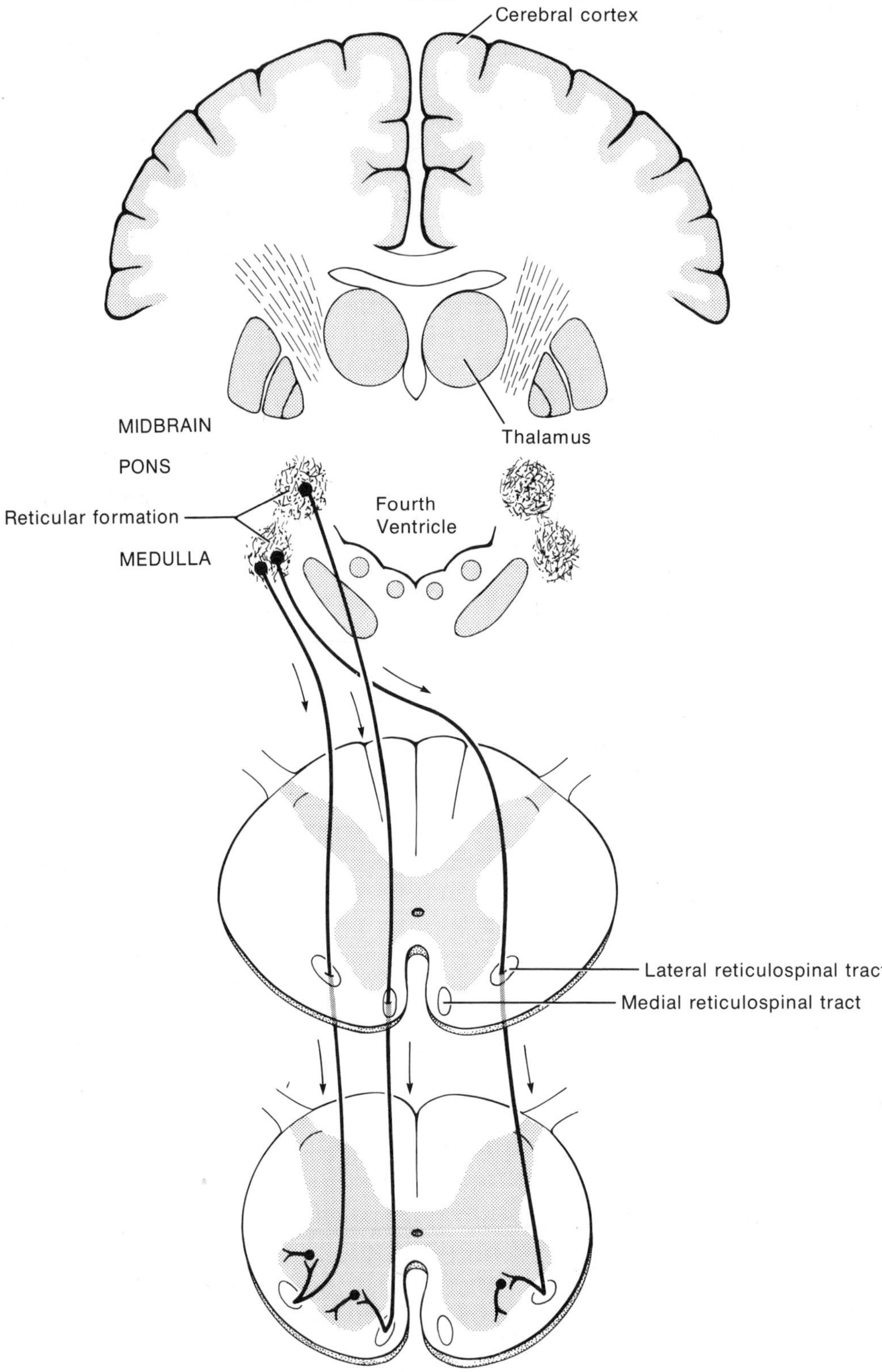

Figure 4–17. The reticulospinal tracts.

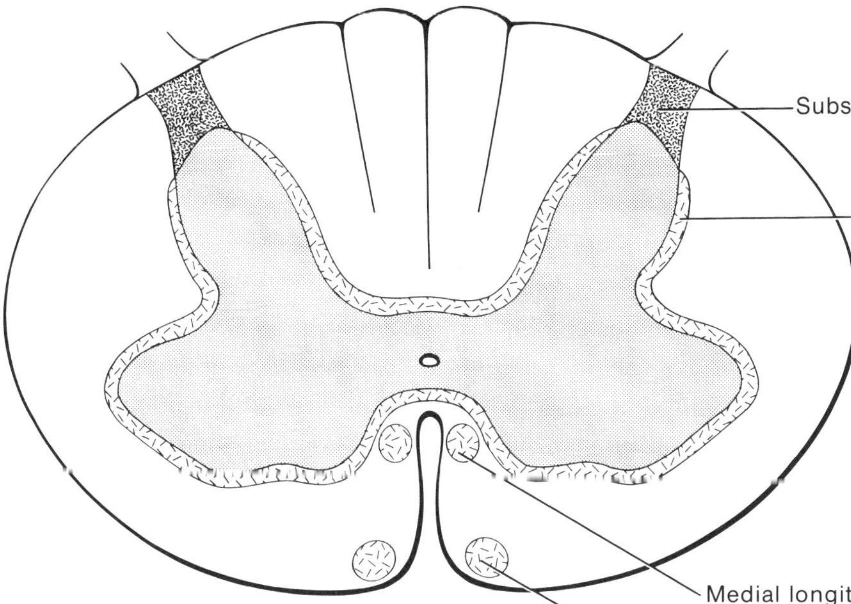

Figure 4–18. A cross-section of the spinal cord illustrating the locations of the tectospinal tract, the medial longitudinal fasciculus and the proprius bundle (nucleus proprius).

motor neurons are primarily by way of interneurons (see Fig. 4–17), although monosynaptic connections have been demonstrated in the cat and rat. In general, those fibers which originate in the pontine reticular formation tend to facilitate gamma activity; those which originate in the medullary reticular formation tend to inhibit gamma activity. In decerebrate animal preparations, the normal inhibitory influence of the cerebral cortex upon reticular formation neurons is absent, in which case the reticulospinal tracts exert an unopposed excitatory influence which facilitates extensor tone and contributes greatly to the condition called *decerebrate rigidity*. This excitatory output is no doubt due to the fact that many of the major afferent systems send collaterals into the brain stem reticular formation, and it is likely that they are responsible in large part for the downward discharge along the reticulospinal tracts.

TECTOSPINAL TRACTS

The tectospinal tracts originate in the superior colliculi of the mesencephalon, *cross* and descend in the anterior funiculi of the spinal cord, anterior to the medial longitudinal fasciculus (see Fig. 4–18). The fibers descend only as far inferior as cervical levels, where they terminate by making polysynaptic connections with motor neurons. Evidence suggests that the tectospinal tracts mediate reflex postural movements of the head, neck and upper extremities in response to visual stimuli. These reactions occur as a result of input to the superior colliculus from both the retinae via the optic nerve, and from cervical spinal segments by way of the spinotectal tract.

MEDIAL LONGITUDINAL FASCICULUS

The medial longitudinal fasciculus (MLF) is a complex brain stem system contributed to by the interstitial nucleus, which is located adjacent to the cerebral aqueduct,* the medial vestibular nucleus, the pontine reticular formation and the superior colliculus via the tectospinal tract. The system is predominantly *uncrossed* and most of the fibers terminate on ventral horn cells at cervical levels, although a few project as far

*Therefore, it is also called the interstitiospinal tract.

caudally as the sacral region. The MLF also projects to cranial nerves III, IV and VI. Its functions are to coordinate movements of the head with visual stimuli and to maintain visual fixation as the neck moves, changing the location of the head.

PROPRIUS BUNDLE (NUCLEUS PROPRIUS)

The proprius bundle consists of neurons that provide connections between adjacent spinal segments. Both ascending and descending fibers are included.

General Points

Some interesting generalizations may be made concerning the descending systems of the spinal cord. The older phylogenetic systems are the vestibulospinal, reticulospinal and tectospinal tracts as well as the medial longitudinal fasciculus. These tracts are located in the ventral and ventrolateral funiculi of the spinal cord, and enter the gray matter from the medial aspect. These pathways tend to be excitatory to extensor motor neurons and inhibitory to flexor motor neurons. The newer phylogenetic systems are the corticospinal and rubrospinal tracts, which are located in the lateral funiculus of the spinal cord and enter the gray matter from the lateral aspect. Whereas the older systems enhance extension and inhibit flexion, the newer systems tend to be excitatory to flexors and inhibitory to extensors.

In the clinical environment, one often hears the terms *upper motor neuron lesions* and *lower motor neuron lesions*. It is important to know what is meant by each of these. Reference to an upper motor neuron lesion indicates that any of the descending CNS tracts, excluding alpha and gamma motor neurons, may be damaged. Symptoms of upper motor neuron lesions are:

1. spastic paralysis (increased resistance to passive movement).
2. increased deep tendon reflexes.
3. muscular atrophy of agonists and antagonists, which may or may not be present.
4. clonus (rapidly alternating muscle contraction in response to stretching a tendon, e.g., the Achilles tendon).
5. a positive Babinski reflex (extension of the hallux in response to stroking the sole of the foot).

It should be understood that a positive Babinski reflex is normal at birth and for approximately the first year of life, which corresponds with the time at which the corticospinal tracts become myelinated.

A lower motor neuron lesion involves trauma to alpha and gamma motor neurons. The symptoms are:

1. flaccid paralysis (decreased resistance to passive movement).
2. areflexia or hyporeflexia (loss of reflexes or diminished reflexes) due to the loss of the efferent limb of the reflex arc.
3. severe muscular atrophy.

There is one important exception to the definition given for upper motor neuron lesions. Pure corticospinal lesions, of which very few have been reported in the literature, do not produce the spectrum of symptoms that other upper motor neuron lesions do. Rather, pure lesions of the corticospinal tracts result in symptoms more typical of a lower motor neuron lesion, involving a flaccid rather than a spastic type of paralysis.

The remaining question is, where are the descending autonomic pathways from the hypothalamus? These are located in the ventral and ventrolateral columns of the spinal cord, but they are diffusely oriented and do not form discrete bundles.

REVIEW QUESTIONS

1. Discuss the types of afferents that enter the spinal cord from the dorsal roots from specific sensory receptors. These afferent neurons will send impulses to higher centers via specific afferent systems. Correlate the information you have absorbed so far and, wherever possible, relate neurons from specific types of receptors with a particular afferent system. Explain the quality of information conveyed to the central nervous system by each of the afferent

systems in terms of receptor adaptability and conduction velocity (due to fiber sizes and numbers of synapses in the pathway).

2. Compare the two ascending pathways that reach consciousness. Trace their routes from their origins in the spinal cord to the somatosensory cortex. How might this sensory information influence motor behavior? Compare the two systems in terms of one of them being an *epicritic* and the other a *protopathic* system.

3. Compare the corticospinal and rubrospinal tracts in terms of their origins, termination, courses, types of connections, function and conduction velocities. If you were working with a patient in whom the corticospinal tracts had been destroyed, would you expect his motor behavior to differ from the normal? If so, how?

4. Compare the symptoms produced by an *upper motor neuron lesion* with those of a *lower motor neuron lesion.*

5. From the information you have been given about the supraspinal influences on gamma motor neurons, does it appear that we consciously control them? What are the implications of this in terms of how we might bias the muscle spindle through gamma motor neurons in treating patients?

CHAPTER 5 • DEVELOPMENT OF THE CENTRAL NERVOUS SYSTEM: SUBDIVISIONS OF THE BRAIN

OBJECTIVES

After reading this chapter, you should: • Have a general understanding of the ontogenetic development of the nervous system. • Be familiar with Volpe's generalizations regarding the effects of teratogenic agents. • Be able to relate specific structures to the subdivisions of the brain (i.e., the thalamus as part of the diencephalon, etc.). • Be familiar with the generalizations about development of the nervous system.

DEVELOPMENT OF THE CENTRAL NERVOUS SYSTEM

Phylogenetic Development

Those who are interested in the details of phylogenetic development are urged to refer to Carpenter's *Human Anatomy* (1976). Here, we will deal only with some generalizations of functional significance.

As evolution has progressed, nerve cells have collected at the rostral end of the spinal cord. The most primitive aggregation of cells was probably equivalent to what has been retained in man as the reticular formation, which is a rather ill-defined area that extends throughout the deep part of the medulla, pons and midbrain. The function of these cells was to regulate the activity of spinal motor neurons, and therefore to control groups of segmental muscles. The reticular formation of man is still capable of modifying reflex activity of the spinal motor neurons. Gradually, additional groups of cells have accumulated, which function as sensory fiber terminals for taste, touch, vision, hearing, equilibrium, reflex centers for control of visceral systems, and in the control of muscles of the eyes and tongue and musculature derived from the branchial arches (see Fig. 7–1). These primitive collections of cells constitute the brain stem, which includes the medulla, pons, mesencephalon, the diencephalon and the deep cerebellar nuclei. The diencephalon and telencephalon are the most recently acquired accumulations of cells. Each additional group of cells has subjected earlier acquired systems to a higher degree of modification of their activities. For example, the spinal cord is capable of segmental reflex activity, but the pons and medulla exert some control over spinal cord activity by way of the reticulospinal tracts. The cerebral cortex, in turn, regulates the activity of the brain stem structures. Many diseases and injuries encountered in clinical practice involve damage to the higher centers of control. In these cases one is dealing with regression in function which is reminiscent of the functional capabilities of species lower on the phylogenetic scale than man.

An important generalization regarding phylogenetic development of the nervous system is that once a structure of the nervous system is developed in the vertebrate brain, it usually remains, even though in higher animals it may be reduced in size and may function only minimally. A good example of this is the olfactory system. It is very important in some of the lower animals such as cats and dogs, and in these the olfactory areas of the brain are very prominent. In man, these areas are very small. This exemplifies the generality that there is a correlation between the size of a structure within the brain and its importance in the life of the animal.

As the cerebral cortex has developed into a more and more complex structure, it has gradually taken over control of the lower centers such as the thalamus, cerebellum, reticular formation and spinal cord. These send sensory information to the cortex which, in turn, integrates and controls the basal ganglia, cerebellum and reticular formation so that smooth, voluntary muscle movements are produced. It should be emphasized, however, that the older systems contribute essential components to movement that may be masked by the cerebral cortex when it is functioning normally. This is why damage to the pathways between the cerebral cortex and the older systems results in regression to poorly controlled activity mediated by the older motor systems.

Ontogenetic Development

During embryonic development in man, phylogenetic development is repeated so that older systems develop first and newer systems, such as the corticospinal tracts, are not fully developed even at birth.

Development of the Spinal Cord

Late in the third week of gestation there is an infolding of posterior ectodermal cells that leads to the establishment of two neural folds. Initially the folds are separated by a neural groove, but they then meet to produce a neural tube, which detaches itself from the surface ectoderm. Some ectodermal cells are not incorporated into the neural tube, but instead remain between the neural tube and the surface ectoderm. This is the primitive neural crest. Concomitant with the appearance of the neural folds, segmentation of adjacent, bilateral strips of mesoderm occurs so that the production of somites begins in a rostrocaudal sequence as the neural tube develops. The tube is formed before the end of the fourth week, closing first in the primitive cervical region and then continuing to close in both rostral and caudal directions. At this time there is an enlarged rostral portion, which will become the brain, and a narrow caudal portion, the primitive spinal cord. Flanking each side of the primitive spinal cord are the neural crests, and the notochord lies ventral to the primitive spinal cord. The somites begin developing during the fourth or fifth week and flank all three of these structures laterally (see Fig. 5–1). It is interesting that the most rostral tip of the developing neural tube consists of the lamina terminalis, but in the mature nervous system the lamina terminalis lies concealed, largely hidden by the gyri of the cerebral cortex. This is instructive in that it shows that extensive migration of cells takes place during development.

The neural crest cells are precursors of sensory neurons (both spinal and cranial) and their ganglia (dorsal root ganglia are illustrated in Fig. 5–1e), Schwann sheath cells, capsule cells (which form a capsule around the bodies of the dorsal root ganglion cells), visceral motor neurons and pigment cells.

The early neural tube consists of a single layer of neuroectodermal cells, but later in development it differentiates into three well-established layers. The layer adjacent to the central canal is called the ependymal or germinal layer. The greatest amount of mitotic division occurs therein, and this layer is the origin of most of the cells that ultimately comprise the central nervous system. The cells that originate here migrate to more superficial layers of the neural tube, and when mitosis ceases the ependymal layer simply becomes the lining of the central canal and cerebral ventricles. As the newly-produced cells migrate out from the ependymal layer they become oriented so that their cell bodies collect close to the ependymal layer, while they send cytoplas-

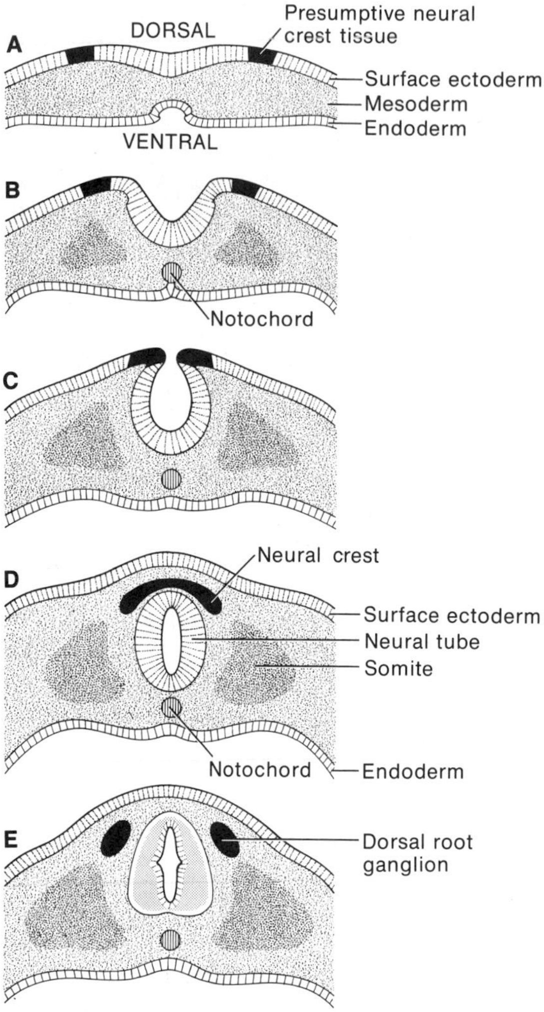

Figure 5–1. The sequence of events during development of the spinal cord and related structures. *A*, The posterior surface ectodermal cells begin to fold in slightly. *B*, Further infolding of the posterior surface ectoderm occurs and the notochord is present. *C*, The ectodermal folds and presumptive neural crest tissue are still separated by a neural groove. *D*, The neural tube has closed; neural crest cells have separated from the surface ectoderm and the somites are well-developed. *E*, The neural crest cells have differentiated into dorsal root ganglion cells.

mic processes out toward the more superficial layers. The layer in which the cell bodies aggregate is called the mantle layer, which is further divided into the intermediate and subventricular layers. The cell bodies aggregate in the intermediate layer after mitosis. The subventricular region is between the ependymal and intermediate region (see Fig. 5–2), and is the region in which cells continue to multiply. The mantle layer is the future gray matter of the spinal cord. The outer layer in which the cytoplasmic processes collect is called the marginal layer. This is the future white matter of the spinal cord.

The neuroectodermal cells may differentiate along two different pathways, either as neuroblasts, which develop into neurons, or as spongioblasts, which differentiate further into glial cells, either astrocytes or oligodendrocytes. The differentiation along the two different pathways may be indicated as follows:

neuroblasts → neurons

spongioblasts → glial cells → astrocytes, oligodendroglial cells

As development of the nervous system progresses, capillaries invade the nervous tissue and from them another type of glial cell migrates, called microglia. The notochord becomes discontinuous as it is engulfed by the developing intervertebral discs. In the adult it may be identified as the white liquid nucleus pulposus within the intervertebral discs.

The spinal cord does not grow in length as rapidly as the vertebral column. Therefore, its caudal end does not reach all the way down to the coccyx, so that at birth the tip of the spinal cord corresponds to the level of the third lumbar vertebra and in the adult it corresponds with the level of the second lumbar vertebra. Because of this ultimate mismatch of vertebrae and spinal segments, the nerve roots run obliquely toward their dorsal root ganglia, which remain located within the intervertebral foramina that corresponded with the spinal segments when development was initiated (see Fig. 5–3). The bundle of nerve fibers that exists within the vertebral canal inferior to the caudal end of the spinal cord (conus medullaris) is called the cauda equina (horse's tail). The area of subarachnoid space in which the cerebrospinal fluid is located, below the level of vertebral segment L2, is the safest place to execute a spinal tap for diagnostic removal of cerebrospinal fluid. A needle inserted in this area will simply move the fibers of the cauda equina aside without damaging them. In areas superior to the level of L2 the spinal cord fills up so much of the vertebral canal that it would be easily damaged by needle insertion.

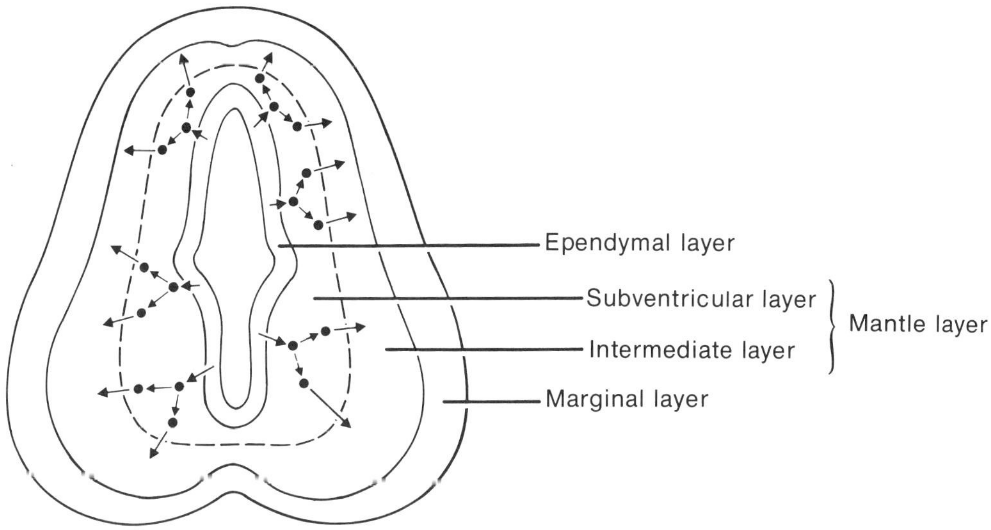

Figure 5–2. The layers of the developing spinal cord. The arrows indicate the migration of developing cells from the ependymal layer. The cells develop in the ependymal layer and migrate into the subventricular layer. After mitosis in the subventricular layer, the cells migrate further into the intermediate layer. The processes of these cells make up the white matter of the marginal layer.

Damage to the nerve fibers of the cauda equina can have very serious repercussions. Figure 5–3 shows that many of the neurons that comprise the cauda equina contribute to the lumbosacral plexus. Therefore, the damage produces a deficit in motor and sensory function in the lower extremities.

One of the most common congenital malformations of the spinal cord is produced by failure of the neural tube to close. This condition is called *spina bifida*. The damage is caused by one of two types of abnormalities. One is the *meningocele*, in which there is herniation of the meninges (dura mater, arachnoid mater and pia mater) through a defective opening in the vertebral column. The other is the *meningomyelocele*. In this condition the spinal cord and meninges may herniate through a defective vertebral column so that the spinal cord is exposed to trauma. The symptoms vary greatly in severity. With a minimal defect associated with a meningocele an individual may live an entirely symptom-free life with only a small tuft of hair over the defect to betray its presence. A patient with a major defect associated with a meningomyelocele may be completely paralyzed below the level of the spinal cord lesion. Until a few years ago patients with such a disability were completely confined to their beds. It was not known how to cope with the paralysis or incompetency in bowel and bladder control. Now, with the increased expertise of the health professions many of these patients can ambulate with crutches and braces and lead meaningful, productive lives. Unfortunately, spina bifida is often associated with hydrocephalus (see discussion after *Development of the brain*) which may involve brain damage. In these cases the prognosis (outlook for improvement) is not as favorable.

Development of the Brain

At the end of the fourth week of gestation there are three dilatations produced at the rostral end of the neural tube. These represent the prosencephalon (forebrain), mesencephalon (midbrain) and rhombencephalon (hindbrain) (see Fig. 5–4). The dilated cavities represent the ventricular system, which is continuous with the central canal of the spinal cord. The roof plates of each of the ventricular cavities are very thin, so that the choroid plexus develops here by invagination of vascular mesenchymal tissue which is derived from the pia mater. Only a layer of ependyma separates the ventricles from the choroid plexus, which latter is important because it is responsible for the elaboration of cerebrospinal fluid.

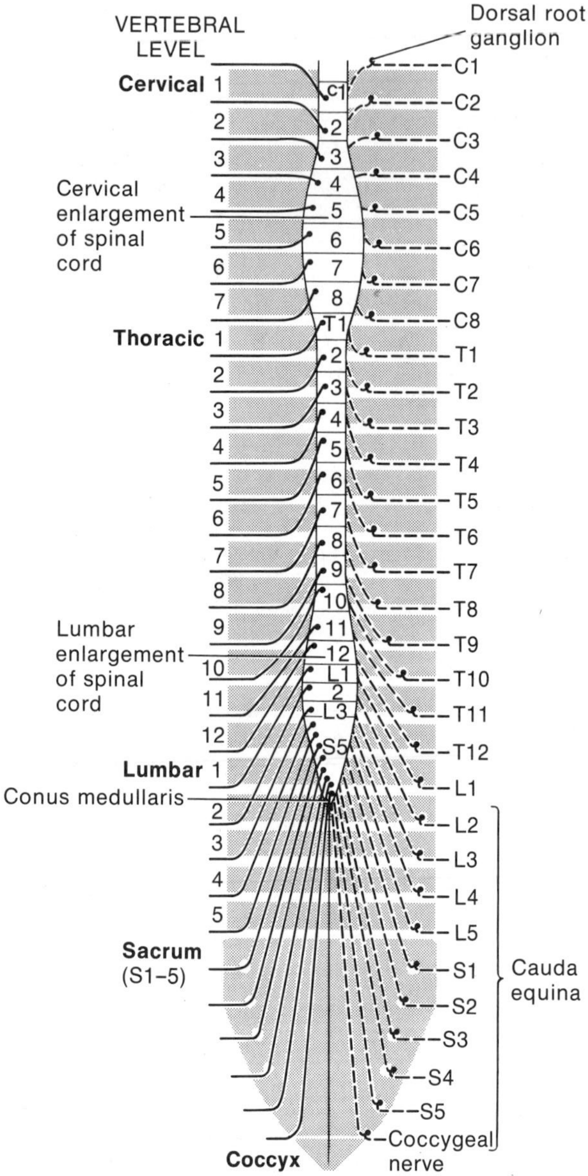

Figure 5–3. A comparison of the segmental levels of the spinal cord with those of the vertebral column. The vertebral levels are labeled on the left and the nerve roots on the right. Notice that the nerve roots course more and more obliquely from superior to inferior as they make their way to the intervertebral foramina through which they exit. Motor nerve roots are illustrated on the left; sensory nerve roots on the right.

By the sixth week the prosencephalon has divided into the telencephalon and the diencephalon. The mesencephalon remains small and does not subdivide further. The rhombencephalon has divided into the metencephalon (the future pons and cerebellum) and the myelencephalon (the future medulla oblongata). Each of these five divisions of the brain undergoes intrinsic organization as growth continues so that each area presents its own special features.

CONGENITAL DEFECTS ASSOCIATED WITH DEVELOPMENT OF THE BRAIN

There are several common developmental defects of the nervous system. One of the most common is *hydrocephalus* ("water head"). In this condition the head becomes enlarged to an extent determined by the amount of accumulation of fluid in the ventricles of the brain. Normally the cerebrospinal fluid is elaborated in the choroid plexuses in all four of the cerebral ventricles. (A few drops a day are elaborated in the central canal of the spinal cord.) The production of cerebrospinal fluid is continuous and under normal conditions is absorbed as rapidly as it is produced, leaving a constant amount within and around the central nervous system. The direction of flow is from the lateral ventricles to the third, then through the cerebral aqueduct to the fourth ventricle. There are three small openings leading from the fourth ventricle into the subarachnoid space. This space is formed by the arachnoid mater, one of the three meningeal layers that completely surround the brain and spinal cord (the dura mater, arachnoid mater and pia mater — see Fig. 5–5). The two lateral openings are called the foramina of Luschka; the midline opening is called the foramen of Magendie.

From the subarachnoid spaces the cerebrospinal fluid is normally absorbed by structures called the arachnoid villi, which are outpouchings of the superior sagittal sinus (a venous channel produced by splitting of the dura mater in the midline — see Fig. 5–5). The cerebrospinal fluid then is drained from the brain through the usual venous channels (see Chapter 13). When more cerebrospinal fluid is produced than is absorbed, hydrocephalus is the result. Usually the causative factor is a blockage of flow of cerebrospinal fluid and this occurs most often at the cerebral aqueduct. As the ventricular system enlarges owing to the collection of cerebrospinal fluid in the ventricles, so does the skull, since the bones of the skull have not yet fused. Eventually, if the condition is not alleviated, there is so much compression on the tissues of the brain that there is destruction of the brain

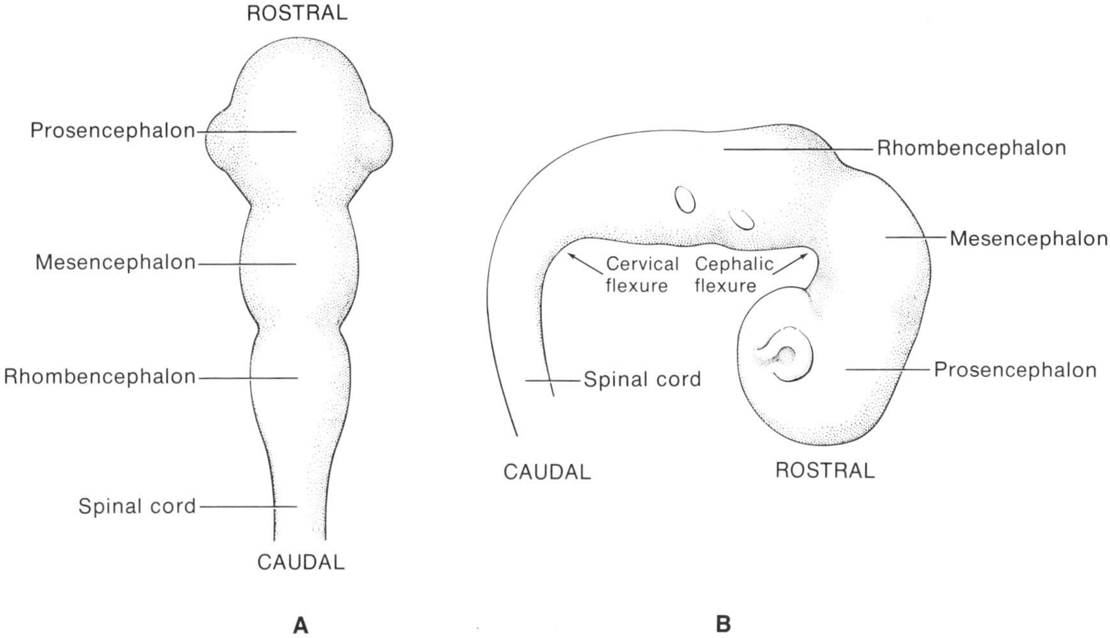

Figure 5–4. The developing nervous system. *A*, Posterior view. *B*, Lateral view at a later stage of development.

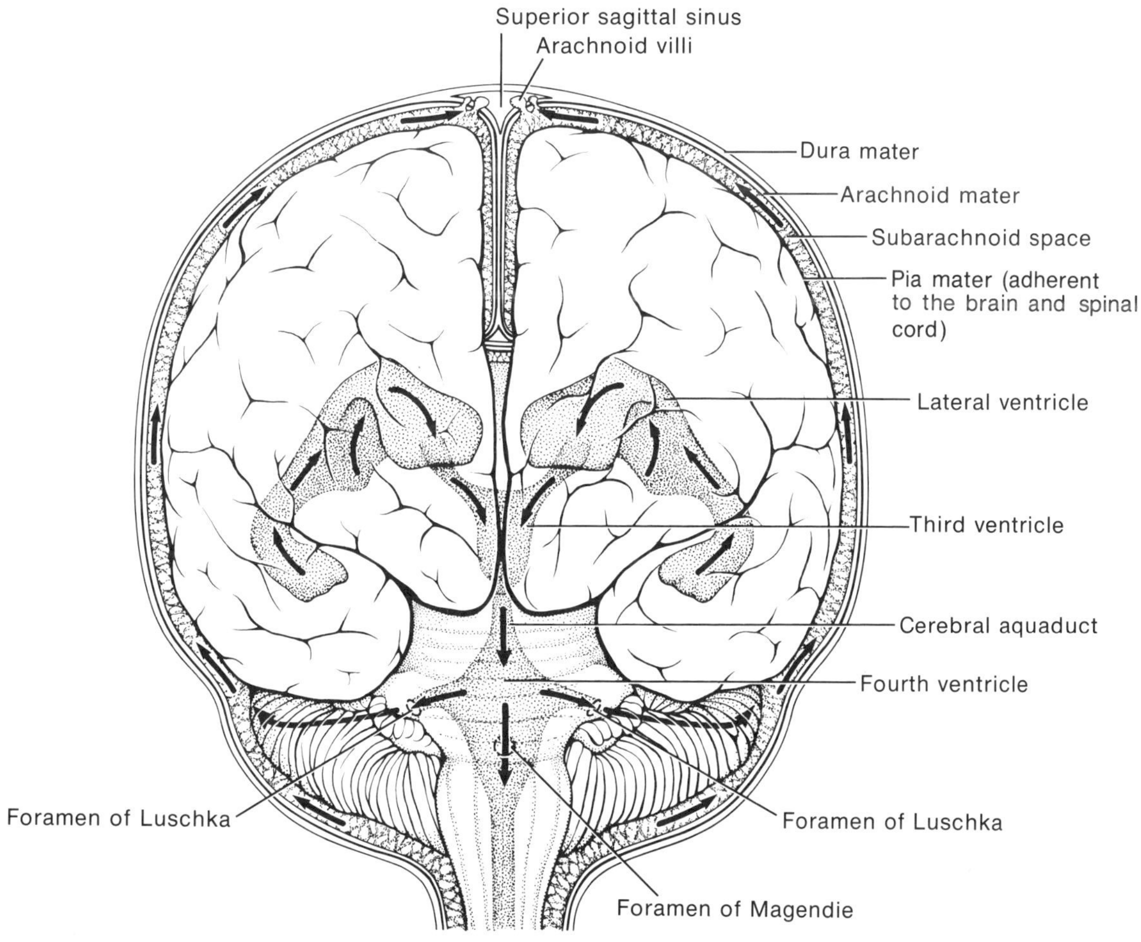

Figure 5–5. The normal direction of cerebrospinal fluid flow (indicated by the arrows) as seen schematically from an anterior view.

tissue which can produce a host of motor and sensory deficits as well as mental retardation. With improved methods of detecting the condition in newborn infants, hydrocephalus now is rarely allowed to progress to that point.

The history of treatment of hydrocephalus is very interesting. Several years ago the use of jugular shunts was initiated, a shunt being placed between the lateral ventricles and the jugular vein. This method was successful in removing the excess cerebrospinal fluid, but the drawback was that with the rapid growth of the infant the shunt would have to be replaced very often. An improvement was the use of intraperitoneal or intrapleural shunts, which were put in place between the lateral ventricles of the brain and the peritoneum or pleural spaces. The advantage of this treatment was that an extra length of tubing could be inserted into the peritoneum or pleural space so that as the infant grew the slack would gradually be taken up, necessitating many fewer replacements of the shunt. More recently, Epstein and his group (1973) reported successful use of a "volume control valve" to eliminate dependency on shunts. The valve permits the passage of fluid only when subjected to transcutaneous compression. Some degree of ventricular dilatation is permitted before the valve is opened so that alternate, spontaneous, absorptive pathways for the cerebrospinal fluid become functional. The shunt extends from the lateral ventricle to the pleural or peritoneal cavity.

The rate of incidence of *anencephalus* (lack of development of the brain) is questionable because many anencephalic embryos abort spontaneously early in gestation. This condition is produced by variable degrees of lack of closure of the rostral end of the developing neural tube (anterior neuropore). Therefore, the extent of the deficiency is dependent on the size of the faulty closure.

German measles (rubella) during the first trimester of pregnancy has been a common cause of congenital deficits in newborn infants. Among the CNS deficits are mental retardation and microcephalus (diminished size of the brain). The earlier in pregnancy that the infection occurs, the greater are the chances of damaging the infant.

Ionizing radiation during pregnancy can also have devastating effects on embryos (first eight weeks of gestation) and fetuses (last seven months of gestation). Infants may become microcephalic idiots after excessive exposure of the mother's pelvic region.

Among the many developmental defects caused by chromosomal abnormalities, *Down's syndrome* (mongolism) is probably the best known. It is caused by an extra 21st chromosome, and is referred to as trisomy 21. Children affected by this syndrome have been described as "unfinished" or 'ill-finished" because their brains do not develop fully and they have poor coordination. Most mongoloids have intelligence quotients betwen 25 and 49, and the great majority are products of mothers over 35 years of age.

Volpe (1971) has made some interesting generalizations regarding the effects of *teratogenic agents*. These are agents that produce congenital abnormalities, e.g., radiation, infections, rubella and other viruses, thalidomide, chemicals such as methyl mercury, malnutrition, hypoxia and acidosis. Some quotations from Volpe follow:

1. "The particular type of fetal malformation is related to the time in development at which the noxious agent is administered or becomes active."
2. "The sensitivity of an organ to a teratogenic influence is greatest during a limited developmental period when the organ or part is undergoing differentiation or growth." It is little wonder, then, that the embryo is so susceptible to injury during the first eight weeks of gestation because all the systems of the body, including the nervous system, are differentiating very rapidly during that time.
3. "A given teratogen produces different malformations when applied at a different time of development." The malformation produced will depend on which structures are actively differentiating when the teratogen is applied.
4. "The potential deleterious effect of a teratogen is influenced by the genetic constitution of the organism." Some individuals may have a genetic constitution that makes them either more susceptible or more resistant to a specific teratogen.

For an in-depth treatment of abnormal development see the book, *Normal and Abnormal Development of the Human Nervous System* by Lemire et al. (1975).

With the development of the nervous system during embryonic and fetal stages some functional activities become possible during prenatal life. In the seventh or eighth week the embryo can respond to cutaneous stimulation, and by ten weeks the fetus is capable of spontaneous activity. Palmar grasp and the Babinski reflex are present at the end of the third prenatal month. These activities represent an increasing integration of the nervous system. For an in-depth treatment of embryonic and fetal development see McGraw, *The Neuromuscular Maturation of the Human Infant,* 1966.

The major subdivisions of the brain are recognized in relation to the ventricles of the brain, as suggested previously, and these relationships can be seen most clearly during the early stages of development.

The *telencephalon* is related to the lateral ventricles. It consists of the cerebral cortex, the olfactory bulbs and the basal ganglia. The latter are a group of subcortical nuclei which include the putamen, globus pallidus, caudate nucleus and amygdaloid nucleus. The term *basal ganglia* is somewhat of a misnomer since we usually think of ganglia as groups of cells located in areas outside the central nervous system, and groups of cells *within* the CNS as nuclei. *Basal nuclei* would be more correct terminology for the basal ganglia, but the literature consistently refers to basal ganglia, and that convention will be followed in this book.

The *diencephalon* is related to the third ventricle and includes the thalamus, epithalamus, subthalamus and hypothalamus.

Included in the *mesencephalon,* which is related to the cerebral aqueduct, are the tectum (corpora quadrigemina), the tegmentum, the crus cerebri, the red nucleus and the substantia nigra.

The *rhombencephalon* is related to the fourth ventricle and may be further subdivided into the *metencephalon* and *myelencephalon*. The former differentiates into the pons and cerebellum and the latter becomes the medulla oblongata.

In the adult there is a distinct functional organization in the spinal cord; i.e., the dorsal portions of the spinal cord contain sensory components and the ventral portions contain motor components. During development the sensory portions are derived from the posteriorly located alar plates of the neural tube. The motor portions are derived from the ventrally located basal plates. Figure 5–6 shows that the alar and

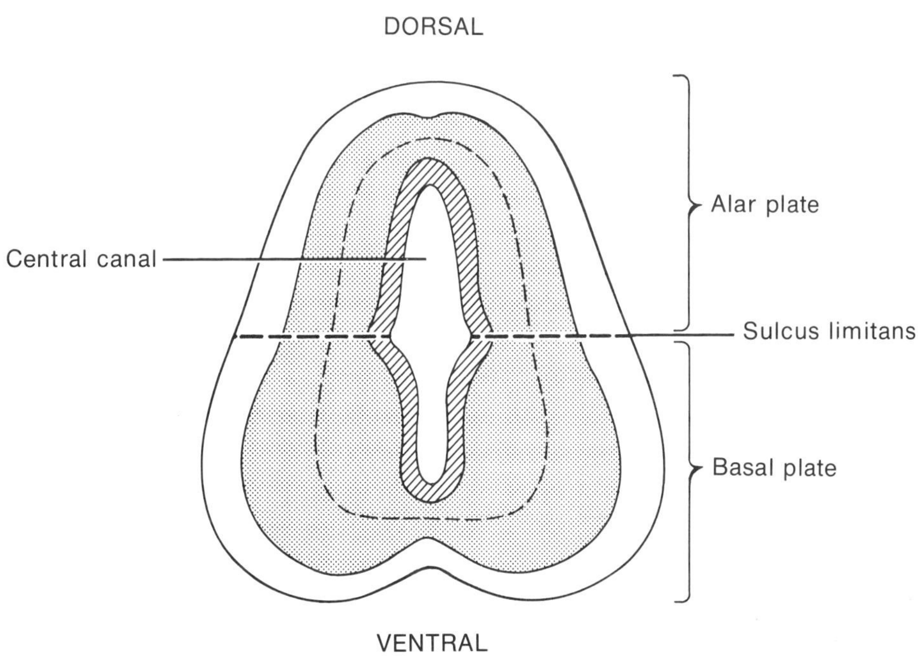

Figure 5–6. A cross-section of the developing spinal cord. The alar plates develop into sensory components; the basal plates differentiate into motor components. These two plates are separated at the level of the sulcus limitans. (The heavy broken lines separate the alar from basal plates.)

basal plates are separated by the sulcus limitans, which extends rostral to the spinal cord and can be identified in the floor of the fourth ventricle in adults. This basic pattern of sensory and motor components exists as far rostrally as the mesencephalon, but is not present in the telencephalon and diencephalon. Therefore, in the spinal cord, medulla, pons and mesencephalon four functional columns exist. They are the somatic sensory, visceral sensory, somatic motor and visceral motor columns. The presence of the cranial nerves modifies the pattern somewhat in the brain stem, but nevertheless it continues to exist.

One of the most interesting questions concerning development of the nervous system is: how do neurons establish the specific connections during development that we know exist in the mature nervous system? Do these connections change during the life of the individual, for example, during learning processes? Very little is known about this subject and there are few answers to questions such as these, but it is an intriguing area of research.

There is much to learn about the development of the nervous system, but from the work that has been done some definite generalizations may be made:

1. Large neurons appear first in a specific region.
2. Small neurons appear later in development and may even appear shortly after birth.
3. Extensive migration of newly formed neurons may occur through regions of previously established neurons. This migration of one type of neuron past another type may provide the basis of specificity of synaptic contact in some instances.
4. More neurons develop in the CNS than are present in the mature CNS. Thus, nerve cell death constitutes a normal part of the maturation process.
5. All nerve cells of the CNS (approximately 10,000,000,000) have developed by the time of birth or shortly thereafter. The fact that nerve cells display no mitotic activity subsequent to this time is an important clinical consideration. It means that nerve cells destroyed by disease or trauma cannot be replaced.

REVIEW QUESTIONS

1. What structures are included in the brain stem?
2. From a developmental point of view, why may damage to the cerebral cortex or its connections with other structures produce lack of coordination and the ability to perform only gross or stereotyped movements?
3. What peripheral structures are derived from the neural tube? From the neural crest?
4. What are the origins of neurons? Astrocytes? Oliogodendroglial cells? Microglia?
5. What is the ultimate fate of the notochord?
6. Locate the safest place to do a spinal tap. Explain.
7. Why can damage to the cauda equina have very serious repercussions?
8. Does a meningocele or a myelomeningocele produce a more severe disability? Why?
9. Explain the cause of hydrocephalus.
10. What types of structures are derived from the alar plates? Basal plates?

CHAPTER 6 • THE BRAIN STEM

OBJECTIVES

After reading this chapter you should: • Have a general understanding of the morphology of the brain stem. • Understand how specific nuclei of the brain stem influence activity and behavior — within the limits of the discussion in this chapter. • Know how the basic structure of the brain stem resembles that of the spinal cord and how it is different. • Know the generalized connections and functions of the brain stem reticular formation. • Be able to trace the route of the feedback circuitry between the cerebral cortex and cerebellum. • Understand the parallelism and the differences between the corticorubrospinal and corticospinal tracts. • Know the interconnections of the substantia nigra. • Know the functions of the superior and inferior colliculi and the interconnections of the superior colliculus. • Know the most frequent symptoms of brain stem damage or disease.

INTRODUCTION

The details concerning most of the structures of the brain stem are dealt with in other chapters as their interconnections with other structures are discussed. The purpose of this chapter is to help the student locate the structures of the brain stem, recognize their relationships to each other, and establish the continuity of the long ascending and descending pathways as they course through this very important area.

BASIC STRUCTURE

The brain stem includes the medulla, pons, midbrain and diencephalon. Many sources include the deep cerebellar nuclei because of their extensive connections with the first three structures. The ten true cranial nerves (III through XII) are contained in the brain stem, as are all of the main afferent and efferent systems with the exception of the olfactory system. The brain stem is a relatively small region, but an extremely important one, since all information relayed between the telencephalon and the spinal cord must travel through it.

The basic structure of the brain stem resembles that of the spinal cord, with the main afferent and efferent cell columns located close to the fourth ventricle; this is similar to their relationship to the central canal in the spinal gray matter. The major pathways lie some distance from the fourth ventricle in the brain stem, as they do from the central canal in the spinal cord. The pattern is basically simple, but is modified by the fourth ventricle, which is larger and not as centrally located as the central canal, so that the pons and medulla lie ventral to it. It is further modified by the presence of the cranial nerve nuclei, which interrupt some of the cell columns, whereas the latter are continuous in the spinal cord. In addition, the

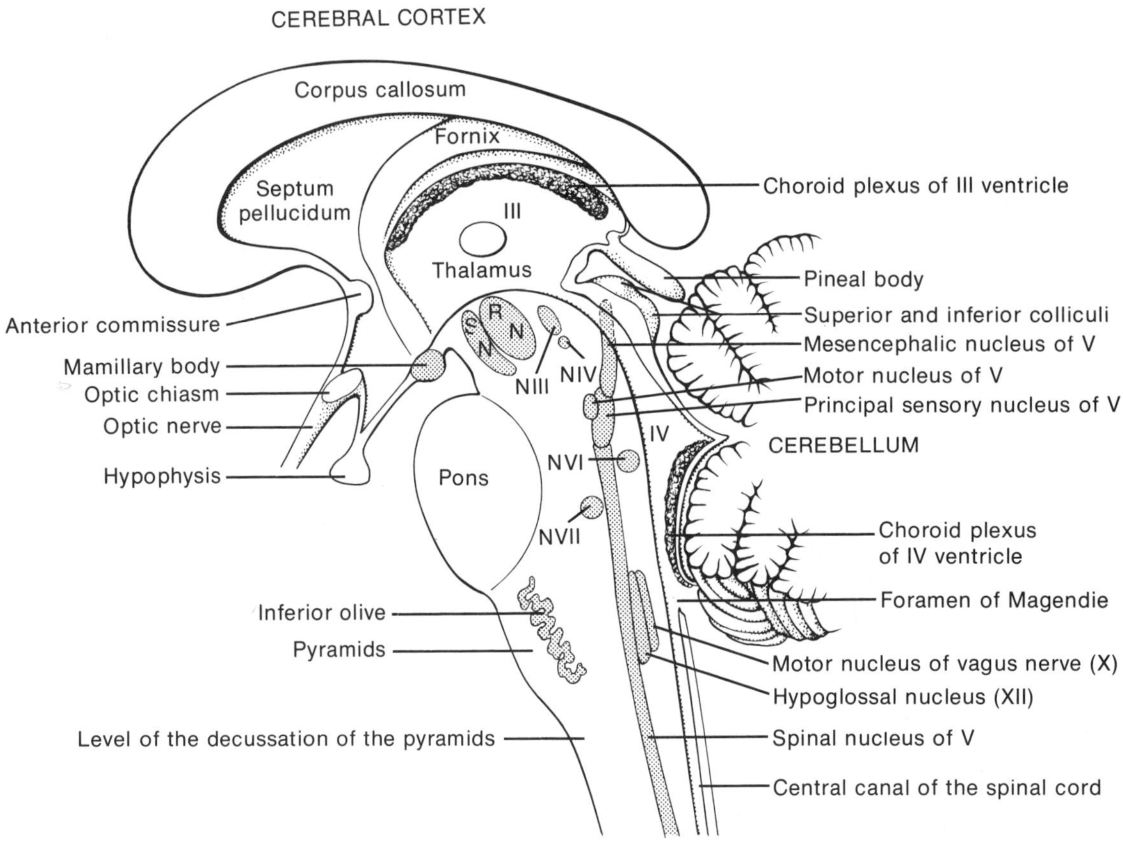

Figure 6–1. A parasagittal section of the brain stem and related areas with all pertinent nuclei and structures indicated and labeled. SN—substantia nigra. RN—red nucleus. NIII—nucleus of the oculomotor nerve. NIV—nucleus of the trochlear nerve. NVI—nucleus of the abducens nerve. NVII—nucleus of the facial nerve. III—third ventricle. IV—fourth ventricle.

ascending and descending pathways are more massive and complex in the brain stem than in the spinal cord, and there are numerous cell groups and fiber pathways located in all parts of the brain stem that are connected primarily with the cerebellum.

Figure 6–3 is a cross-section of the spinal cord in the high cervical region. It illustrates the major tracts of the spinal cord so that they can be related to the locations of brain stem structures in the following Figures.

*The Medulla Oblongata**

Some of the important structures located in the medulla are the following.

*See Figures 6–4 through 6–6.

CORTICOSPINAL AND CORTICOBULBAR TRACTS

These are continuous with the cell bodies of these tracts which originate in the cerebral cortex and descend through structures that can be identified in Figures 6–4 through 6–14, i.e., the internal capsule, crus cerebri and corticospinal tracts as they descend within the pons. The corticobulbar fibers descend in close association with the corticospinal fibers, but terminate on cranial nerve nuclei rather than continuing to descend to spinal cord levels.

MEDULLARY PYRAMIDS

The descending corticospinal fibers are grouped together in the medulla to form the anteriorly located medullary pyramids

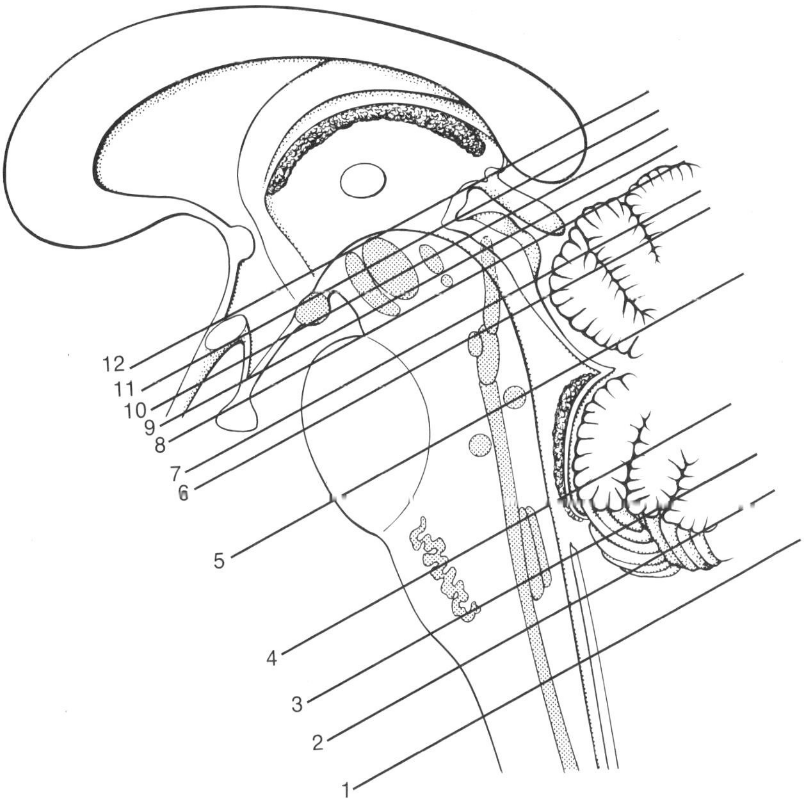

Figure 6–2. The same parasagittal section as in Figure 6–1, indicating the levels from which each of the following sections are taken.

(Figs. 6–4, 6–5 and 6–6). Most of the fibers of these tracts cross in the caudal medulla, constituting the decussation of the pyramids (Fig. 6–4).

NUCLEUS GRACILIS, NUCLEUS CUNEATUS AND ACCESSORY CUNEATE NUCLEUS.

Nucleus gracilis and nucleus cuneatus provide the first relay in the dorsal column (medial lemniscal) system, and are located in the posteromedial portion of the caudal medulla (Figs. 6–4 and 6–5). It should be recalled that some of the fibers of the corticospinal tracts terminate on these nuclei to inhibit unneeded information that is en route to the cerebral cortex. The accessory cuneate nucleus is located anterolateral to the cuneate nucleus (Fig. 6–5). This may be thought of as the homologue of Clarke's column in the spinal cord because it is a relay for subconscious proprioceptive information that enters the spinal cord superior to Clarke's column.

SPINAL NUCLEUS AND TRACT OF THE TRIGEMINAL NERVE

This nucleus and tract are located in the posterolateral portion of the brain stem (Figs. 6–4 through 6–8). The nucleus is continuous caudally with the substantia gelatinosa of the spinal cord and the tract is continuous caudally with Lissauer's tract (Fig. 6–3). The nucleus and tract extend from the level of the second cervical segment of the spinal cord to the pons, where the trigeminal nerve emerges from the brain stem. The connections of the trigeminal complex of nuclei will be dealt with in the section on cranial nerves, as will those of the other cranial nerve nuclei of the brain stem.

THE MAJOR ASCENDING AND DESCENDING TRACTS

All of these except the olfactory tract can be found in Figures 6–3 through 6–14.

Text continued on page 88

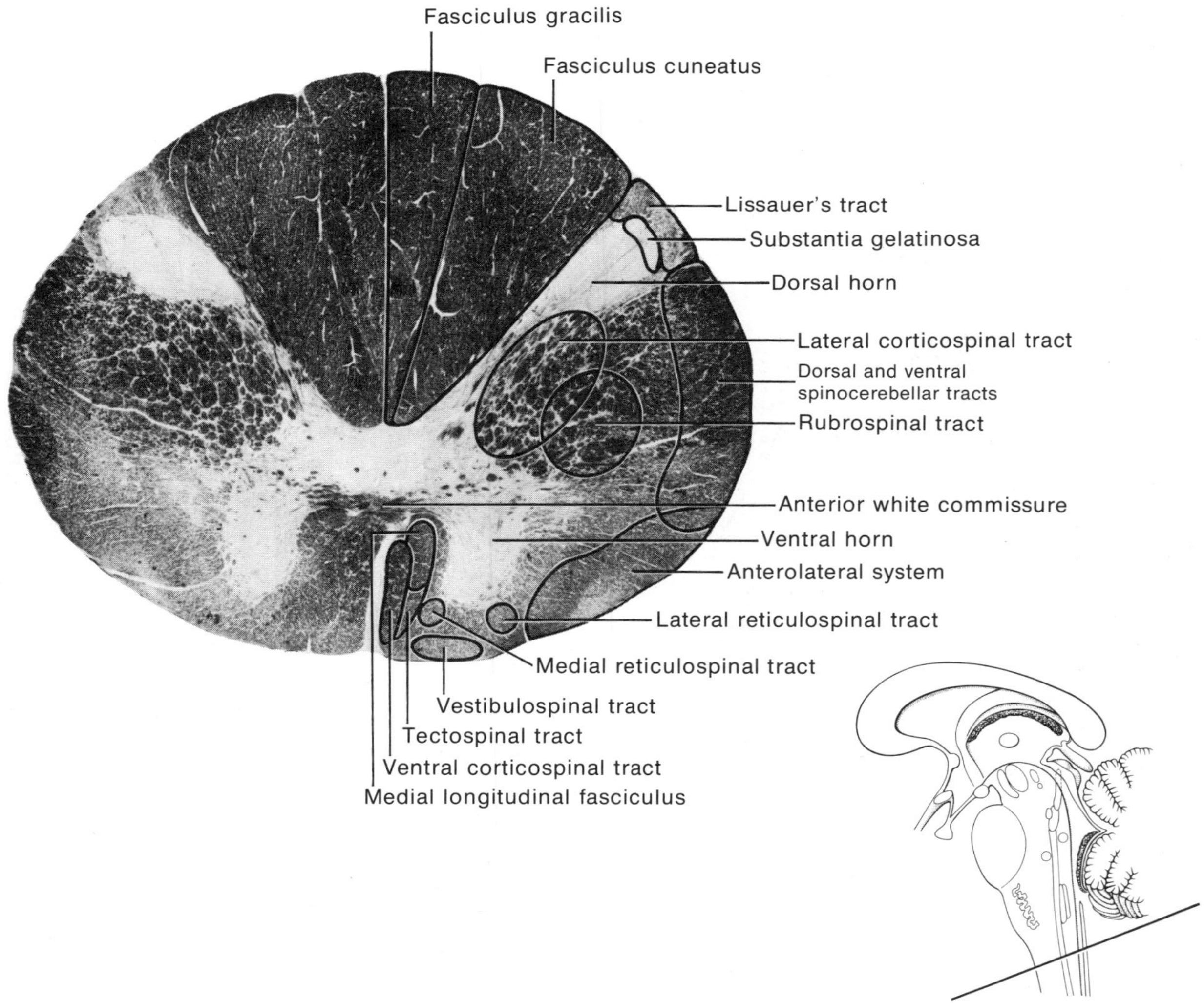

Figure 6–3. Cross-section of the spinal cord—high cervical region.

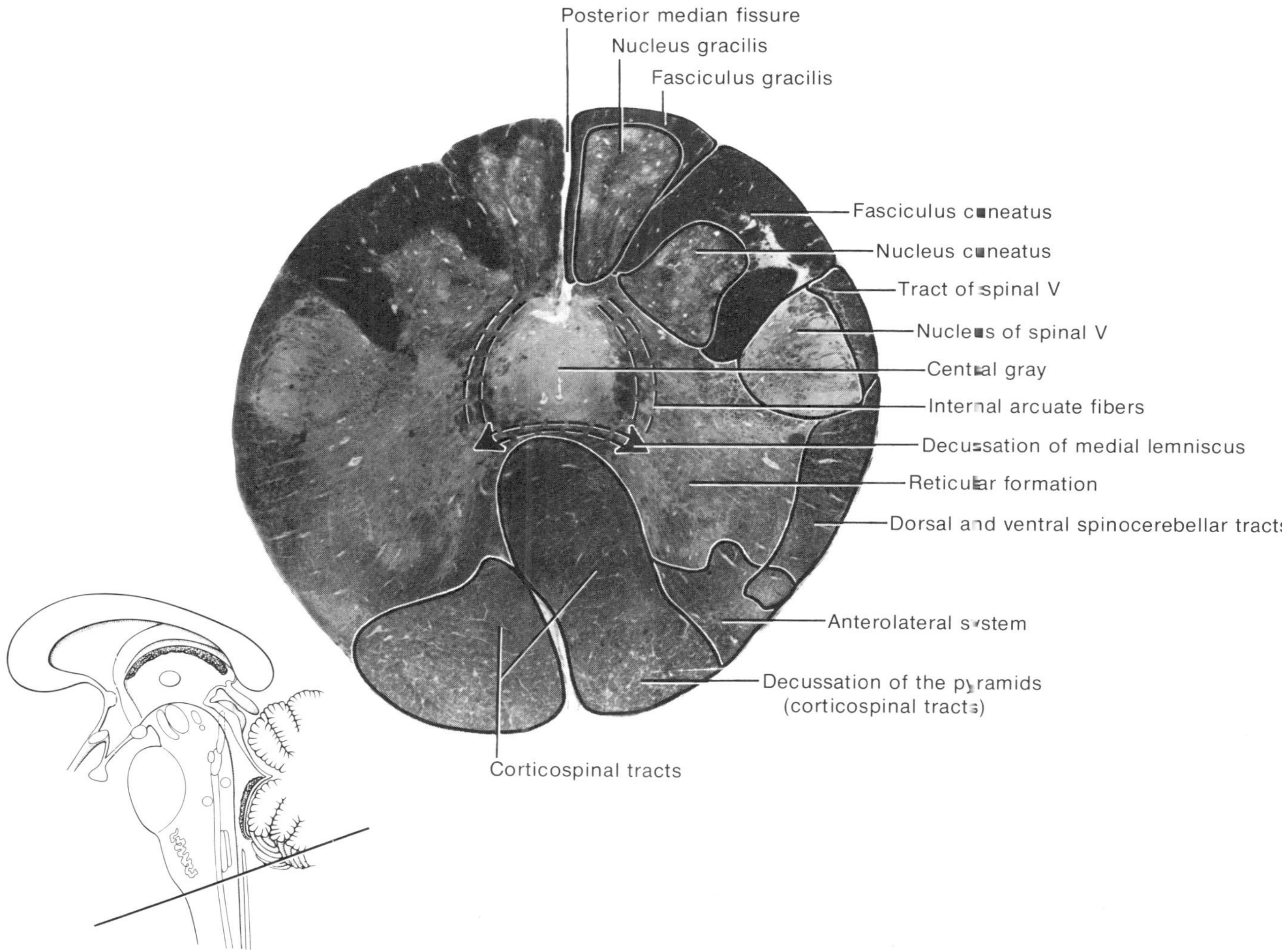

Figure 6–4. Cross-section of the medulla – level of the decussation of the pyramids – beginning of the decussation of the medial lemniscus.

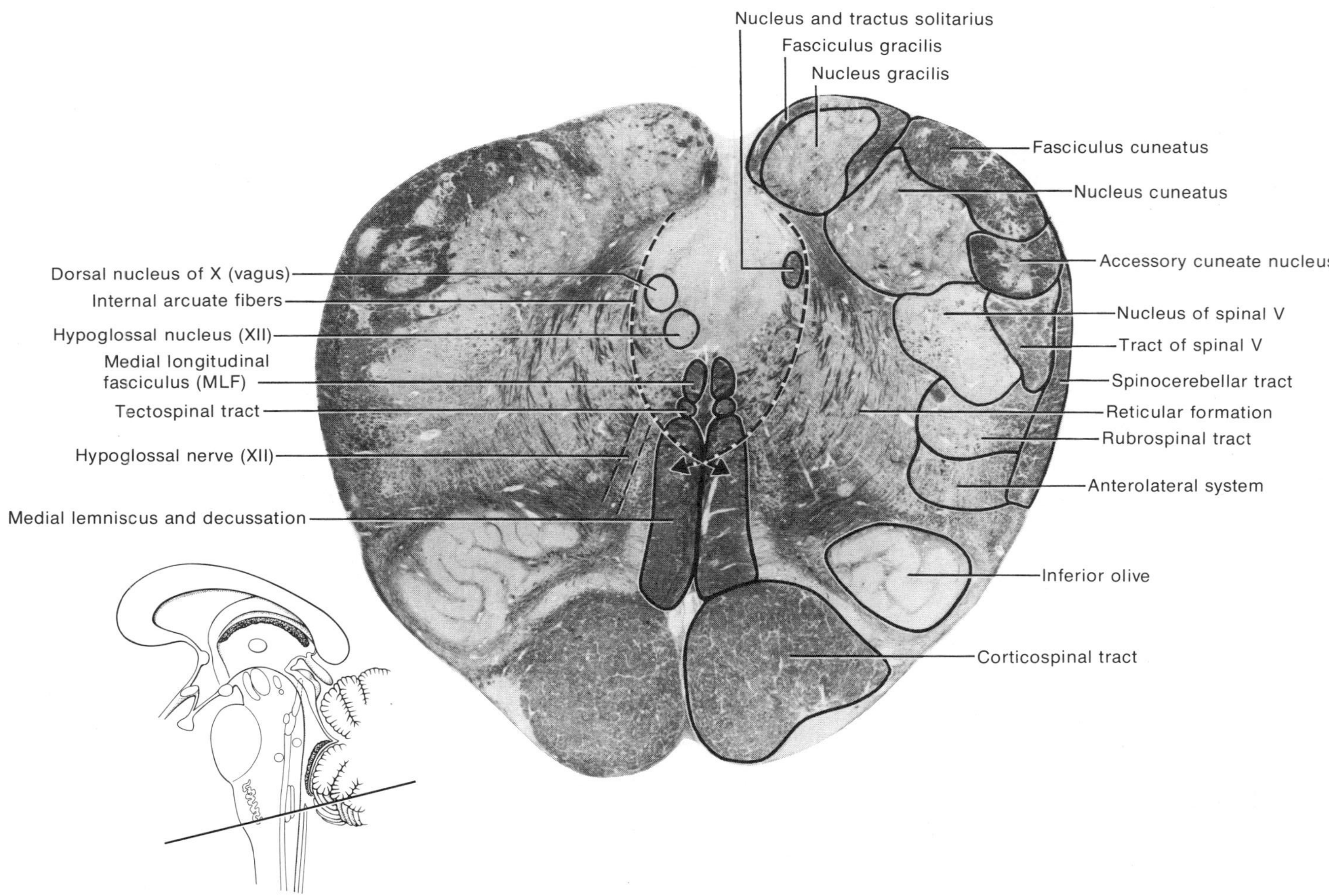

Figure 6–5. Cross-section of the medulla – level of the medial lemniscus – above the pyramidal decussation.

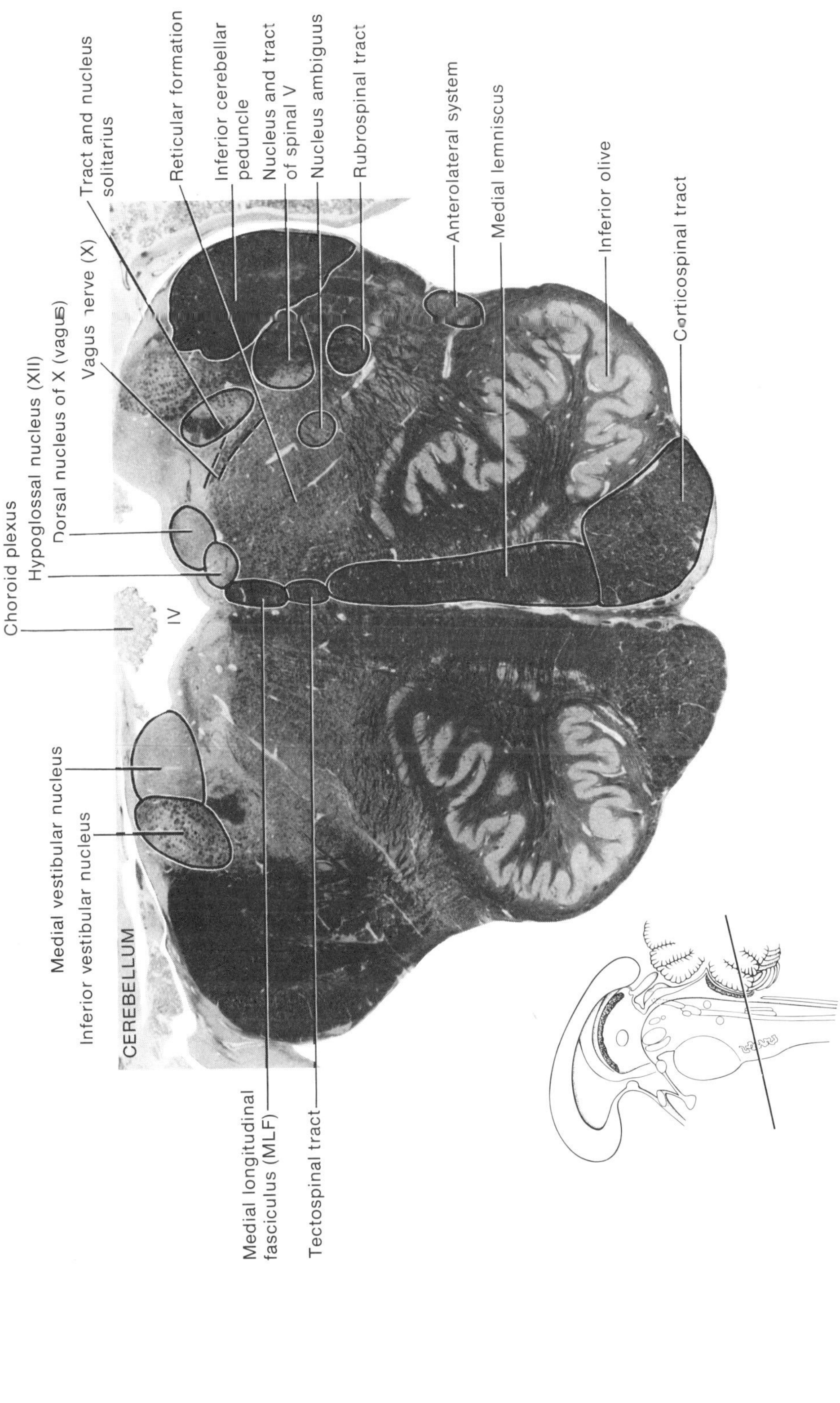

Figure 6–6. Cross-section of the midregion of the medulla.

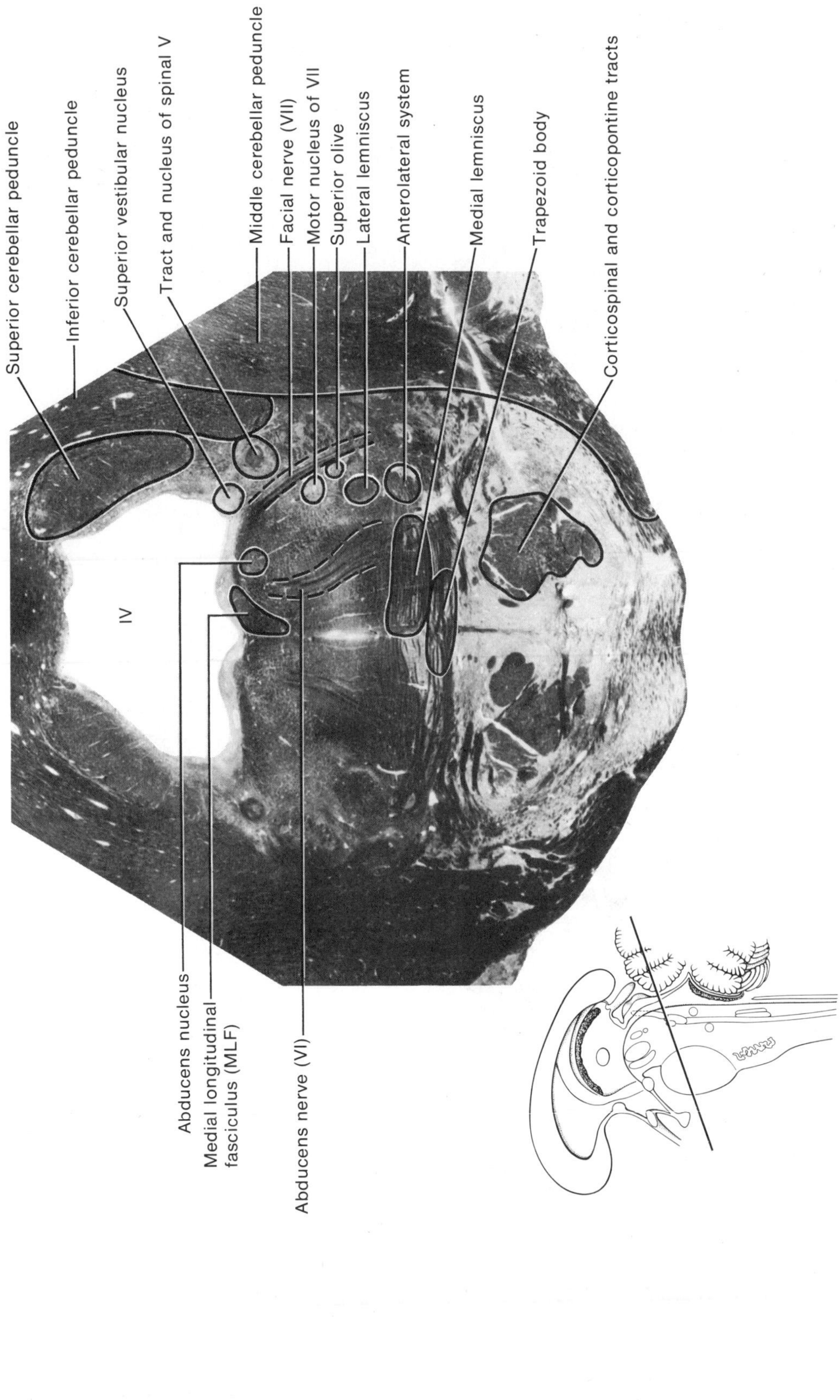

Figure 6–7. Cross-section of the lower pons.

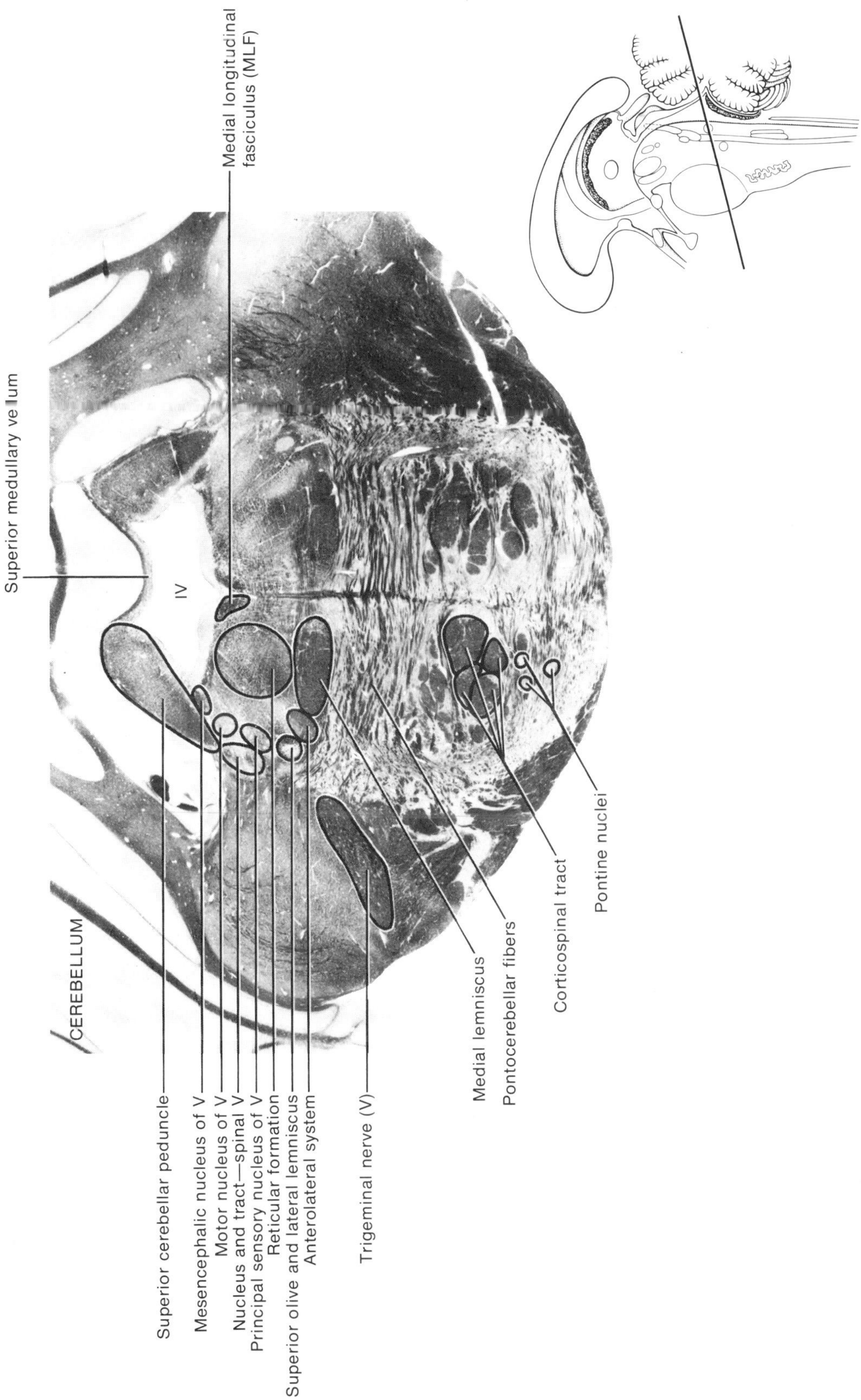

Figure 6–8. Cross-section of the mid/upper pons.

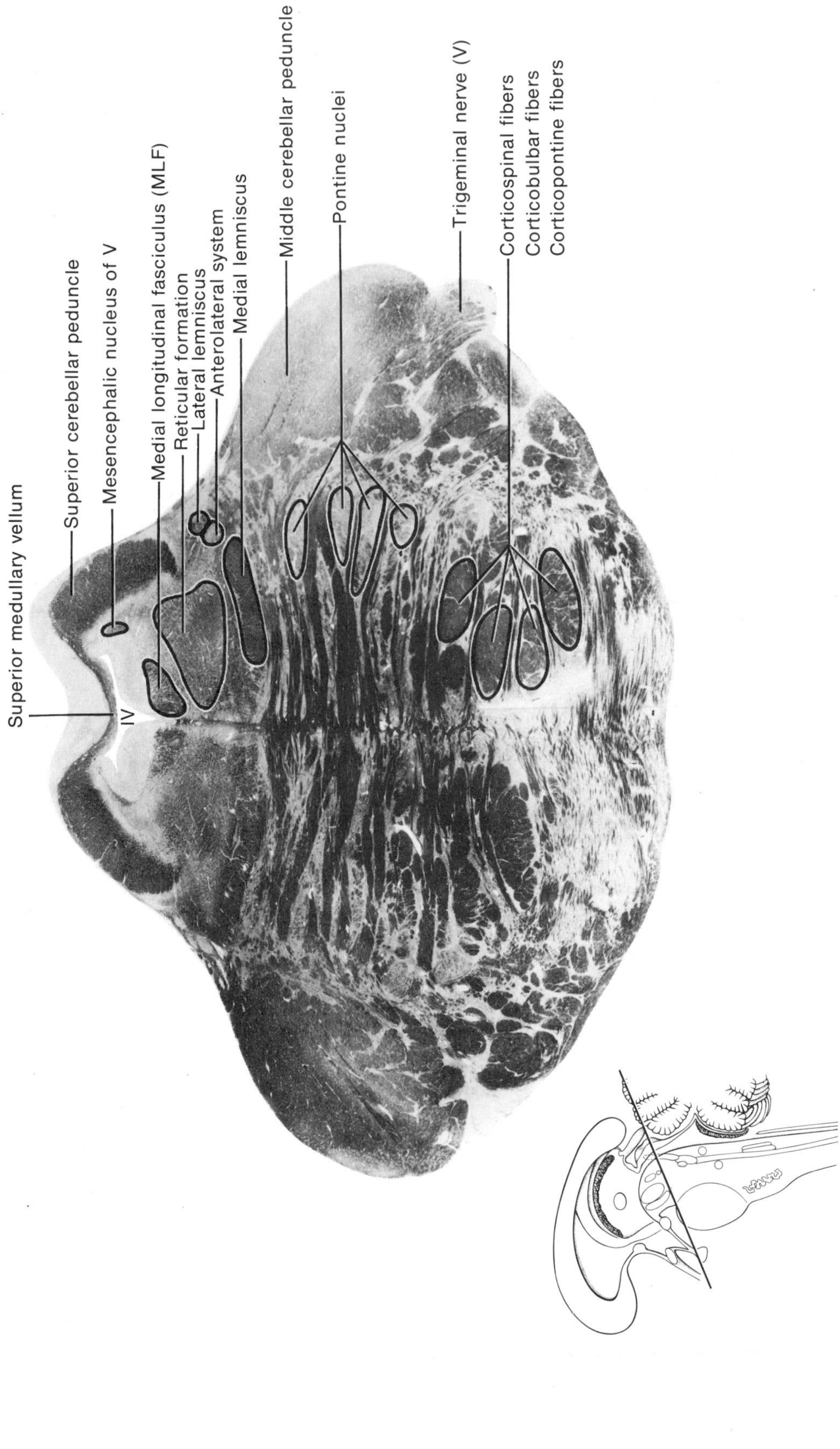

Figure 6–9. Cross-section of the upper pons.

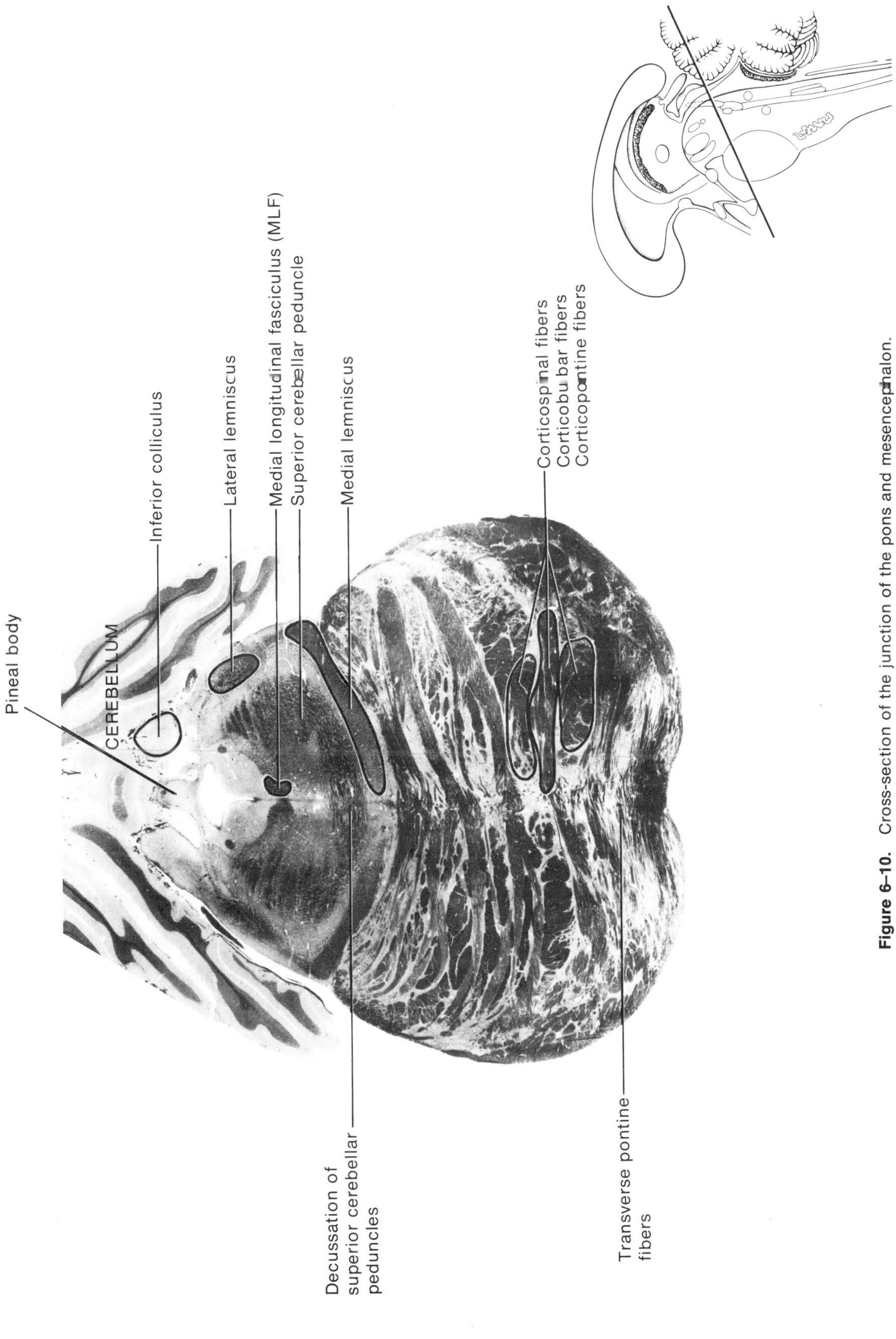

Figure 6–10. Cross-section of the junction of the pons and mesencephalon.

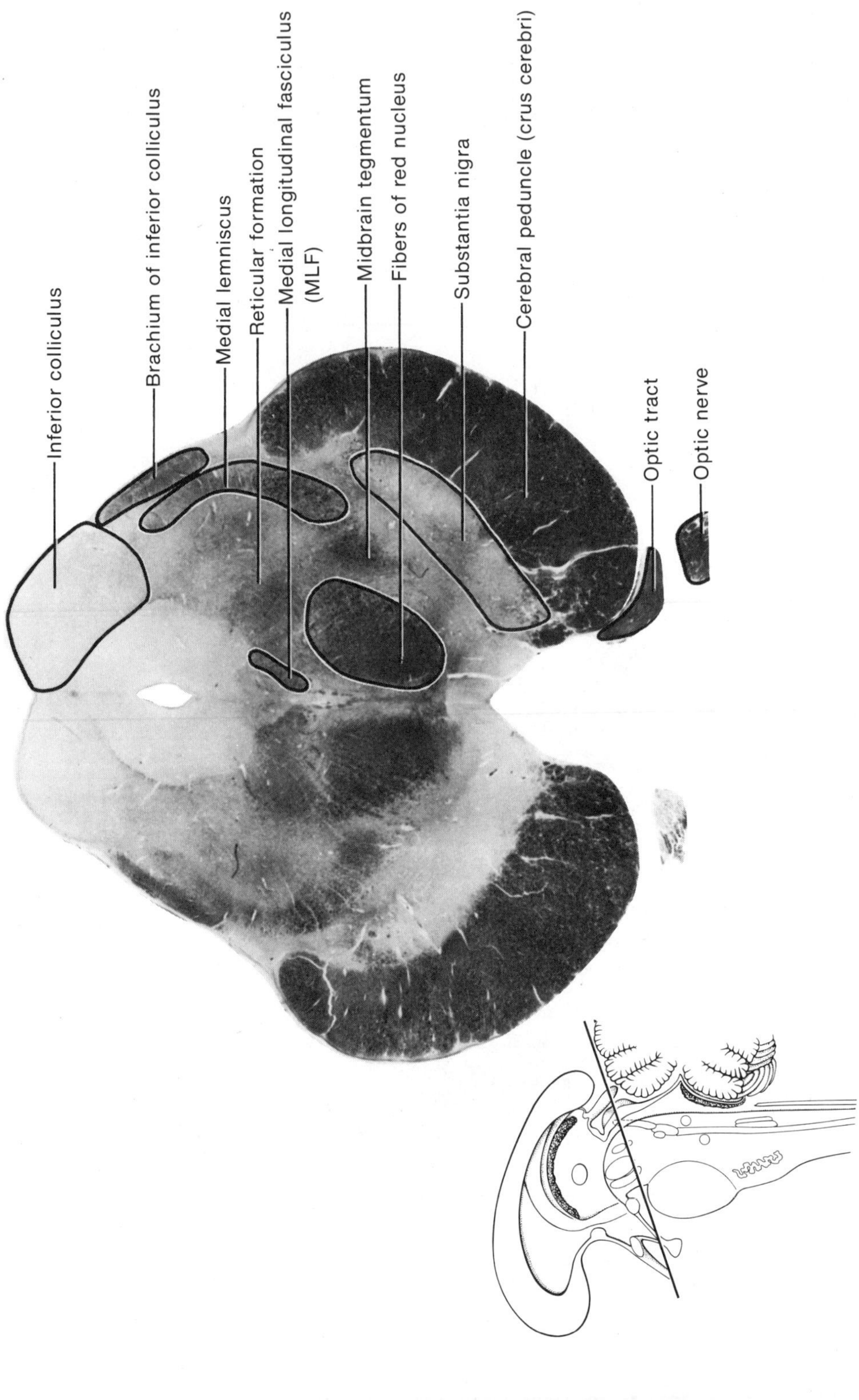

Figure 6–11. Cross-section of the mesencephalon—level of inferior colliculus.

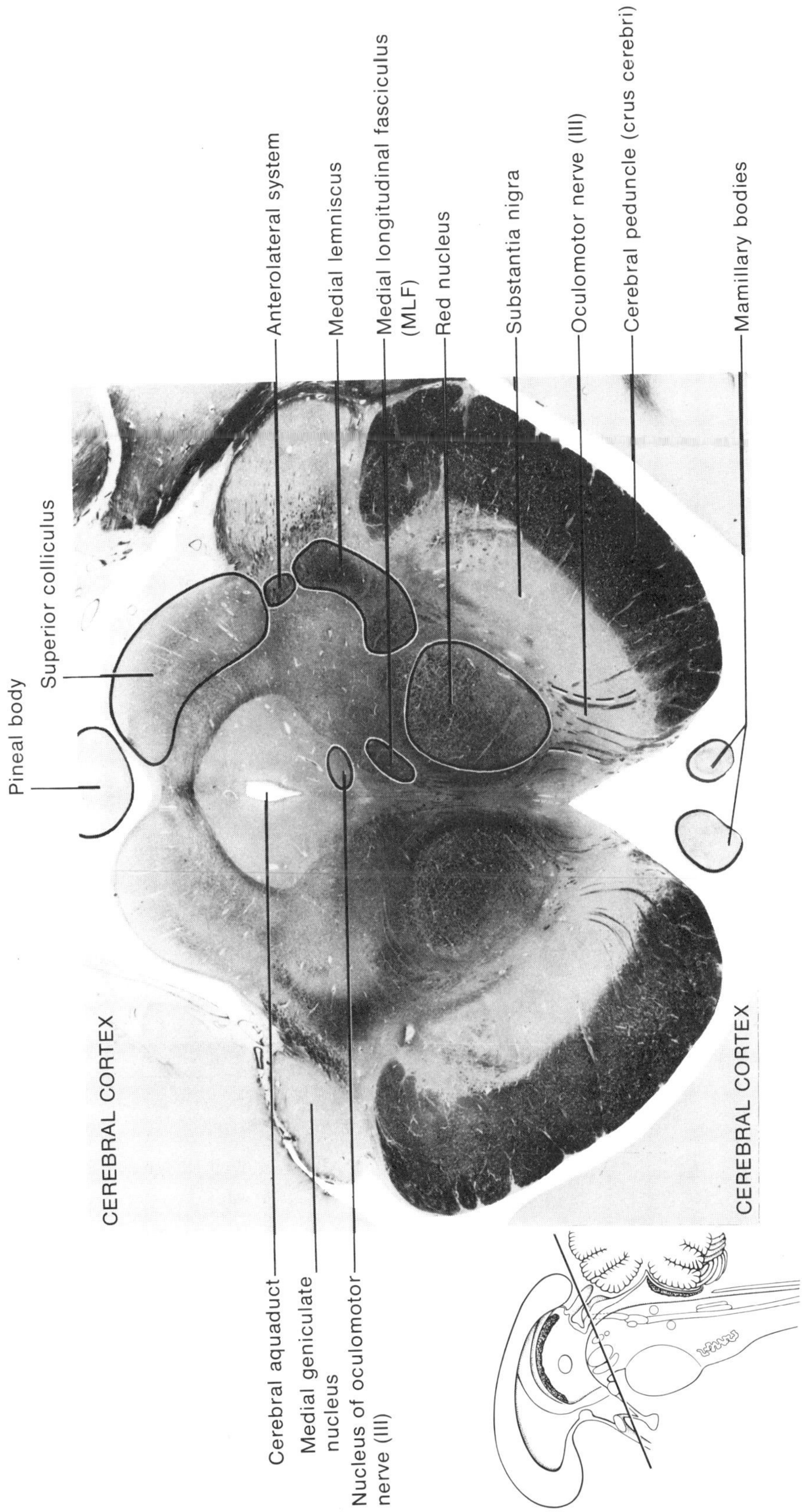

Figure 6–12. Cross-section of the upper mesencephalon.

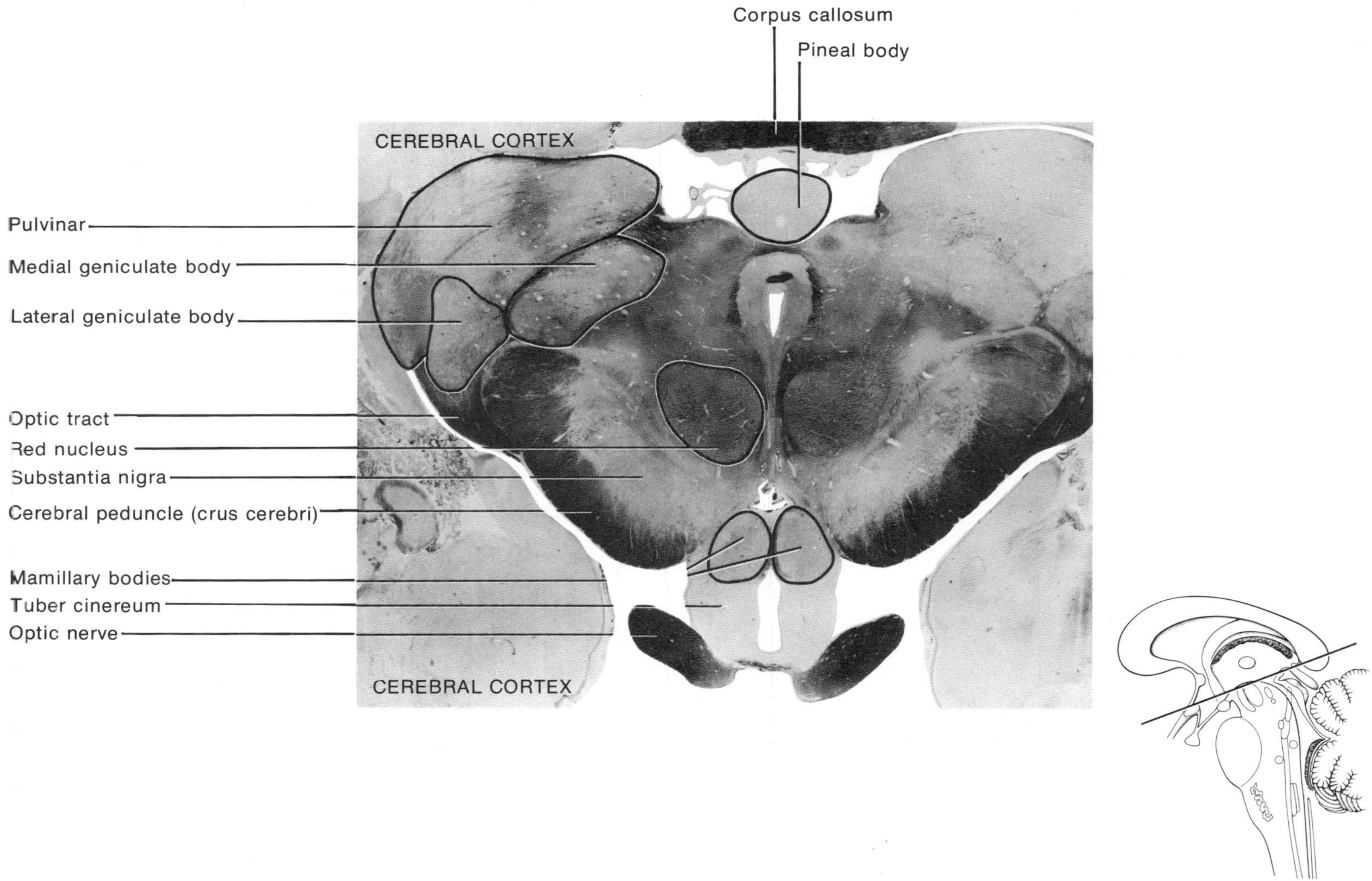

Figure 6–13. Cross-section of the junction of the mesencephalon and the diencephalon.

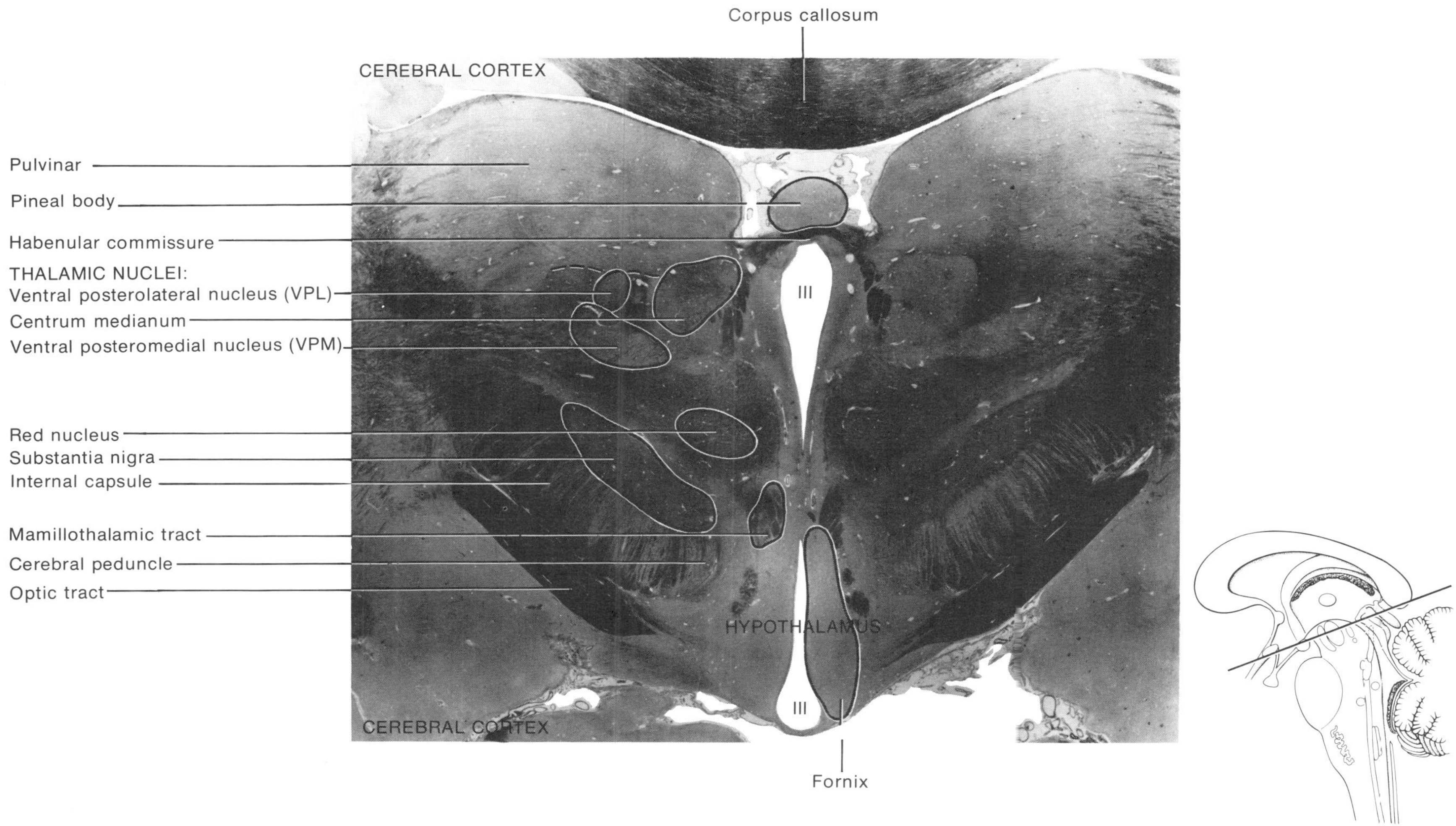

Figure 6–14. Cross-section of the caudal diencephalon.

CRANIAL NERVE NUCLEI OF THE VAGUS, CRANIAL PORTION OF THE SPINAL ACCESSORY AND HYPOGLOSSAL NERVES

The dorsal nucleus of the vagus nerve can be seen in the midregion of the medulla in Figure 6–6. The cranial portion of the spinal accessory nerve originates in the nucleus ambiguus (Fig. 6–6) and the nucleus of the hypoglossal nerve is shown in Figures 6–5 and 6–6.

INFERIOR OLIVE

This structure is recognizable grossly as a bilateral protuberance situated just posterolateral to the rostral portion of the medullary pyramids. Its internal structure is illustrated in Figures 6–5 and 6–6. The inferior olive receives afferent fibers from all regions of the cerebral cortex; from the red nucleus, spinal cord, basal ganglia and reticular formation. It sends efferent projections to the spinal cord by way of the cerebellum, and to the reticular formation. Therefore, the inferior olive is influenced by many regions of the central nervous system and in turn can influence the spinal cord, cerebellum and diffuse areas by means of its connections with the reticular formation. Presumably, it is concerned with integration of muscular activity, but surprisingly, large lesions in the inferior olive produce only instability of the soft palate. Probably the reason why more severe symptoms are not produced by such a lesion is that there are several alternative pathways responsible for the control of muscular activity, and the olivary route may function as a supplementary pathway when others are not working normally.

VESTIBULAR NUCLEI

These four nuclei (Figs. 6–6 and 6–7) are located in both the pons and the rostral medulla, in the lateral part of the floor of the fourth ventricle. Recall that these nuclei are involved with vestibulo-ocular reflexes through their connections with cranial nerves III (oculomotor), IV (trochlear), VI (abducens) and VII (facial), and with spinal cord reflex activity by way of the vestibulospinal tracts.

INFERIOR CEREBELLAR PEDUNCLES

These connect the rostral part of the medulla with the cerebellum. They are illustrated in Figures 6–6 and 6–7. Several important afferent systems project to the cerebellum via these peduncles, some of which have been discussed earlier, and they are listed below.

Dorsal Spinocerebellar Tracts. These project to the anterior lobe of the cerebellum (paleocerebellum).

Cuneocerebellar Tracts. These originate in the accessory cuneate nucleus and distribute primarily to the same areas of the cerebellum as the dorsal spinocerebellar tracts.

Crossed Olivocerebellar Tracts. These are the largest constituents of the inferior cerebellar peduncles. They originate in the inferior olive and project to all parts of the cerebellum.

Reticulocerebellar Fibers. These originate in the reticular formation and project the great majority of fibers to the ipsilateral anterior lobe of the cerebellum.

Vestibulocerebellar Fibers. These project from the vestibular nerve and nuclei to the flocculonodular lobe of the cerebellum (archicerebellum).

Quintocerebellar Tracts. These project from the mesencephalic nucleus of the trigeminal nerve to the anterior lobe of the cerebellum.

RETICULAR FORMATION

This extends from the thalamus to and through the medulla (see Figs. 6–4 through 6–12). The literature deals with three levels of the reticular formation — mesencephalic, pontine and medullary, which will be considered together for the most part in this discussion. The term *reticular formation* is often used to give a functional rather than an anatomic meaning, and largely applies to brain stem nuclei that do not fit readily into any other category. Only one of the reticular nuclei, the lateral reticular nucleus of the medulla, has a characteristic structure.

The reticular formation has important connections with the cerebellum and spinal cord (spinoreticular and reticulospinal tracts), and very diffuse connections with the cerebral cortex. In general, it is a complex region that is not well understood, but we do know that when stimulated it produces changes in the electroencephalogram that reflect cortical arousal, that it influences activity in the autonomic nervous system, and that it changes spinal cord reflex activity. The pontine reticular formation tends to facilitate activity, and the medullary reticular formation to inhibit activity, in gamma motor neurons.

The small neurons of the reticular formation are extremely sensitive to metabolites and anesthetics and this information can be put to practical clinical use. For example, when working with hyperexcitable children, it may be beneficial to begin by giving the child a glass of orange juice or something to eat. This may reduce the excitatory influence that the reticular formation may be exerting on the cerebral cortex.

The Pons and Midbrain

The important structures of the pons and midbrain are listed below.

NUCLEI OF CRANIAL NERVES III (OCULOMOTOR), IV (TROCHLEAR), V (TRIGEMINAL), VI (ABDUCENS), VII (FACIAL) AND VIII (VESTIBULOCOCHLEAR)

These can be identified in Figures 6–6 through 6–9 and 6–12, and details thereof will be examined in the discussion on cranial nerves (Chapter 7).

STRUCTURES INVOLVED WITH THE AUDITORY SYSTEM

These include the trapezoid body (Fig. 6–7), the superior olivary complex (Figs. 6–7 and 6–8), the lateral lemniscus (Figs. 6–7 through 6–10) and the inferior colliculus (Fig. 6–11).

PONTINE NUCLEI

These are huge, important relay stations in the pathway between the cerebral cortex and the cerebellum (Figs. 6–8 and 6–9). Fibers that synapse in the pontine nuclei originate in most parts of the cerebral cortex, and descend in the posterior limb of the internal capsule and the crus cerebri to the pontine nuclei. From the latter, fibers cross to the contralateral side where they form the massive middle cerebellar peduncle (Figs. 6–7 through 6–9) and terminate in all parts of the cerebellar cortex.

SUPERIOR CEREBELLAR PEDUNCLES

The superior cerebellar peduncles (Fig. 6–10) contain the major portion of the efferent fibers that leave the cerebellum. Efferents project to the cerebral cortex, completing the feedback circuitry between the cerebral cortex and the cerebellum. This entire circuitry consists of the pathway from the cerebral cortex to the pontine nuclei that has just been described as terminating in all parts of the cerebellar cortex, projections from the cerebellar cortex to the deep cerebellar nuclei, which in turn project fibers via the superior cerebellar peduncles to the contralateral side by way of the decussation of the superior cerebellar peduncles. These fibers either terminate in the red nucleus or ascend to the ventrolateral and ventroanterior nuclei of the thalamus, which in turn project to the motor area of the cerebral cortex. This complete pathway provides a cortico-ponto-cerebello-thalamo-cortical feedback system which presumably has to do with control of movement.

The superior cerebellar peduncles also contain efferent neurons that project to the reticular formation, and these projections are reciprocal. Therefore, the cerebellum influences the spinal cord and cranial nerve nuclei through the corticospinal and corticobulbar tracts, reticulospinal tracts, and rubrospinal and rubrobulbar tracts. The details of cerebellar structure, function and interconnections are dealt with in Chapter 8.

RED NUCLEUS

The red nucleus (Figs. 6–11 through 6–14) is a large, round cell mass located mainly in the mesencephalon. In addition to receiving afferent projections from the deep cerebellar nuclei, it receives a somatotopically organized projection from the ipsilateral motor cortex. The red nucleus, in turn, sends somatotopically organized, crossed projections to all spinal cord levels. This means that the red nucleus provides a corticorubrospinal link that closely parallels the corticospinal system. The parallelism results from the fact that the motor cortex projects directly to the spinal column and is under the influence of afferent projections from the deep cerebellar nuclei. Neurons from the motor cortex also project to the spinal cord after synapsing in the red nucleus, which is also influenced by projections from the deep cerebellar nuclei. The greatest difference in the corticospinal system and the corticorubrospinal systems is that rubrospinal neurons do not make monosynaptic connections with alpha motor neurons in the ventral horns of the spinal cord, so that there are more synapses involved in the corticorubrospinal system, both at spinal cord levels and in the red nucleus. This means that the corticospinal system is a much more rapidly conducting system, with more direct control over fine, coordinated types of movement than the corticorubrospinal system.

SUBSTANTIA NIGRA

The substantia nigra (Figs. 6–11 through 6–14) lies in the mesencephalon, just dorsal to the crus cerebri, and extends through the entire rostrocaudal dimension of the midbrain. Because it is so inaccessible, it has been difficult to study the effects of isolated lesions, and therefore its connections have not been well defined. The information available provides evidence that it receives afferent projections from the motor and sensory cortices and from the striatum (putamen and caudate nucleus). It sends efferent projections back to the striatum, to the ventrolateral and ventroanterior nuclei of the thalamus, and perhaps to the reticular formation. The fibers that project from the substantia nigra to the striatum are extremely fine and rich in dopamine. There is strong evidence that this projection is implicated in Parkinson's disease.

MIDBRAIN TECTUM

The tectum is located dorsal to the cerebral aqueduct and forms the roof of the midbrain. It consists of the corpora quadrigemina or two paired superior and inferior colliculi (see Figs. 6–11 and 6–12). The superior colliculi are reflex centers concerned with sight, and the inferior colliculi are relay stations for auditory information that will terminate in the auditory cortex.

The importance of the superior colliculus in vision varies greatly from species to species. In submammalian species the superior colliculi comprise the main visual centers and there is little or no representation in the cerebral cortex. However, in man the superior colliculi represent a small part of the visual system. Rather, in man, vision has a very large representation in the cerebral cortex and the tectum appears to be concerned only with relatively simple reflex movements that occur in response to visual stimuli. The most important efferent projections of the superior colliculi are to the spinal cord via the tectospinal tracts and to the nuclei of cranial nerves III (oculomotor), IV (trochlear) and VI (abducens). *There are no fibers that project from the superior colliculi to the cerebral cortex in man.* Thus, visual stimulation evokes reflex control of neck and eye movements, but the reflex control is modified by very heavy afferent projections to the superior colliculi from the cerebral cortex. In fact, the responses of the tectum are more profoundly influenced by an intact cerebral cortex than they are by the retina. The interconnections of the superior colliculi may be represented very simply in diagrammatic form as follows:

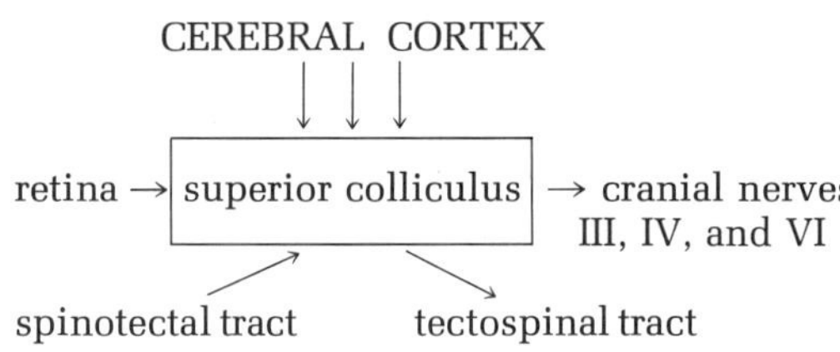

The inferior colliculus will be considered again in the discussion on the vestibulocochlear nerve in Chapter 8.

THE CEREBRAL PEDUNCLES

These are major constituents of the midbrain (see Figs. 6–11 through 6–13). They are located anteriorly, and actually consist of the crus cerebri, of which the major constituents are the descending corticobulbar and corticospinal pathways, the substantia nigra and the midbrain tegmentum (Fig. 6–11). Many sources use the term *cerebral peduncles* interchangeably with the *crura cerebri*, but it should be understood that the crus cerebri comprise only a part of the cerebral peduncle.

Within the crus cerebri the corticobulbar and corticospinal systems are somatotopically organized. The lower extremity is represented laterally, the face medially and the upper extremity in an intermediate position.

The most frequent symptoms of brain stem damage or disease are diplopia (double vision), dysphagia (difficulty with swallowing), nausea, vomiting and vertigo (dizziness). In addition there may be sensory and motor deficits due to disruption of the long ascending and descending pathways, the cranial nerves and their nuclei, and the cerebellar connections, or damage to any of the structures that constitute the brain stem. The extent and nature of the disability will depend on the location of the lesion. For detailed descriptions of symptoms produced by specific brain stem lesions see Patten's *Neurological Differential Diagnosis*, 1977, pp. 114–118.

The figures in this chapter represent an atlas of Weigert stained cross-sections of the brain stem. Each figure is accompanied by an inset which indicates the level from which that section was taken. (Weigert stained cross-sections, compliments of the Department of Physiology, University of Wisconsin Medical School, Madison.)

REVIEW QUESTIONS

1. In what brain stem structures do the corticospinal and corticobulbar fibers course en route to their terminations?
2. What is the function of the accessory cuneate nucleus?
3. Which cranial nerve nuclei are located in the medulla? In the pons? In the midbrain?
4. What is the assumption regarding the role of the inferior olive? Why do large lesions of this nucleus produce only mild symptoms?
5. Which important afferent systems project to the cerebellum by way of the *inferior* cerebellar peduncles?
6. The massive middle cerebellar peduncles are comprised of fibers that originate and terminate where?
7. The superior cerebellar peduncles contain fibers that terminate where?
8. What are the generalized functions of the reticular formation?
9. How does the red nucleus provide a corticorubrospinal link that parallels the corticospinal tract? How are the two systems different? A diagrammatic representation of the circuitry involved will be helpful.
10. What brain stem structures are implicated in Parkinson's disease? Explain.
11. Draw a diagram to show how the superior colliculus functions in the control of movement and how its responses are influenced by other CNS structures.
12. What are the most frequent symptoms of brain stem damage or disease?

CHAPTER 7 • THE CRANIAL NERVES

OBJECTIVES

After reading this chapter you should: • Understand the functions of the cranial nerves well enough to enable you to identify symptoms that occur when the nerves are damaged. • Understand how the cranial nerves interact to produce reflex activity and how the corticobulbar system acts to influence cranial nerve nuclei.

FUNCTION, COMPOSITION AND LOCATION

In contrast to typical spinal nerves, there is a great deal of variability in the functional constituents of cranial nerves. Typical spinal nerves contain four functional types of neurons:

1. *General somatic efferents,* which innervate striated somatic musculature derived from the mesodermal somites.
2. *General visceral efferents,* which innervate viscera and vascular smooth muscles.
3. *General somatic afferents,* which convey information from somatic structures to the central nervous system. Somatic structures are those innervated by the exteroceptors and proprioceptors (muscle spindles, joint receptors, etc.)
4. *General visceral afferents,* which project to the central nervous system from the viscera by way of interoceptors.

Cranial nerves differ from spinal nerves in that they may contain as few as one, or as many as five, functional constituents. In other respects, cranial and spinal nerves have much in common in that the cell bodies of motor neurons of both cranial and spinal nerves are located within the CNS (cranial nerve cell bodies in nuclei of the brain stem and spinal nerve cell bodies in ventral horns of the spinal cord), and in most cases the cell bodies of sensory neurons of both cranial and spinal nerves are located in ganglia outside of the CNS.

Cranial nerves may contain three functional components in addition to those contained in spinal nerves. They are:

1. *Special visceral efferents,* which innervate special visceral muscles that are derived from the branchial arches (see Fig. 7–1). These latter appear in about the fourth week of gestation and resemble the gill slits of fish. They are the precursors of the neck, jaws, face and external ear, and the associated musculature is innervated by these special visceral efferents. The muscles include muscles of the pharynx and larynx, and those of facial expression and mastication, as well as the sternocleidomastoideus and trapezius muscles.
2. *Special visceral afferents,* which subserve the modalities of taste and olfaction (detection of odors).
3. *Special somatic afferents,* which subserve the special senses of hearing, equilibrium and vision.

The nuclei of the cranial nerves are locat-

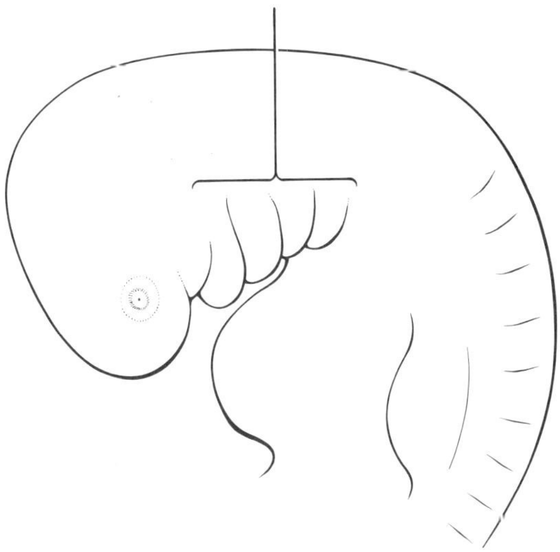

Figure 7–1. The location of the embryonic branchial arches.

ed in the brain stem (medulla, pons and midbrain), and the nerves emerge at the locations shown in Figure 7–2. The functional organization in the brain stem is similar to that in the spinal cord: i.e., afferent systems are associated with dorsal regions and efferent systems with ventral regions. Therefore, in general, the four functional afferent columns are located dorsolateral to the sulcus limitans (see Fig. 5–6), and the three functional efferent columns are located ventromedial to the sulcus limitans at brain stem levels. All of these functional columns receive fibers from the cerebral cortex via corticobulbar fibers, the origins and functions of which are the same as the corticospinal fibers. The only difference between corticobulbar and corticospinal fibers is their level of termination. Whereas corticospinal fibers terminate at levels of the spinal cord, corticobulbar fibers terminate in the brain stem, which in older terminology was called the *bulb* (hence the term cortico*bulbar*). It is important to understand that the corticobulbar fibers project not only to motor nuclei of cranial nerves, but also to sensory nuclei of cranial nerves. Their function parallels that of the corticospinal fibers which project to the dorsal column nuclei and the dorsal horns of the spinal cord, i.e., they filter out information of no value to the cerebral cortex.

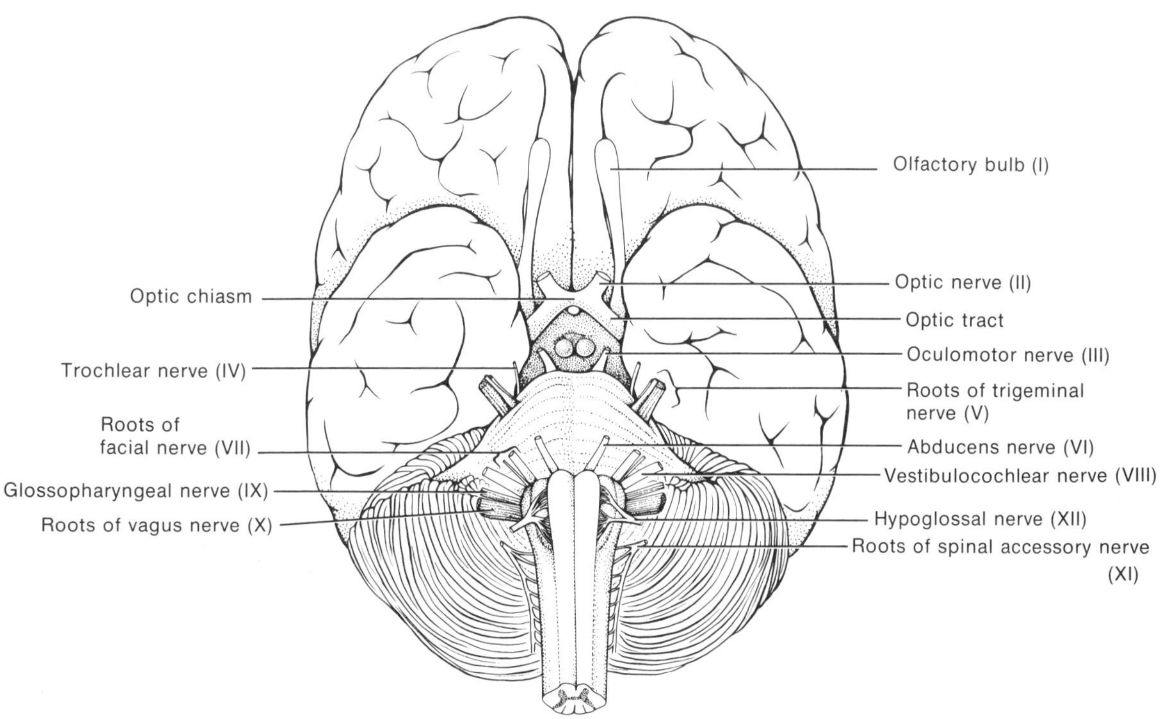

Figure 7–2. The cranial nerves as they emerge from the brain stem.

Olfactory Nerve

The cell bodies of the first order neurons in the olfactory system are located in the mucous membranes of the upper part of the nasal passages. The axons are very fine, unmyelinated special visceral afferent fibers that project through the cribriform plates of the anterior cranial fossa and terminate by synapsing with the second order neurons in the olfactory bulbs, which rest upon the cribriform plates. The fibers of the tract may or may not synapse again and their primary projections are: (1) to the region of the prepyriform cortex, a phylogenetically old part of the brain located on the anterior dorsal portion of the parahippocampal gyrus (olfactory cortex) of the temporal lobe; and (2) to the amygdaloid nucleus, which is located in the dorsomedial portion of the temporal lobe. The amygdaloid nucleus is continuous with the uncus, which is just medial to it.

There is no evidence to indicate that discrimination of odors is based on structurally distinct types of receptors, but some evidence suggests that some odors may be distinguished by their relative effectiveness in stimulating specific regions of the olfactory epithelium.

The olfactory system is unique among the sensory systems in that it is the only one which does not relay through the thalamus en route to the cerebral cortex.

Optic Nerve

The visual receptors consist of the rods and cones of the retina, which is actually an outgrowth of the diencephalon. The cell bodies of the optic neurons are located in the retinal ganglion cell layer and their axons exit from the retina at the optic disc. The axons that subserve vision are myelinated special somatic afferents, which enter the skull as the optic nerve via the optic foramina to form the optic chiasm. In the optic chiasm the fibers that originate from the nasal hemiretina (half of the retina) cross, but those that originate from the temporal hemiretina do not cross. This partial decussation results in the left cerebral hemisphere seeing the right half of the visual field, and the right cerebral hemisphere seeing the left half of the visual field (see Fig. 7–3).

With the pattern of these projections in mind one can determine whether a lesion is anterior or posterior to the optic chiasm. If the optic nerve is sectioned completely on one side anterior to the optic chiasm, there will be loss of vision on the side of the lesion. If the optic tract is lesioned unilaterally posterior to the optic chiasm, it will produce loss of vision in the visual field on the contralateral side (i.e., if the lesion is on the left, vision will be lost in the right half of the visual field). Loss of vision which is restricted to a single peripheral visual field is called *homonymous hemianopia.* It is not uncommon for a patient who has had a cerebral vascular accident to have concomitant involvement of the optic tract. In this case he may have a spastic hemiplegia or hemiparesis (hemiplegia = complete paralysis, hemiparesis = partial paralysis) in combination with an ipsilateral homonymous hemianopia.

The visual loss that these patients experience is amazingly discrete in its localization. It can be detected easily by having the patient focus on an object straight ahead, and moving an object in from the periphery of normal vision from one side and then the other. If the patient has homonymous hemianopia, he will not see the object on the side of the deficit until it reaches the exact midline of the total visual field, in other words, until it is placed exactly in front of him. This disability can be a devastating one. The patient may bump into things on the side of the deficit, he may deny the existence of the side of the body on which the deficit has occurred, and his visual impressions of the world may be severely distorted. It is extremely important to recognize homonymous hemianopia when it is present in order to work with the patient effectively. He can be helped to adjust movements of the head to avoid bumping into things; personnel should be instructed not to carry on conversations or give instructions from the side of the deficit; the bed and/or seating arrangements in his hospital room should be such that he can see into the hallway. All too often the author has seen the room arrangement neglected so that the patient has the impression of living in a vacuum.

There are other types of hemianopia as well as other types of visual defects (see *Neurological Differential Diagnosis*, Patten, 1977, pp. 11–25), but homonymous hemianopia is the form most frequently encoun-

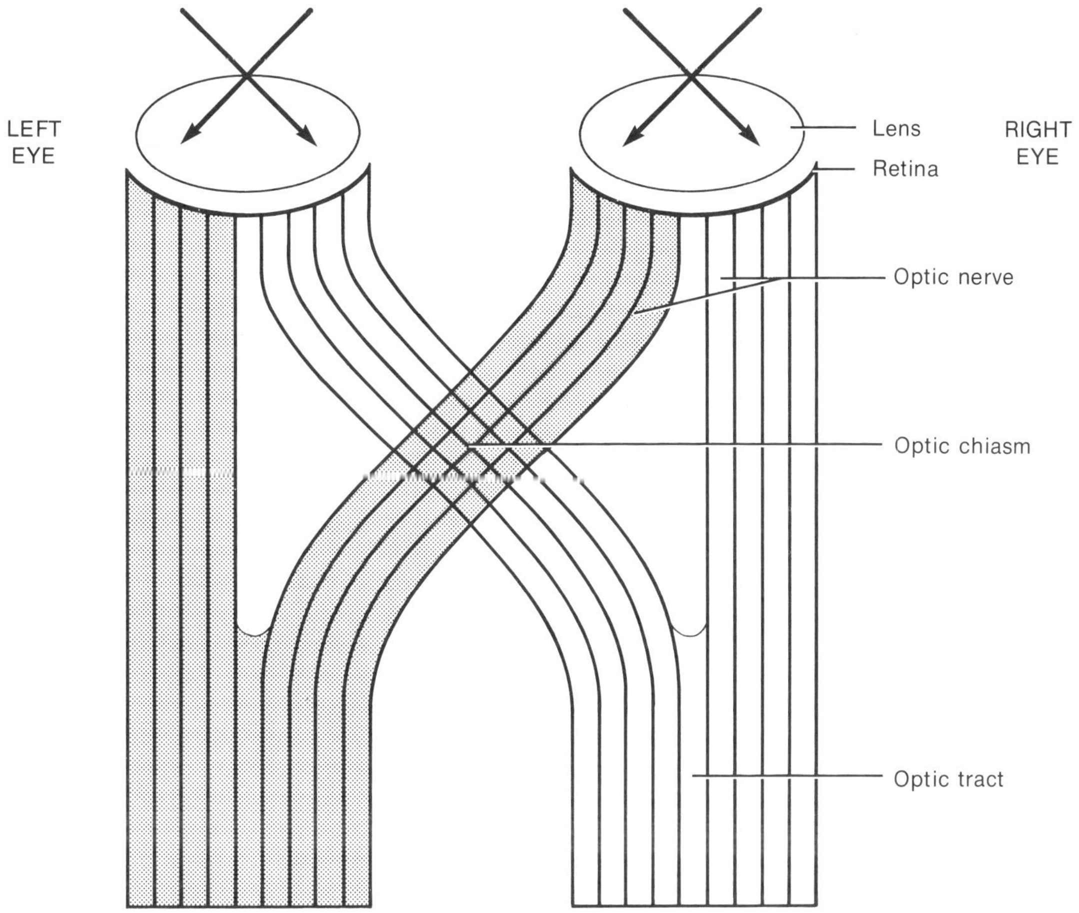

Figure 7–3. The arrangement of nerve fibers in the optic chiasm. The arrows indicate the direction in which the rays of light penetrate the lenses. The shaded nerve fibers from the left temporal hemiretina and the right nasal hemiretina carry information from the right visual field, and the unshaded fibers from the left nasal hemiretina and right temporal hemiretina carry information from the left visual field. Therefore, the right cerebral cortex sees the left visual field and the left cerebral cortex sees the right visual field.

tered when working with the rehabilitation of patients.

Posterior to the optic chiasm the optic neurons course posteriorly in the optic tracts and may terminate in one of three areas.

1. They may terminate in the superior colliculus where they participate in reflex arcs that involve movements of the neck region via the tectospinal tract and movements of the eyes via cranial nerve nuclei III (oculomotor), IV (trochlear) and VI (abducens).
2. They may project to the pretectal area, which is just rostral to the superior colliculus. This projection provides the afferent link of the pupillary light reflex (pupillary constriction in response to light). Axons of the pretectal area project bilaterally to the Edinger-Westphal nucleus, which is part of the oculomotor nerve nuclear complex. Fibers from the Edinger-Westphal nucleus project to the ciliary ganglion and from there to the smooth muscle of the sphincter of the iris, to complete the reflex arc.
3. The largest component of the optic tract projects to the lateral geniculate nucleus of the thalamus, which is the last relay en route to the visual cortex. The latter is located on either side of the calcarine fissure of the occipital lobe, and thus the last portion of this tract is called the geniculocalcarine tract. Whereas the first

two projections have to do with a variety of optic reflexes, the lateral geniculate nucleus receives fibers which are concerned with visual perception.

Oculomotor Nerve

The cells of origin of the third nerve are located in the mesencephalon, ventral to the cerebral aqueduct at the level of the superior colliculus. It contains the following.

GENERAL SOMATIC EFFERENTS

These supply all of the extraocular eye muscles except the lateral rectus and superior oblique muscles. They also supply the levator palpebrae superioris muscle, which elevates the upper eyelid. These fibers leave the skull via the superior orbital fissure.

GENERAL VISCERAL EFFERENTS

These are preganglionic parasympathetic fibers that arise specifically in the Edinger-Westphal nucleus. They project to the ciliary ganglion and on to the sphincter of the iris. This projection was described in connection with the second cranial nerve. These fibers function to constrict the pupils. If light is shown into one eye only, both pupils constrict because fibers from one optic tract project to the pretectal nuclei of both sides by way of the posterior commissure (a small mass of fibers that connects the two cerebral hemispheres, located rostral to the superior colliculus at the junction of the cerebral aqueduct and the third ventricle). Control of pupillary dilatation is a function of the sympathetic nervous system. These postganglionic sympathetic fibers originate in the superior cervical ganglion.

There are also projections from the Edinger-Westphal nucleus that control the ciliary muscles of the eye. These produce alterations in the shape of the lens so that the eye can accommodate to visualize objects at different distances.

Very recent evidence (Saper et al. 1977) indicates that the Edinger-Westphal nucleus also projects to the medulla and spinal cord. The functional implications of these connections have not been explored, but we may have to start thinking of this nucleus as more than just a parasympathetic preganglionic nucleus, as it has been traditionally regarded.

Lesions of the third cranial nerve may produce an ipsilateral lower motor neuron paralysis, with the following symptoms:

1. External strabismus (the eye is turned laterally), due to the unopposed action of the lateral rectus muscle, which results in diplopia (double or blurred vision).
2. Inability to move the eye vertically.
3. Ptosis (drooping of the eyelid).
4. Loss of the pupillary light reflex.
5. Loss of the ability of the lens to accommodate.

Because of the close proximity of the third nerves to the crus cerebri as they emerge from the midbrain, both the corticospinal and extrapyramidal tracts along with the third nerve are often included in a single lesion. When such a lesion occurs, the result is an ipsilateral lower motor neuron paralysis of the muscles innervated by the third nerve, combined with a contralateral hemiplegia or hemiparesis.

The function of the third nerve also may be impaired in conjunction with lesions of the brain stem because of the location of its nucleus and emerging fibers ventral to the cerebral aqueduct.

Trochlear Nerve

The nucleus of the fourth cranial nerve is also located in the mesencephalon just caudal to the nuclear complex of the third cranial nerve, near the midline. This is the only one of the cranial nerves to emerge from the posterior aspect of the brain stem. After emerging from the nucleus, the fibers decussate in the superior medullary velum (which forms part of the roof of the fourth ventricle), curve around the lateral aspect of the brain stem and enter the cavernous sinus. Coursing anteriorly from the cavernous sinuses the nerves exit from the skull through the superior orbital fissures, along with the third nerves and the ophthalmic divisions of the fifth cranial nerves. The fourth cranial nerve contains *general somatic efferent* fibers that supply the superior oblique muscles.

Isolated lesions of the trochlear nerve are rare, and when they do occur the symptoms are difficult to detect.

Trigeminal Nerve

The fifth cranial nerve contains both motor and sensory components.

GENERAL SOMATIC AFFERENTS

These convey:

1. exteroceptive impulses from
   a. the skin of the face and forehead;
   b. mucous membranes of the nose, nasal sinuses and mouth;
   c. the teeth;
   d. extensive portions of the cranial dura mater.
2. proprioceptive impulses from
   a. muscles of the face;
   b. temporomandibular joint receptors.

SPECIAL VISCERAL EFFERENTS

These control:

1. muscles of mastication;
2. tensor tympani muscles;
3. tensor veli palatini muscles;
4. mylohyoid muscles;
5. the anterior belly of the digastric muscles.

All of the afferent fibers of the trigeminal complex except those that subserve proprioception have their cell bodies in the trigeminal (semilunar) ganglion, which is located on the petrous portion of the temporal bone. The peripheral processes enter the ganglion through the three divisions of the fifth cranial nerve: (1) the ophthalmic (enters the skull via the superior orbital fissure); (2) the maxillary (enters the skull via the foramen rotundum); and (3) the mandibular nerve (enters the skull via the foramen ovale). The ophthalmic and maxillary divisions of the nerve both contain only sensory neurons. The entire motor root is incorporated into the mandibular division, which is the sole nerve supply of the muscles of mastication.

The central processes of the sensory neurons which have their cell bodies located in the trigeminal ganglion enter the brain stem at the level of the pons. They then terminate in one of two nuclei. Some of them ascend for a short distance to terminate in the *principal sensory nucleus* of nerve V; these fibers primarily subserve the modalities of touch, pressure and two-point discrimination. Some of the sensory fibers descend for long distances to make up the *spinal trigeminal tract,* which along with its nucleus extends from upper cervical segments to the point of entry of the fifth nerve into the pons. The modalities of pain and thermal sense are handled exclusively by this part of the trigeminal complex. There is also some representation of proprioception from the extraocular muscles located in the rostral part of the spinal nucleus of V. Fibers that enter the spinal tract of nerve V terminate at all levels of the spinal nucleus. The spinal trigeminal nucleus also receives fibers that subserve pain and temperature from cranial nerves VII (facial), IX (glossopharyngeal) and X (vagus), as well as from corticobulbar tracts. The spinal tract is somatotopically organized, with fibers from the ophthalmic division in a ventral position, those from the mandibular division in a dorsal position and those from the maxillary division in an intermediate position.

The *mesencephalic nucleus* of the fifth nerve consists of very large cells that appear to represent dorsal root ganglion cells within the central nervous system. (This is an exception to the rule that nerve cell bodies of sensory neurons are located outside the CNS.) This nucleus, as its name implies, is located in the caudal portion of the mesencephalon. It receives impulses from proprioceptors located in the muscles of mastication and facial expression, and may be thought of as the homologue of Clarke's column for the face area. Afferents to this nucleus are found only in the mandibular division of the fifth nerve and are probably concerned with the reflex control of the force of biting.

The fibers that originate in the *motor nucleus* of the fifth nerve emerge from the pons along with the sensory portions of the nerve, but they do not enter the trigeminal ganglion. Instead they bypass the ganglion by coursing inferior to it, and then become incorporated into the mandibular division. The motor portion accompanies the sensory portion of the mandibular nerve through the foramen ovale, but then diverges from the sensory portion to innervate the muscles of mastication in addition to several other muscles mentioned previously. The motor nucleus receives afferents from all three of the sensory nuclei of the fifth nerve complex. The projections from the mesencephalic nucleus provides an arc for reflex control of the muscles of mastication in response to stretch and/or contraction of those muscles. Fibers that project to the motor nucleus from the principal sensory nucleus and the spinal nucleus provide reflex control of the muscles of mastication in response to stimulation of superficial or cutaneous receptors, especially from the lingual and oral mucous membranes. The motor nucleus also receives crossed projections from the cerebral cortex so that the musculature of the jaw is under direct cortical control.

The *principal sensory* and *spinal trigeminal nuclei* both project ipsilaterally to the motor nuclei of cranial nerves VII and XII, and provide the afferent limb of reflexes associated with the muscles of facial expression (efferent link is via nerve VII) and intrinsic muscles of the tongue (efferent link is via nerve XII) in response to stimulation of superficial receptors in the distribution of nerve V. In addition, the principal sensory and spinal nuclei both send projections to the contralateral medial lemniscus, thus providing the head for the headless man represented in the dorsal column system (see Fig. 4–7). These fibers then project, along with the dorsal column system, to the ventrobasal complex of the thalamus and on to the somatosensory cortex. The modalities of pain and temperature from the seventh, ninth and tenth cranial nerves accompany these fibers en route to the cerebral cortex. The spinal trigeminal nucleus also sends projections to the reticular formation.

The central projections of the *mesencephalic nucleus* are obscure, but it is reasonable to assume that they terminate in the cerebellum via some route, since other pathways subserving subconscious proprioception terminate there.

Irritation of the fifth cranial nerve, which is called *trigeminal neuralgia* or *tic douloureux,* is a condition sometimes encountered clinically in which there is excruciating pain over the distribution of part of or the entire nerve. The pain is not constant but rather is transient in nature. It can be triggered by a variety of stimuli, such as smiling, yawning, chewing, hot or cold foods, brushing one's teeth, draughts on the face or sudden noises.

There are several factors involved in the presence of tic douloureux:

1. Compression of the sensory root of the trigeminal nerve by the petrous bone, aberrant arteries or tumors.
2. Chronic trauma
3. Herpes simplex virus (frequent cold sores).
4. It is often associated with multiple sclerosis owing to plaques of demyelination of branches of the trigeminal nerve.
5. It tends to be more common in women and older people. Most often, however, tic douloureux is idiopathic in origin, i.e., its etiology (history leading to its cause) is unknown.

If the pain is intractable (cannot be alleviated), surgery may be indicated. There are several surgical procedures now being utilized, but one of them, called *trigeminal tractotomy,* serves well to emphasize the anatomy of the spinal trigeminal complex. It consists of cutting the spinal tract in the brain stem at the level of the obex of the fourth ventricle, where the tract is located very superficially. The pain is thus eliminated or at least reduced without loss of other qualities of sensation to any extent. Figure 7–4 illustrates the relationships of the central nuclei of the trigeminal complex to each other and the location at which trigeminal tractotomy may be done.

Another surgical procedure available is *avulsion of the cutaneous branches* that supply the area involved. However, according to Loeser (1977), it produces total anesthesia, rarely provides more than one year of pain relief and is less likely to succeed when repeated.

Percutaneous (through unbroken skin) *radiofrequency trigeminal gangliolysis* (destruction of the ganglion) is one of the safest, least expensive and most reliable surgical procedures for the relief of neuralgic pain. It can be done under a local anesthetic and can be repeated if the pain recurs.

Janetta (1975) has introduced a surgical procedure that involves *decompression of the trigeminal nerve.* This is effective when tic douloureux is produced by an aberrant blood vessel or a tumor impinging upon the trigeminal root in the region of the brain stem. It is a major surgical procedure in which a suboccipital craniectomy (excision of the skull in the suboccipital region) is done, and a small piece of nonabsorbable sponge is placed between the aberrant blood vessel and the nerve. Janetta has had a high rate of successful long-term cures with this

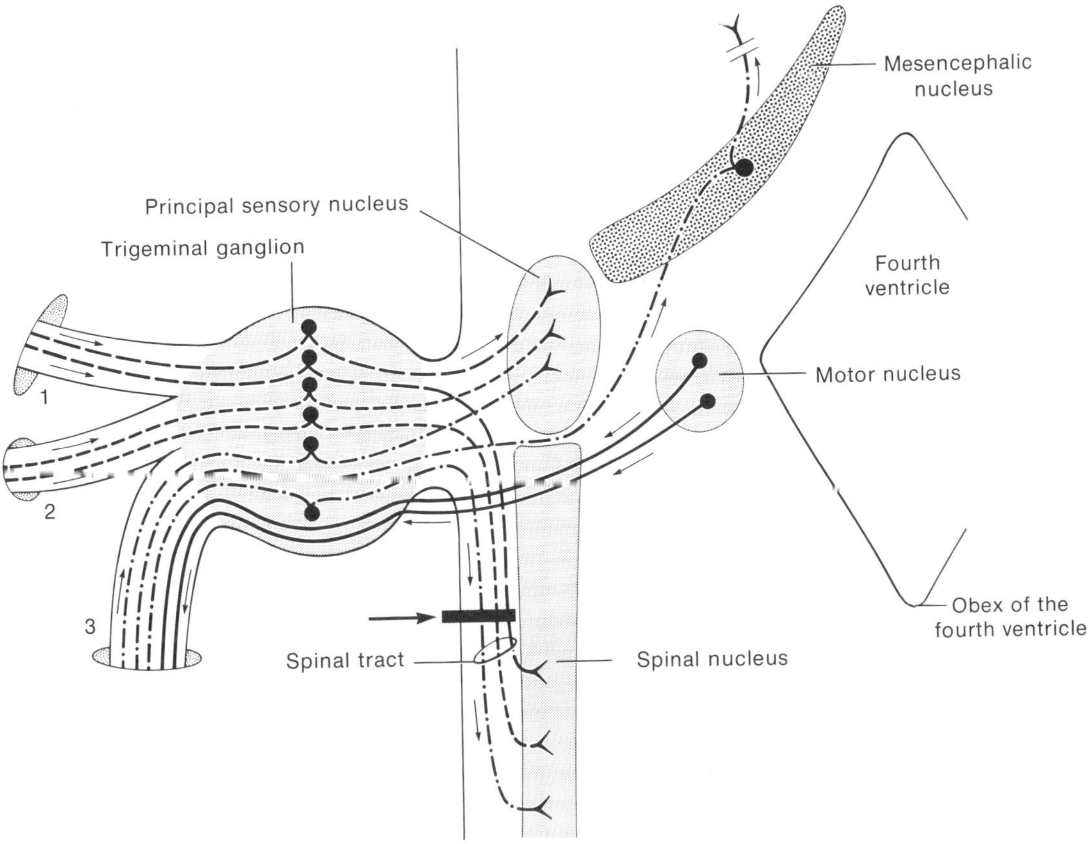

Figure 7–4. The central nuclei of the trigeminal complex. *1*, The ophthalmic division; *2*, the maxillary division; *3*, the mandibular division. The arrow indicates the level at which trigeminal tractotomy may be done for relief of pain from trigeminal neuralgia. In this procedure the neurons that convey the modalities of pain and thermal sense to the spinal nucleus are cut without interruption of the other neurons of the system.

procedure, but it requires a highly skilled surgeon to manipulate carefully the necessary cranial nerves and blood vessels.

There is one drug (carbamazepine) which is particularly effective for the relief of neuralgic pain, especially on a short-term basis. In addition, the pain may be blocked temporarily by injection of local anesthetics such as alcohol in the region of the trigger area, but relief from the pain is not long-lasting and the nerve block produces complete anesthesia in the distribution of the anesthesized nerve. Loeser (1977) believes that alcohol injections and peripheral nerve avulsions are outdated procedures that should be used only rarely, and takes the sensible conservative view that a trial of drug therapy should be given to the patient before surgery is attempted.

Damage to the motor root of the trigeminal nerve may be evaluated by having the patient move the mandible from side to side. This determines whether or not the pterygoid muscles are functioning. Protrusion to the right tests the left pterygoid muscles and protrusion to the left tests the right pterygoid muscles. The strength of the masseter and temporal muscles may be determined by placing a tongue depressor between the teeth and having the patient bite it enthusiastically.

One of the most important reflexes involving the sensory side of the trigeminal nerve is the corneal reflex. This may be elicited normally by mechanical stimulation such as touching the cornea with a piece of cotton. The afferent limb of the reflex arc is provided by the ophthalmic division of cranial nerve V, which projects to the motor nucleus of the facial nerve. The efferent link of the reflex consists of innervation of the orbicularis oculi by the facial nerve. The response to stimulation is bilateral blinking. If the ophthalmic division of the trigeminal nerve is damaged the reflex is lost on the side of the lesion. The projections of the ophthalmic division of cranial nerve V to the motor nucleus of the facial nerve are bilateral, so that if the cornea is stimulated on the normal side when the nerve on the other side has been damaged, the response is still bilateral blinking. Obviously, the normal response to corneal stimulation is dependent on a normal motor component of the facial nerve which innervates the orbicularis oculi. If the nerve supply to the latter is damaged on one side the corneal reflex cannot be elicited on that side owing to elimination of the efferent component of the reflex arc, but corneal stimulation on the side of the lesion does produce blinking of the normal contralateral eye because the afferent bilateral sensory projections of the ophthalmic division of the trigeminal nerve are still intact.

Some of the reflex connections of the trigeminal nerve provide the basis for Rood's therapeutic use of perioral stimulation for improvement of abnormal feeding patterns in infants. The stimulus is light moving touch to the perioral area to facilitate and integrate sucking, swallowing and respiration. The afferent link of the reflex arc is composed of the maxillary and mandibular divisions of the trigeminal nerve, and the efferent links are composed of the facial and hypoglossal nerves that control the muscles of facial expression and the tongue.

Abducens Nerve

The abducens nerve nucleus is located in the floor of the fourth ventricle, deep to the facial colliculus (a protuberance in the floor of the fourth ventricle produced by motor fibers of the facial nerve) at the level of the pons. It emerges from the brain at the caudal level of the pons, and after a long intracranial course it leaves the skull via the superior orbital fissure to innervate the *lateral rectus muscle*. The sixth nerve contains only *general somatic efferent* fibers, since the lateral rectus muscle is the sole structure which it innervates.

The nucleus receives crossed and uncrossed fibers from the vestibular nuclei via the medial longitudinal fasciculus, and therefore is involved with vestibular control of eye movements, as are cranial nerves III and IV. It also receives bilateral projections from the cerebral cortex by way of the corticobulbar tracts.

Because this nerve has a very long intracranial course, it is subject to trauma, especially when there is an increase in intracranial pressure. The symptoms of sixth nerve involvement are medial deviation of the eye caused by weakness of the lateral rectus muscle, which leads to diplopia (blurred or double vision). As the fibers from the sixth nerve emerge from the pons, they are in very close approximation to the corticospinal and extrapyramidal tracts, so that often a lesion will involve both systems. The result is an ipsilateral lower motor neuron paralysis of the lateral rectus muscle combined with a contralateral hemiplegia or hemiparesis.

The third, fourth and sixth cranial nerves all course through the cavernous sinus between their origins and the superior orbital fissure. If the cavernous sinus is subjected to compression for any reason the integrity of these nerves is at risk. In addition, the ophthalmic division of the fifth cranial nerve is in very close approximation to the sinus and may also be subject to damage.

Facial Nerve

The facial nerve emerges from the brain stem at the level of the lower pons. It contains several functional components.

GENERAL SOMATIC AFFERENTS

These fibers from the posterior auricular nerve supply the skin posterior to the ear and the external meatus along with nerves IX and X; they are contained in the nervus intermedius and terminate in the spinal trigeminal nucleus. They provide the afferent limb of a reflex arc which produces responses in the muscles of mastication to cutaneous stimulation. The efferent limb of the reflex is provided by projections from the spinal trigeminal nucleus to the motor nucleus of the fifth nerve, from whence efferent fibers reach the muscles of mastication by way of the mandibular division of the fifth nerve.

SPECIAL VISCERAL AFFERENTS

These subserve taste on the anterior two-thirds of the tongue, and are contained in the *chorda tympani* branch of the facial nerve. The nerve enters the stylomastoid foramen along with the general somatic afferents of the seventh cranial nerve and, after synapsing in the geniculate ganglion, which is located within the internal acoustic meatus, it enters the middle cranial fossa via the internal acoustic meatus along with the remainder of the facial nerve and the vestibulocochlear nerve. The fibers then project to the tractus solitarius and terminate in the nucleus solitarius (see Fig. 6–6). From there, fibers project to the ventrobasal complex of the thalamus, and the last order neurons project to the cerebral cortex.

SPECIAL VISCERAL EFFERENTS

These supply the muscles of facial expression, the stapedius muscle, the posterior belly of the digastric muscle and the stylohyoid muscle. These neurons arise from the motor nucleus of the seventh nerve at the level of the pons, and emerge from the brain stem at the level of the caudal pons after taking a tortuous course dorsally between the abducens nucleus and the floor of the fourth ventricle. This arrangement produces the facial colliculus (see Fig. 7–5).

GENERAL VISCERAL EFFERENTS

These originate from the superior salivatory nucleus (see Fig. 7–5), which is located just rostral to the nucleus ambiguus. The general visceral efferents are preganglionic parasympathetic fibers, which after synapsing in peripheral ganglia supply the submaxillary, sublingual and lacrimal glands.

The facial motor nucleus receives projections from a number of sources, one of which is the spinal trigeminal nucleus. Sensory fibers of the trigeminal nerve provide the afferent link of a reflex arc, of which the special visceral efferent fibers of the facial nerve supply the efferent link to provide for

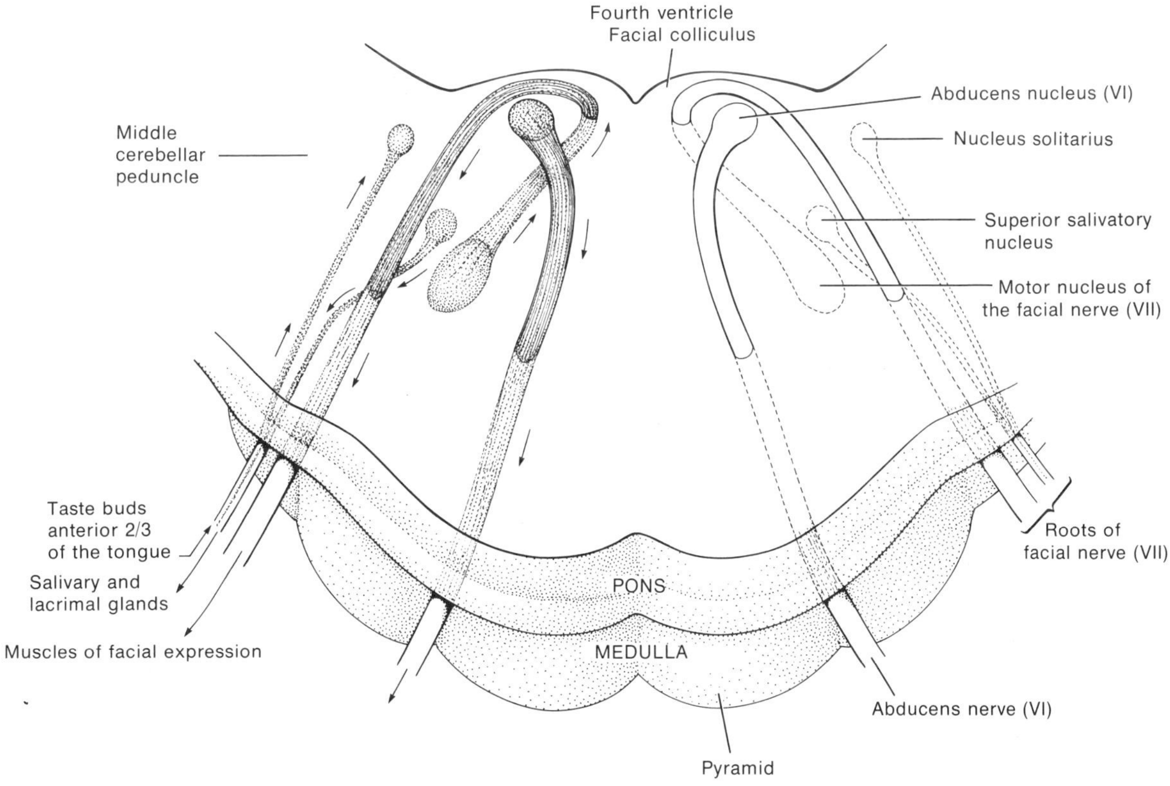

Figure 7–5. The nuclei and nerves closely associated with the facial nerve complex area. This figure may be helpful in interpreting atlas number 6–7 in Chapter 6 and clarifying the relationship between the facial and abducens nerves. The structures shown by solid lines in the right half of the drawing are in the plane of section. Other structures (*dashed lines*) are below the plane of section.

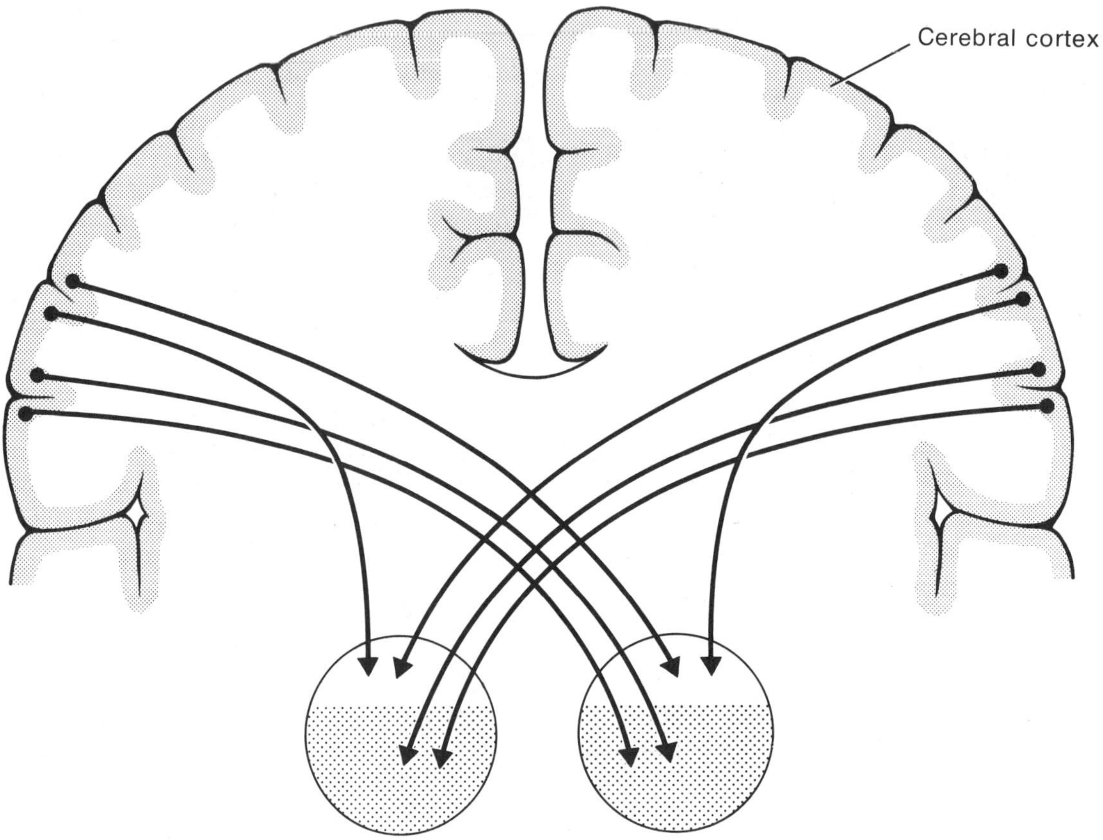

Figure 7–6. The corticobulbar projections to the motor nucleus of the facial nerve. The shaded areas in the nuclei control muscles of the lower two-thirds of the face. The nonshaded areas control the muscles of the upper one-third of the face. The muscles of the lower two-thirds are under only contralateral control of the cerebral cortex, whereas the muscles of the upper one-third are under bilateral control of the cerebral cortex.

corneal and trigeminal–facial reflexes. In addition, the nucleus receives fibers from the corticobulbar system, the rubrobulbar system, and presumably from the mesencephalic reticular formation and the auditory and visual systems. Projections from the auditory system probably mediate certain acousticofacial reflexes, such as closing one's eyes in response to loud noises. Those from the visual system produce squinting in response to bright light.

The control of the facial musculature by the cerebral cortex shows regional differences in different areas of the face. The muscles of the upper one-third of the face are innervated by a part of the facial motor nucleus which is controlled bilaterally by the cortex; those of the lower two-thirds are innervated by a part of the nucleus controlled by the contralateral hemisphere of the cerebral cortex only (see Fig. 7–6). This is important clinically. If the corticobulbar projections to the motor nucleus of the seventh cranial nerve are damaged unilaterally there will be little or no weakness of the muscles of the upper one-third of the face, but there will be contralateral paralysis of the muscles of the lower two-thirds of the face.

If the facial nerve is damaged peripheral to the motor nucleus of nerve VII, all muscles on the ipsilateral side will be paralyzed.

Accompanying such a lesion there may also be a disturbance in the ability to taste and in glandular secretory function. Occasionally in such cases aberrant regrowth of the parasympathetic fibers may result in tearing in response to a salivary stimulus (crocodile tears) or in salivation in response to an emotional stimulus. Lower motor neuron lesions of the facial nerve are referred to clinically as *Bell's palsy*.

Patients with paralysis of the muscles of facial expression have difficulty with eating and particularly with drinking. They are also painfully aware of the cosmetic effects of the condition. The corner of the mouth droops and they can only smile in a one-sided fashion. Often it is advisable to splint up the corner of the mouth with a hook device between that and the ear. Along with electrical stimulation of the muscles and re-education, this often produces good results depending on the cause of the paralysis.

Vestibulocochlear Nerve

The eighth cranial nerve, as its name indicates, consists of two parts, both of which contain *special somatic afferent* fibers. The cochlear division conveys auditory impulses from the organ of Corti, and the vestibular division conveys impulses from the utricle, saccule and semicircular canals.

COCHLEAR DIVISION

The centrally directed fibers of the cochlear nerve originate within the spiral ganglion of the cochlea, and from there project to the dorsal and ventral cochlear nuclei via the internal acoustic meatus. The dorsal and ventral cochlear nuclei, which are located on the external surface of the inferior cerebellar peduncle, are thus the first relay stations in the auditory system. Both of these nuclei contain complete tonotopic organization, i.e., they both receive the entire spectrum of auditory frequencies, from the highest, projected from the basilar part of the cochlea, to the lowest, projected from the apical portion of the cochlea.

From the cochlear nuclei some fibers enter the ipsilateral superior olive or lateral lemniscus, or cross to the contralateral superior olive or lateral lemniscus and ascend to the inferior colliculi bilaterally. From the inferior colliculus fibers are relayed to the medial geniculate nucleus of the thalamus and on to the auditory cortex in the temporal lobe (see Fig. 7–7). It should be emphasized that auditory representation in the cerebral cortex is bilateral, since some fibers cross and some do not en route to the cortex. Therefore, loss of hearing in one ear indicates a peripheral lesion, and loss of hearing in both ears indicates a central lesion or bilateral involvement of both ears. One symptom of cochlear nerve lesions may be buzzing or ringing in the ears (tinnitus), which usually precedes diminution in hearing.

VESTIBULAR DIVISION

The vestibular nerve is concerned with orientation of the head in three-dimensional space and with equilibrium. The cell bodies are located in Scarpa's ganglion, which lies in the internal acoustic meatus. Impulses from the utricle, saccule and semicircular canals reach the four vestibular nuclei, but some impulses proceed directly to the ipsilateral cerebellum by way of the inferior cerebellar peduncle (vestibulocerebellar tracts).

From the vestibular nuclei fibers project to the cerebellum (also the vestibulocerebellar tracts), the medial longitudinal fasciculus and to the spinal cord via the vestibulospinal tracts. The latter originate from the lateral vestibular (Deiters') nucleus only. There are also important reciprocal connections between the cerebellum and the vestibular nuclei, and between the reticular formation and the vestibular nuclei. The connections with the reticular formation are responsible for the vomiting and cardiovascular reactions associated with Meniere's diesease. In addition, the vestibular nuclei project to the contralateral cerebral cortex close to the area in which the face is represented in the primary somatosensory cortex. The exact location of the pathway is not known, but it is responsible for conscious knowledge of spatial orientation.

The vestibular nuclei play an important role in cerebellar mechanisms and in control of movement by way of the medial longitudinal fasciculus, which projects to cervical spinal cord levels as well as to cranial nerves III, IV and VI, and by way of the vestibulospinal tracts which project to all levels of the spinal cord. The connections of

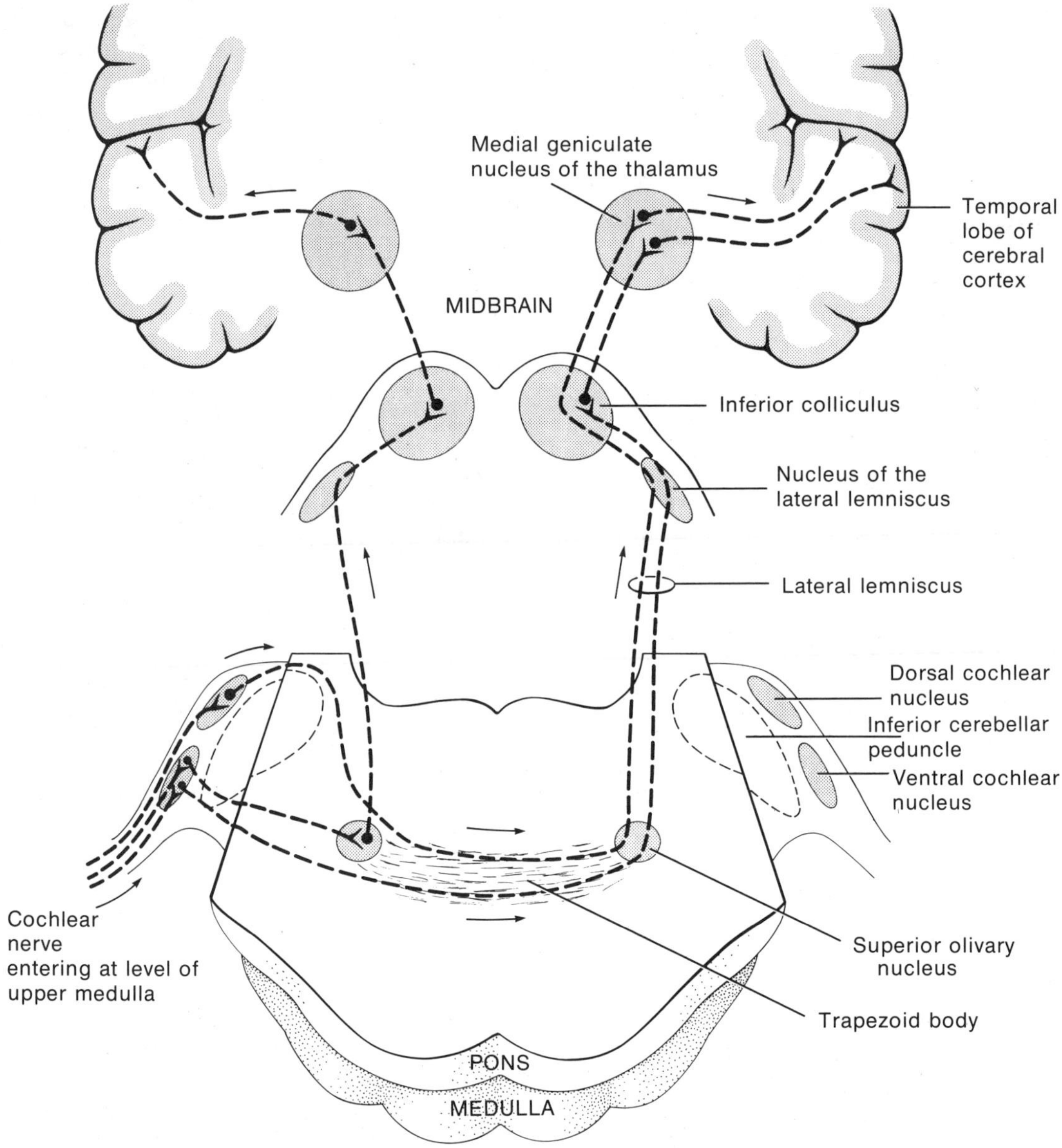

Figure 7–7. The auditory system. The important point to observe is that this system is represented bilaterally in the cerebral cortex.

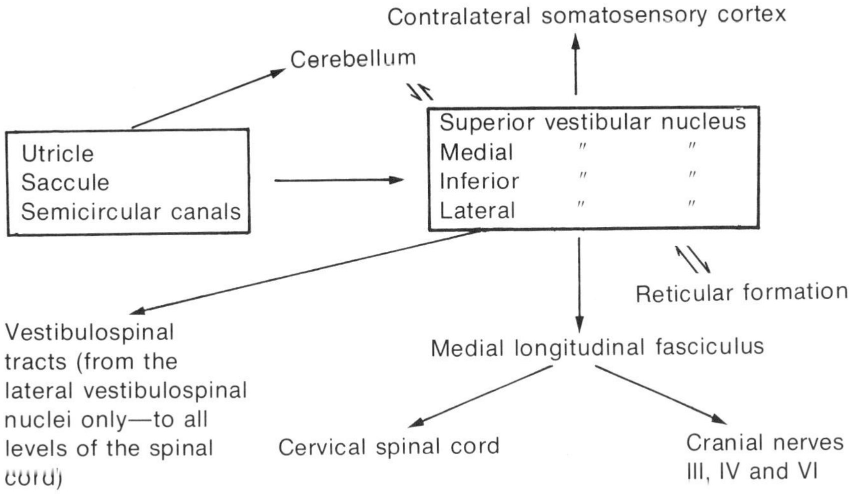

the vestibular nuclei may be summarized as follows and are illustrated above.

If the vestibular nerve is damaged the symptoms are:

1. vertigo (dizziness), which may result in nausea and vomiting.
2. nystagmus (rotary, horizontal or vertical rhythmic movements of the eye). The horizontal variety is the most common. This type of nystagmus has a slow and a quick component, the latter occurring toward the normal side. It is named for the direction in which the quick component occurs: i.e., if the quick component is toward the right and the slow component toward the left, the left side is the abnormal side but it is called a right nystagmus. This condition ceases during sleep.
3. A tendency to fall toward the abnormal side, which is also true of patients with cerebellar damage. Therefore, this symptom cannot be used to differentiate between vestibular and cerebellar damage.

Within the substance of the brain stem the cochlear and vestibular divisions are separated, so that a lesion in that area could damage one of the divisions selectively. However, in the internal acoustic meatus, both divisions course together, along with the seventh cranial nerve, so that a lesion in that area could involve both divisions of the eighth nerve along with the facial nerve.

Tumors or other lesions, such as aneurysms of the basilar artery in the area of the cerebellopontine junction, can damage several of the cranial nerves. A vestibulocochlear nerve tumor is signaled initially by symptoms of damage to the cochlear division of the nerve, i.e., tinnitus, followed by a gradual loss of hearing. Vertigo, due to involvement of the vestibular division of the nerve, usually occurs later. The facial nerve may also be involved in any kind of lesion to this area and the damage is reflected early by twitching of the muscles of facial expression, which may progress to a complete facial nerve paralysis. If the trigeminal nerve is involved there may be a diminution or complete absence of the corneal reflex, and there may also be some numbness over the area of the cutaneous distribution of the nerve. Only rarely will there be complete sensory loss or motor weakness of the muscles of mastication.

If the lesion is a tumor its growth may compress the brain stem and cerebellum, thus giving rise to symptoms such as ataxia, severe attacks of vertigo and increased deep tendon reflexes. If the tumor is not surgically removed the symptoms will gradually increase in severity, and destruction of brain stem structures that are essential to life may eventually lead to death.

Glossopharyngeal Nerve

The ninth cranial nerve contains both afferent and efferent fibers and emerges from the skull at the jugular foramen. It contains several functional components.

GENERAL SOMATIC AFFERENTS

These supply the skin posterior to the ear and the external acoustic meatus via the posterior auricular nerve in common with cranial nerves VII and X. The cell bodies of these fibers are located in the superior ganglion of the ninth nerve, which is found within the jugular foramen. From the superior ganglion the axons project to the tract and nucleus of the spinal division of the trigeminal nerve, and the pathway terminates in the somatosensory cortex after relaying through the ventrobasal complex of the thalamus.

SPECIAL VISCERAL AFFERENTS

These subserve taste on the posterior one-third of the tongue. They terminate in the nucleus solitarius along with the gustatory fibers of cranial nerves VII and X. Through pathways that are not well-established subsequent fibers terminate in the cerebral cortex after a synapse in the thalamus.

GENERAL VISCERAL AFFERENTS

These convey touch, pain and temperature senses from the mucous membranes of the posterior portion of the tongue, tonsils and eustachian tubes. Their cells of origin are located in the inferior ganglion of the glossopharyngeal nerve, which is located in the petrous portion of the temporal bone. These fibers terminate in the nucleus of the spinal division of the trigeminal nerve and the pathway then joins the medial lemniscus, as do other fibers that terminate in that nucleus.

There is also a special sensory branch of the ninth cranial nerve that carries information from the carotid sinus and carotid body, which are located at the bifurcation of the common carotid artery into the internal and external carotid arteries. Impulses are sent to the dorsal motor nucleus of the vagus nerve in the medulla. The efferent link of the reflex arc consists of vagal fibers that terminate in the sinoatrial and atrioventricular nodes as well as in atrial muscle fibers of the heart. The effective stimulus for impulse transmission in this branch of the glossopharyngeal nerve is an increase in blood pressure. Through this reflex arc, the vagus nerve reduces both heart rate and blood pressure.

GENERAL VISCERAL EFFERENTS

These originate in the inferior salivatory nucleus of the medulla and are responsible for secretory activity in the parotid gland.

SPECIAL VISCERAL EFFERENTS

These originate in the nucleus ambiguus, which is located in the reticular formation approximately halfway between the spinal trigeminal nucleus and the inferior olive. These fibers innervate the stylopharyngeus muscle, which elevates the pharynx during swallowing and speech.

Selective lesions of the ninth cranial nerve are rare, but when they do occur the following symptoms may be produced.

1. Loss of the gag reflex.
2. Loss of the carotid sinus and carotid body reflexes.
3. Loss of taste on the posterior one-third of the tongue.
4. Excruciating pain over the sensory distribution of the nerve (the areas posterior to the ear, in the external acoustic meatus and part of the pharynx). Some clinicians refer to this condition as "tic douloureux" associated with the glossopharyngeal nerve.

Vagus Nerve

The vagus nerve accompanies the glossopharyngeal and spinal accessory nerves through the jugular foramen, and also contains several afferent and efferent components.

GENERAL SOMATIC AFFERENTS

These arise by way of the posterior auricular nerve, which distributes in common with cranial nerves VII and IX. The central pathways are the same as those described for cranial nerves VII and IX (i.e., to the tract and nucleus of the spinal division of the trigeminal nerve, through the thalamus and on to the somatosensory cortex).

GENERAL VISCERAL AFFERENTS

From the pharynx, larynx, trachea, esophagus and thoracic and abdominal viscera, these fibers project to the caudal portion of the nucleus solitarius (Fig. 6–6) and from there some terminate in the reticular formation of the medulla, where they function in the central regulation of respiratory, cardiovascular and emetic activities. Other fibers terminate in the motor nuclei of the facial and glossopharyngeal nerves for control of lingual and secretory functions.

SPECIAL VISCERAL AFFERENTS

From taste buds on the epiglottis these fibers project to the nucleus solitarius, as do gustatory neurons from the facial and glossopharyngeal nerves. The ensuing pathways to the ventral basal nucleus of the thalamus and the cerebral cortex are as described for the seventh and ninth cranial nerves.

GENERAL VISCERAL EFFERENTS

These are preganglionic parasympathetic neurons which innervate all thoracic and visceral structures as far inferior as the level at which the transverse and descending colons meet. Structures inferior to that level are innervated by parasympathetic fibers from spinal nerves S2, S3 and S4. The preganglionic parasympathetic fibers of the vagus nerve originate in the dorsal nucleus of the vagus, which is located in the floor of the fourth ventricle.

SPECIAL VISCERAL EFFERENTS

These originate in the nucleus ambiguus, and innervate the muscles of the larynx and the pharynx.

If the vagus nerve is destroyed bilaterally, death follows very rapidly owing to the loss of respiratory reflexes and uncontrolled cardiac acceleration. The accompanying complete laryngeal paralysis is of little consequence. If the vagus nerve is damaged unilaterally the most common symptoms are deviation of the soft palate and uvula to the normal side, hoarseness due to weakness in the laryngeal muscles, and dysphagia (difficulty with swallowing) caused by weakness of the pharyngeal constrictors.

Spinal Accessory Nerve

The spinal accessory nerve is divided into cranial and spinal components. The cranial root contains special visceral efferent fibers with their cell bodies located in the nucleus ambiguus. From their origin in that nucleus, they join the vagus nerve to innervate the intrinsic muscles of the larynx. The spinal root originates in the anterior horns of spinal segments extending rostrally from the pyramidal decussation to as far caudally as cervical segments 5 or 6.

The cranial portion of the nerve exits from the medulla posterior to the inferior olive, as do the glossopharyngeal and vagus nerves. The spinal portion enters the skull via the foramen magnum, joins the cranial portion, and both parts leave the skull via the jugular foramen. The spinal portion of the nerve innervates the sternocleidomastoideus and trapezius muscles.

The spinal accessory nerve receives projections from the medial longitudinal fasciculus and other systems involved with eye–head–neck coordination, as well as from the cerebral cortex via corticobulbar fibers.

The major symptoms produced by lesions of the spinal accessory nerve are weakness in rotation of the head to the opposite side owing to dysfunction of the sternocleidomastoideus muscle, and in shoulder girdle elevation and retraction as a result of dysfunction of the trapezius muscle.

Hypoglossal Nerve

The hypoglossal nerve is known to contain only general somatic efferent fibers, although it may have some general somatic afferent fibers that innervate muscle spindles of the tongue. The general somatic efferent fibers originate in the hypoglossal nuclei, which are located in the medial portion of the caudal end of the floor of the fourth ventricle. The fibers emerge from the medulla in the anterolateral sulcus anterior to the inferior olive. They leave the skull by way of the hypoglossal canal.

The hypoglossal nucleus receives projections from the reticular formation, from corticobulbar fibers and from cranial nerves V, IX, and X. These cranial nerves mediate reflex tongue movements in response to stimulation of the mucous membranes of the lingual, oral and pharyngeal areas. The hypoglossal nucleus also receives some afferent fibers from visceral centers.

Unilateral lesions of the XIIth nerve produce a lower motor neuron paralysis of the

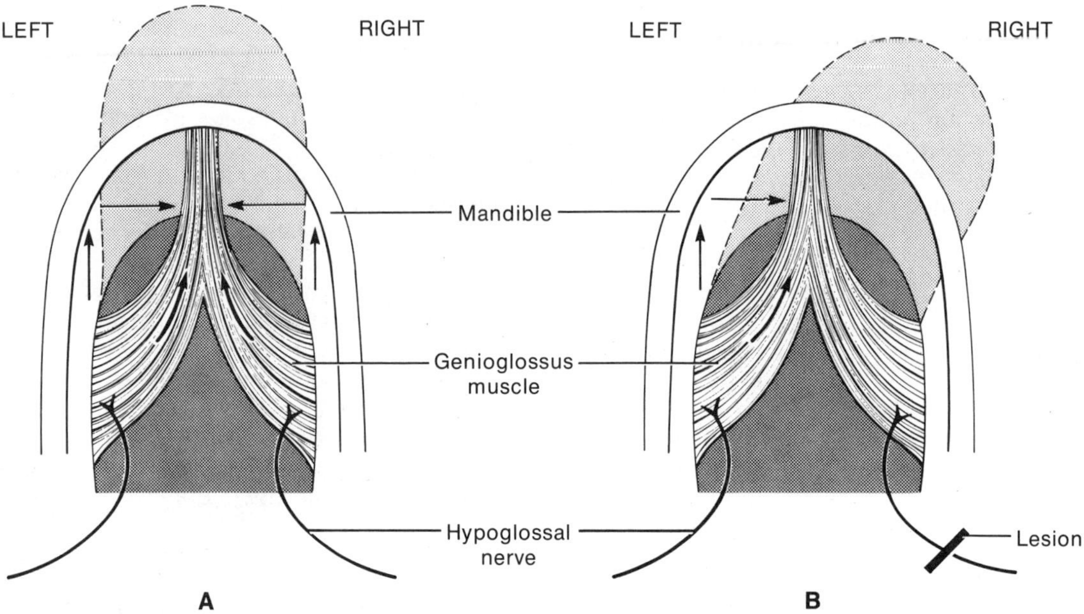

Figure 7–8. An inferior view of the tongue and mandible. *A* illustrates the normal resting position of the tongue within the mouth (*darkly shaded area*). When the tongue is protruded, there is no deviation to the left or to the right because the pulls of the left and right genioglossus muscles offset each other. The protruded tongue is indicated by the lighter shaded areas in both *A* and *B*. In *B* the hypoglossal nerve has been damaged on the right side so that the right genioglossus muscle is not functioning. The left genioglossus muscle exerts an unopposed medial pull as it shortens toward the symphysis menti of the mandible, and therefore the tongue deviates to the weak side as it is protruded. In *A* the arrows indicate the direction of pull of both genioglossus muscles; in *B* the arrows indicate the directions of pull of the intact left genioglossus muscle only.

ipsilateral one-half of the tongue, which includes loss of tone and movement as well as atrophy. When the tongue is protruded it *deviates to the weak side* owing to inactivity of the genioglossus muscle on that side (see Fig. 7–8). The root of the XIIth cranial nerve emerges in close association with the corticospinal tracts, and thus both may be involved in a common lesion. Ipsilateral weakness of the tongue with a contralateral hemiplegia or hemiparesis may then be produced.

TABLE 7–1.

	SVA	SSA	GSA	GVA	SVE	GSE	GVE
I	×						
II		×					
III						×	×
IV						×	
V			×		×		
VI						×	
VII	×		×		×		×
VIII		×					
IX	×		×	×	×		×
X	×		×	×	×		×
XI					×	×	
XII						×	

If the corticobulbar fibers that project to the hypoglossal nucleus are damaged, an upper motor neuron paralysis of the contralateral side of the tongue may be produced, since the corticobulbar fibers which control that nucleus are crossed.

The functional constituents of the cranial nerves are summarized in Table 7–1.

REVIEW QUESTIONS

1. Explain what is meant, in terms of types of structures innervated, by:
   a. general somatic efferent.
   b. general visceral efferent
   c. special visceral efferent.
   d. general somatic afferent.
   e. general visceral afferent.
   f. special visceral afferent.
   g. special somatic afferent.
2. List the similarities and differences between spinal and cranial nerves.
3. A condition called homonymous hemianopia is sometimes encountered in the clinic, particularly when working with patients who have had a cerebral vascular accident. Is the lesion anterior or posterior to the optic chiasm? Explain what homonymous hemianopia is and diagram the morphologic basis for it.
4. Why are the oculomotor nerve and the corticospinal tract so often both involved in a single lesion? When this happens, what specific symptoms may present themselves? (Remember that extrapyramidal tracts are usually damaged as well as corticospinal tracts.)
5. Irritation of which cranial nerve is most frequently responsible for the clinical entity known as "tic douloureux"? Locate the area in which surgical tractotomy may be done successfully for the relief of pain in this condition. Explain why this surgical procedure eliminates or at least reduces the pain without impairing the sense of two-point discrimination, pressure, vibration, etc.
6. Different parts of the trigeminal nerve complex function homologously with the major ascending systems of the spinal cord. Explain which parts of the trigeminal complex correspond functionally with specific ascending systems.
7. What is symptomatic of a lesion of the VIth cranial nerve? What other tracts are often included in a lesion of this nerve? Why?
8. Explain by diagram the distribution of loss of function or weakness of the muscles of facial expression after: a. a unilateral lesion of the corticobulbar fibers which terminate on the VIIth nerve nuclei. b. a lesion of the VIIth cranial nerve, peripheral to the motor nucleus.
9. Diagram the connections by which the vestibular nuclei influence posture and movement. What symptoms are produced by lesions of the vestibular portion of the VIIIth cranial nerve?
10. What muscles are innervated by the XIth cranial nerve? What movements are impaired when this nerve is damaged?
11. If the XIIth nerve is cut on the right, to which side will the tongue deviate? Why?

CHAPTER 8 • THE CEREBELLUM

OBJECTIVES

After reading this chapter, you should know in detail the: • Functional divisions of the cerebellum. • Intrinsic circuitry of the cerebellum. • Interconnections of the cerebellum with other central nervous system structures. • Influence of the cerebellum upon movement and posture.

STRUCTURE AND FUNCTION

The cerebellum is concerned primarily with mechanisms that influence coordination of somatic motor activity, equilibrium and muscle tone. It is interconnected with several areas of the central nervous system by way of the superior, middle and inferior cerebellar peduncles. Very little is understood concerning the mechanisms that underlie cerebellar function, but we do know that lesions of the cerebellum produce characteristic disorders of coordinated movement and muscle tone as well as loss of equilibrium.

The cerebellum can be split into three distinct divisions, based on both function and location. The *paleocerebellum* or *anterior lobe* is located between the primary fissure and the rostral limit of the cerebellum (see Fig. 8–1). In man, this is the principal area to which information about subconscious proprioception from muscle spindles and Golgi tendon organs projects, so that the paleocerebellum is concerned with regulation of muscle tone. The information regarding subconscious proprioception arrives in the cerebellum by way of the dorsal and ventral spinocerebellar tracts, the cuneocerebellar tracts and the quintocerebellar tracts.

The *neocerebellum* or *posterior lobe* is the newest part of the cerebellum phylogenetically, and includes the area between the primary fissure and the flocculonodular lobe (Fig. 8–1). It is the largest part of the cerebellum and is primarily related to coordination of skilled movements which are initiated at cortical levels.

The *archicerebellum* or *flocculonodular lobe,* which consists of the paired flocculi and the nodule, is the oldest phylogenetic part of the cerebellum and is located anteriorly between the anterior and posterior lobes (Fig. 8–1). The archicerebellum is closely associated with the vestibular nerve and nuclei, and functions primarily in equilibrium and the righting responses.

There is auditory and visual representation in the midline region of the cerebellum, and this is called the *vermis.* These projections probably function in the involuntary startle responses to auditory and visual experiences.

Imbedded within the white matter of each cerebellar hemisphere are four nuclear masses, the fastigial, globose, emboliform and dentate nuclei (see Fig. 8–2). These will be discussed along with the internal circuitry of the cerebellum.

The cerebellar cortex is a three-layered structure throughout its entire extent (see

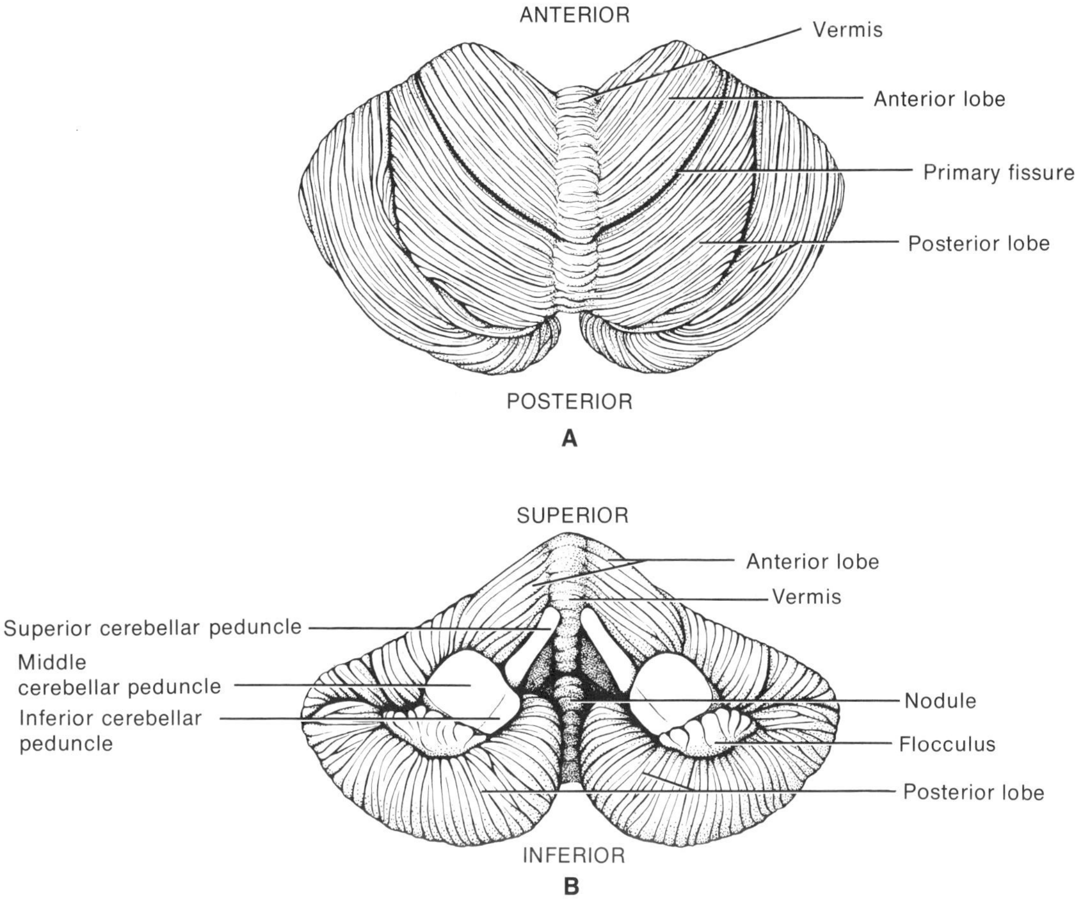

Figure 8–1. *A*, Superior view of the cerebellum. *B*, Anterior view of the cerebellum. The cerebellar peduncles have been cut.

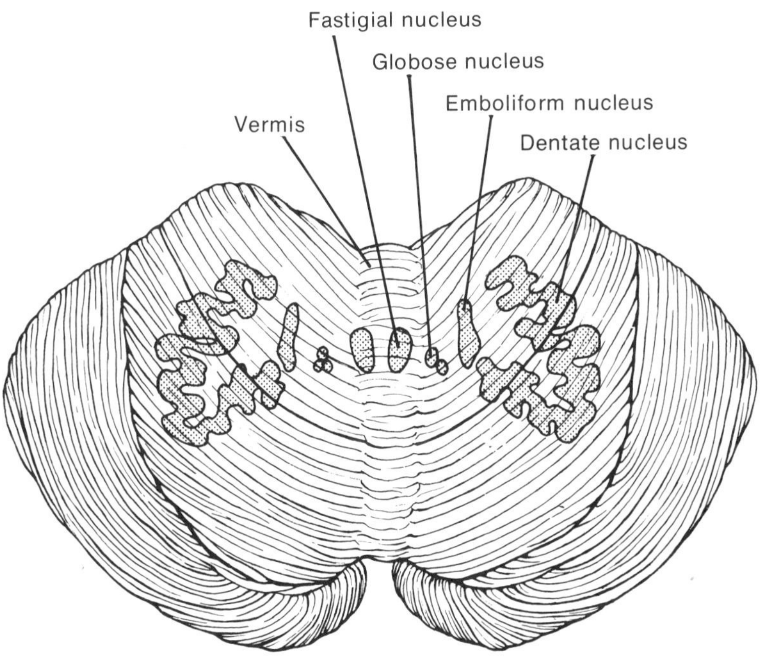

Figure 8–2. A horizontal section through the cerebellum, showing the locations of the deep cerebellar nuclei.

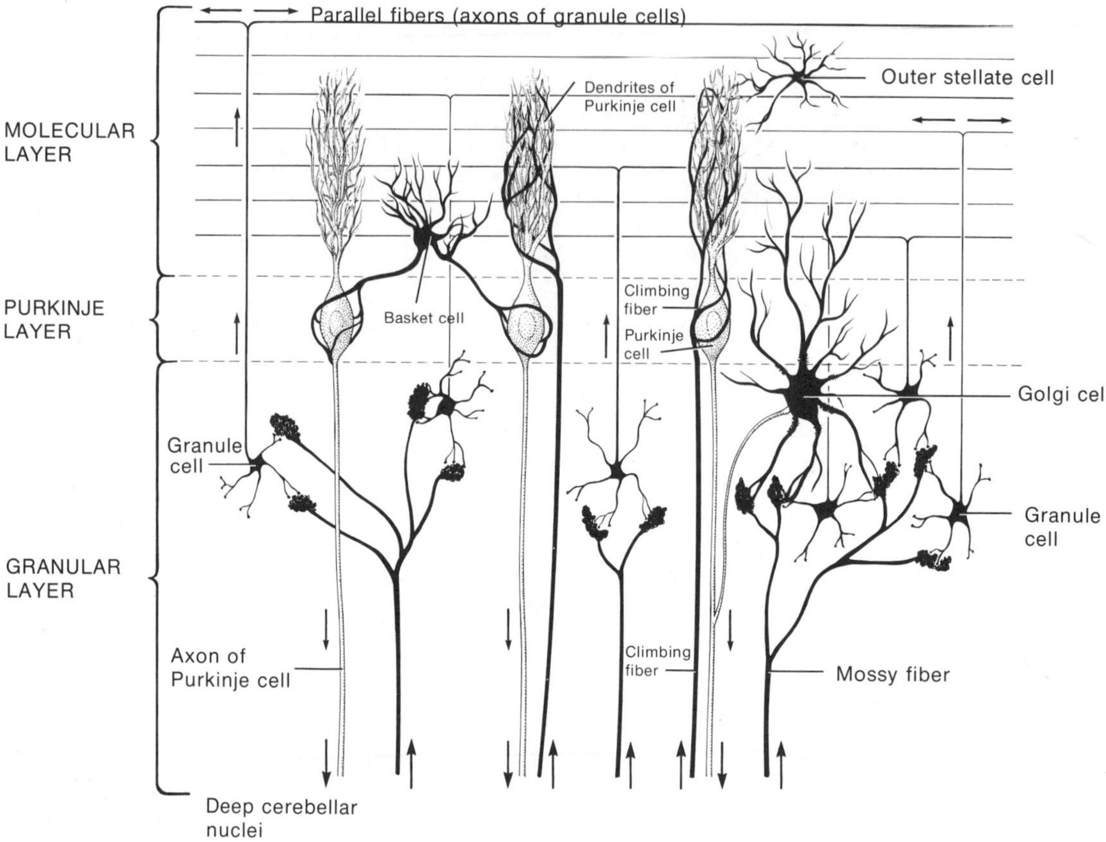

Figure 8–3. A diagrammatic representation of the constituents of the three layers of the cerebellar cortex. Notice the arrows that indicate afferent projections to the cerebellar cortex by way of mossy and climbing fibers, and arrows that indicate the sole efferent projections by Purkinje axons.

Fig. 8–3). The outer layer is called the *molecular layer* and contains the dendritic trees of Purkinje cells, basket cells, outer stellate cells and parallel fibers. The middle layer, the *Purkinje layer,* consists primarily of Purkinje cell bodies. The inner layer, or *granular layer*, contains many, many small granule cells, Golgi cells and mossy fiber terminals.

There are two types of afferent nerve fibers that project to the cerebellar cortex: the mossy fibers and the climbing fibers. It has been thought traditionally that the mossy fibers projected from all the afferent systems that terminate in the cerebellum *except* those which project from the inferior olive of the medulla. However, recent electrophysiologic and neuroanatomic studies have provided evidence that climbing fibers stem from a number of sources, and that both mossy and climbing fibers may originate from the same nuclei.

The climbing fibers synapse with the cell bodies and dendrites of Purkinje cells, stellate cells, dendrites of granule cells and with Golgi cells. Those climbing fibers that synapse upon Purkinje cells are distributed on a one-to-one basis and have an *excitatory* influence. The mossy fibers synapse with the dendrites of innumerable granule cells and also exert an excitatory influence upon those cells.

The systems that project to the cerebellum may be subdivided on the basis of the lobe to which they project and on the basis of their functions.

1. Fibers which terminate in all lobes of the cerebellum project from the inferior olive. These *olivocerebellar tracts* project to the contralateral cerebellar cortex by way of very heavy crossed projections that enter the cerebellum via the inferior cerebellar peduncles. The inferior olive receives ascending projections from the

spino-olivary tracts and descending projections from the cerebral cortex, red nucleus and basal ganglia. The olivary pathways function in the regulation of muscle tone.

2. Nerve fibers which terminate in the archicerebellum (flocculonodular lobe) originate from the vestibular nerve and nuclei. The *vestibulocerebellar tracts* project primarily to the ipsilateral side, although some cross to the contralateral side of the cerebellum after entering via the inferior cerebellar peduncles. The flocculonodular lobe and the vestibulocerebellar tracts function in equilibrium reactions.
3. The fiber systems which terminate in the paleocerebellum (anterior lobe) function in regulation of muscle tone.
   a. *Dorsal spinocerebellar tracts* project to the ipsilateral side (on the side on which the first order neurons of the system enter the spinal cord) via the inferior cerebellar peduncles.
   b. *Cuneocerebellar tracts* from the accessory (also called lateral or external) cuneate nucleus project to the ipsilateral side by way of the inferior cerebellar peduncles.
   c. *Quintocerebellar tracts* from the three sensory nuclei of the trigeminal complex project to the cerebellum. Those from the mesencephalic nucleus enter by way of the superior cerebellar peduncles, and those from the principal sensory and spinal nuclei enter via the inferior cerebellar peduncles. It is known that some of these fibers project to the deep cerebellar nuclei, but the areas in which all of the fibers terminate is not known. It may be safe to assume that those fibers from the mesencephalic nucleus terminate in the paleocerebellum since they convey information from muscle spindles located in the muscles of mastication, and information regarding the tension of the musculature from other systems projects to the paleocerebellum.
   d. *Ventral spinocerebellar tracts* enter the cerebellum by way of the superior cerebellar peduncles. Most of these fibers cross within the cerebellum and terminate in the paleocerebellum on the side on which the impulses were originally generated.
   e. Reticulocerebellar tracts originate in the lateral reticular nuclei, which receive projections from the spinoreticular tracts, the red nucleus and the fastigial nucleus of the cerebellum. Carpenter (1976) suggests that the projections from the lateral reticular nucleus appear to mediate tactile impulses, and perhaps some other types, to the cerebellum, and that those fibers from the fastigial nucleus function in a cerebelloreticular feedback system. The reticulocerebellar tracts terminate in the ipsilateral cerebellar cortex after entering through the inferior cerebellar peduncles.
4. Fibers which terminate in the neocerebellum (posterior lobe) function in coordination of movement and enter the cerebellum via the middle cerebellar peduncles. These fibers consist of the *corticopontocerebellar* pathways that were discussed in an earlier chapter. This input makes up by far the most massive afferent system of the cerebellum in primates.

After the mossy fibers synapse with the granule cells, the latter in turn send their axons to the molecular layer of the cerebellar cortex. Their axons are the parallel fibers, which synapse with the dendrites of Purkinje, basket, Golgi and outer stellate cells. The granule cell input to Purkinje cells is excitatory, and therefore the excitatory input to Purkinje cells is both direct, via climbing fibers, and indirect via mossy fibers and granule cells by way of the parallel fibers.

Basket, outer stellate and Golgi cells are inhibitory to Purkinje cells in the following ways. The basket cells receive information from granule cells, and in turn transmit impulses to Purkinje cells. These impulses are strongly inhibitory. Golgi cells receive information from both climbing fibers and parallel fibers of granule cells. The Golgi axons terminate on mossy fibers, inhibiting them and damping the excitatory effect of the mossy fibers on the granule cells, which results in relative inhibition of the Purkinje cells. The complex of mossy fiber terminals, granule cell dendrites and Golgi cell axons is called a cerebellar glomerulus. Outer stellate cells receive information from granule cell parallel fibers and synapse with Purkinje cells to inhibit them.

One might at this point ask, why is so

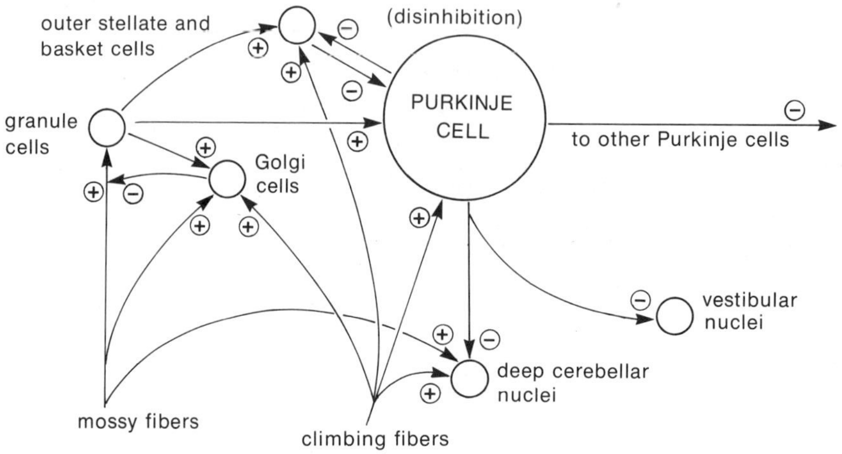

much emphasis placed on the influences of all the cell types on the Purkinje cells? The reason is that the Purkinje cells constitute the only efferent output of the cerebellar cortex. Purkinje cell axons project to the vestibular nuclei and to the four deep cerebellar nuclei (fastigial, globose, emboliform and dentate). The influence of the Purkinje cells on the vestibular and deep cerebellar nuclei is always inhibitory, so that their function is to modulate ongoing activity in these nuclei. It is necessary to assume, then, that the deep cerebellar nuclei are either spontaneously active or that there is excitatory input to them from other sources. Evidence has been provided that these excitatory inputs originate from collaterals of both mossy and climbing fibers.

The internal circuitry of the cerebellum may be summarized diagrammatically as followed in the illustration above.

The neurophysiologists have done a masterful job in sorting out all the excitatory and inhibitory influences exerted within the cerebellum, but it is difficult to understand the functional significance of this complicated circuitry. The extent to which the Purkinje cells inhibit the deep cerebellar and vestibular nuclei must be dependent on the extent to which the Purkinje cells are being excited by the granule cells and climbing fibers at a given moment. It seems that the more the Purkinje cells are excited by these cells the more they will exert their inhibitory capabilities. In addition the Purkinje cells can inhibit the inhibitory influences of the outer stellate and basket cells (disinhibition that is shown on the diagram), and this further enhances the potency of the inhibitory influence of the Purkinje cells. In summary, it can be said that the degree to which the efferent outflow of the Purkinje cells inhibits their target nuclei depends on the balance between those excitatory and inhibitory neurons that impinge upon them at any given time.

There are several efferent projections from the three functional parts of the cerebellum. Those that do not project directly to the vestibular nuclei project to their terminations after synapsing in the deep cerebellar nuclei.

THE ARCHICEREBELLUM

Purkinje cell axons from the archicerebellum are responsible for the direct projections to the vestibular nuclei that have been mentioned previously. In addition, the archicerebellum projects to the ipsilateral vestibular nuclei after synapsing in the fastigial nucleus. These axons exit from the cerebellum through the inferior cerebellar peduncles to exert important influences on the vestibulospinal tracts and cranial nerves III, IV and VI, the nuclei of which receive projections from the vestibular nuclei. The archicerebellum therefore exerts its influence on spinal cord activity and the muscles that control the eyes.

THE PALEOCEREBELLUM

Purkinje cell axons which originate in the paleocerebellum project to the globose and

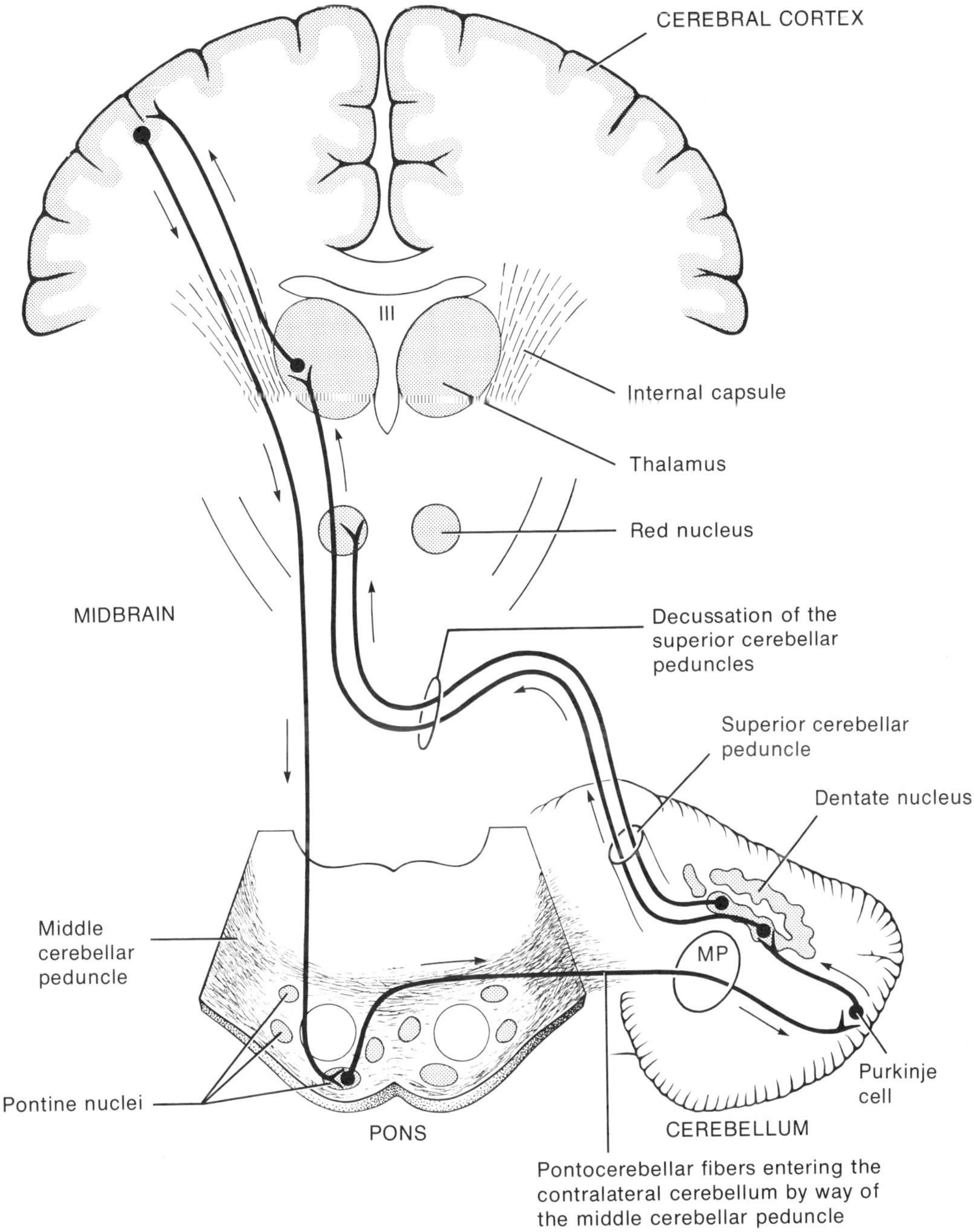

Figure 8–4. The cortico-ponto-cerebello-thalamo-cortical feedback loop. Neurons that originate in the cerebral cortex project to the ipsilateral pontine nuclei, synapse and cross to the contralateral side. These project to the neocerebellar cortex by way of the middle cerebellar peduncle (MP). Purkinje cell axons project primarily to the dentate nucleus (one of the deep cerebellar nuclei) where they synapse with neurons that exit the cerebellum by way of the superior cerebellar peduncle. These cross in the decussation of the superior cerebellar peduncle, after which they terminate in either the red nucleus or the thalamus. Those that terminate in the thalamus synapse with neurons that project back to the cerebral cortex. Notice that those fibers that terminate in the red nucleus in the midbrain are not a part of the feedback loop. These cerebellorubral fibers exert an influence on the rubrospinal and rubrobulbar systems.

fastigial nuclei. From these nuclei fibers project to the reticular formation, the red nucleus and the lateral vestibular nuclei bilaterally via the superior cerebellar peduncles. By way of these connections the paleocerebellum influences spinal cord reflex activity through the vestibulospinal, rubrospinal and reticulospinal tracts.

THE NEOCEREBELLUM

This is the site of origin of Purkinje cell axons that project to the dentate and emboliform nuclei. Via the superior cerebellar peduncles, these nuclei send some axons to the contralateral red nucleus to exert their influence on the rubrospinal system, and some axons by way of the ventrolateral and ventroanterior nucleus of the thalamus to the motor area of the cerebral cortex. The fibers that project to the motor cortex complete a feedback loop between the cerebral cortex and the cerebellar cortex. Fibers from the motor cortex project to the pontine nuclei, which in turn project to the neocerebellum by way of the middle cerebellar peduncles (the corticopontocerebellar pathway described earlier). The fibers that project from the neocerebellar cortex to the motor area of the cerebral cortex provide the other one-half of the loop, so that we have a cortico-ponto-cerebellar-thalamo-cortical feedback loop by which the cerebral cortex can influence the cerebellum, which in turn can influence the cerebral cortex. These connections are illustrated in Figure 8–4.

It is important to understand that the connections between the cerebellum and cerebral cortex are crossed because this arrangement makes good teleologic sense. The cerebellum receives the vast majority of its information from the ipsilateral side of the body; the motor cortex controls the contralateral side. Therefore, the cerebral cortex is receiving the cerebellar information from the side of the body which it controls, and can respond by exerting its influence on the side of the body from which the information originated.

Thus, the cerebellum receives information from the skin, muscles and vestibular system in addition to monitoring impulses from wide regions of the cerebral cortex. It then projects by way of complex pathways to the spinal cord, reticular formation, vestibular nuclei, basal ganglia, thalamus, red nucleus and cerebral cortex, providing extensive interconnections with many important structures of the nervous system. There follows on the opposite page a simplified diagrammatic representation of the afferent and efferent projections of the three divisions of the cerebellum.

A diagrammatic representation such as this may be misleading because it separates the functional divisions of the cerebellum a little too neatly. The reader should be cautioned that there is some overlap in function between the three divisions.

DISORDERS

The cerebellum is extremely important in the control of movement, so that cerebellar lesions are characterized by a constellation of disorders of movement. Specific symptoms are produced by selective lesions in various parts of the cerebellum.

Damage to the *archicerebellum* produces:

1. *Nystagmus,* which is probably an expression of impairment of cerebellar mechanisms that control the synergy and tone of the extraocular muscles.
2. *Loss of equilibrium.*
3. *Ataxia,* which is a distortion of basic movement patterns, and results in unsteady movements such as a weaving gait. If the lesion is unilateral, the patient veers toward the side of the lesion.

Damage to the *paleocerebellum* may result in *hypotonia.* The muscles become flabby and tire easily owing to interruption of afferent input from the stretch receptors and/or destruction of efferent pathways that facilitate the fusimotor system.

Damage to the *neocerebellum* may produce a number of symptoms:

1. *Asynergia,* or incoordination (lack of ability of parts that normally act in unison to do so). One way of testing for asynergia is to use what is known as the "rebound phenomenon." This entails the patient practicing elbow joint flexion against resistance. When the resistance is suddenly discontinued, the normal response is to remain in the same degree of flexion as when the resistance was exerted. Patients with neocerebellar damage will immediately flex further when the

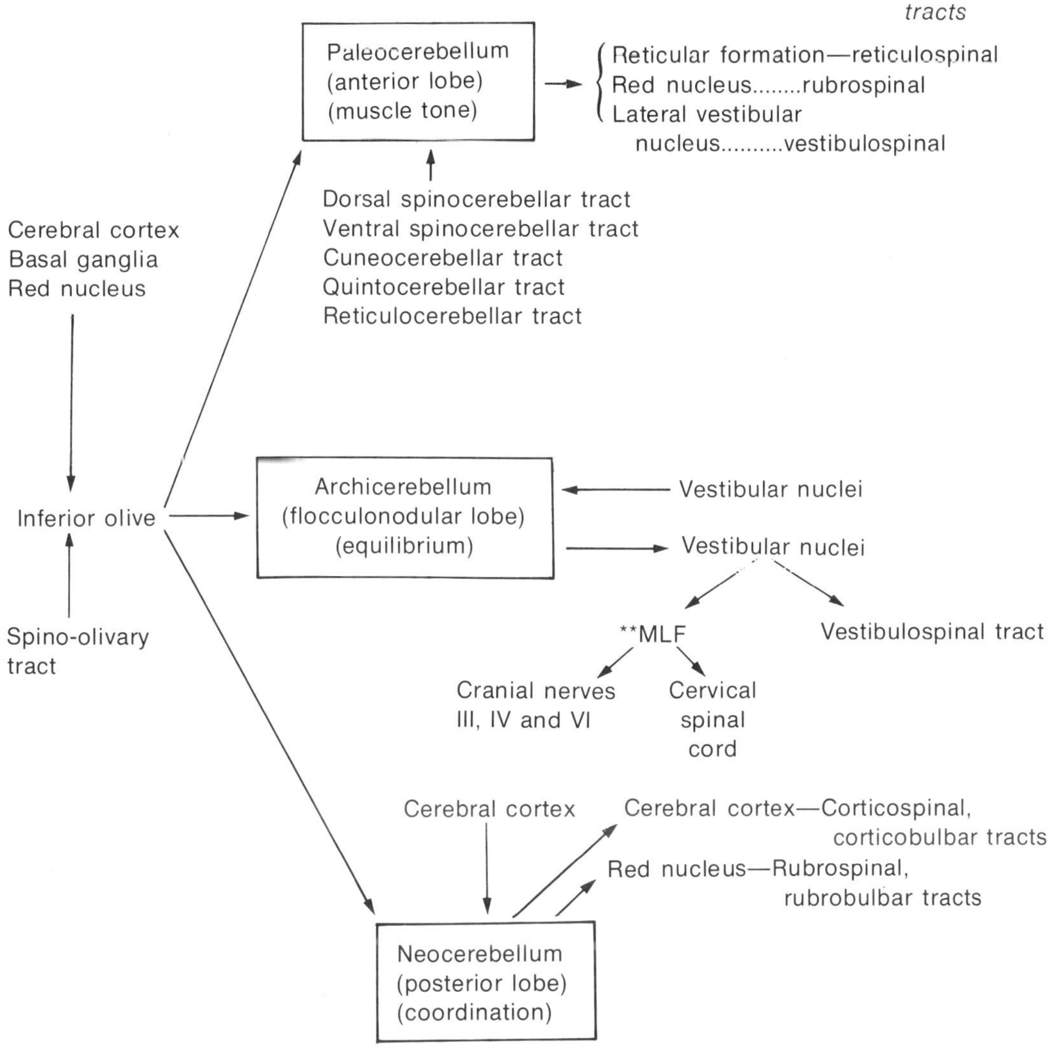

resistance is removed and may even hit themselves in the face. Be careful!

2. *Ataxia.*
3. *Adiadokokinesia,* or the inability to perform rapid, alternating movements. One way to test for adiadokokinesia is to have the patient flex his elbows to 90 degrees and ask him to rapidly pronate and supinate at the radioulnar joints. Normally this can be performed easily, but with neocerebellar damage it cannot be done. As the patient attempts the task he will go into varying degrees of shoulder joint abduction and will not be successful.
4. *Dysmetria,* or the inability to gauge distances accurately. Tests for this include having the patient (1) touch his nose with the index finger with the eyes open or shut and (2) run the heel of one foot lightly along the opposite anterior border of the tibia.
5. *Intention tremor,* which is a coarse, irregular tremor evident only during voluntary movements.

Since the connections of the cerebellum are primarily with those systems that project from or control the ipsilateral side of the body, the signs of cerebellar damage always involve the side of the body ipsilateral to the site of the lesion. The most severe symptoms are produced when there is damage to the connections of the cerebellum with the brain stem or the cerebral cortex.

**MLF = medial longitudinal fasciculus

REVIEW QUESTIONS

1. What are the functions of the cerebellum?
2. Correlate the functions of the cerebellum with its specific morphologic divisions.
3. Diagram the entire afferent input to the cerebellum according to the functional divisions in which they terminate.
4. Show which cell types, i.e., granule cells, climbing fibers, stellates, etc., exert an excitatory and which an inhibitory influence on Purkinje cells.
5. What influence do the Purkinje cells have on the deep cerebellar nuclei? Trace the efferent outputs from the deep cerebellar nuclei.
6. What is the functional significance of the crossed feedback loop between the cerebellum and the cerebral cortex?
7. List and define the symptoms of lesions of: a. the archicerebellum. b. the paleocerebellum. c. the neocerebellum.
   Are the symptoms of lesions ipsilateral or contralateral to the site of the lesion?

CHAPTER 9 • MOTOR SYSTEMS

OBJECTIVES

After reading this chapter you should: • Understand how the motor systems interconnect to produce meaningful movement. • Understand the underlying mechanisms responsible for the production of decerebrate rigidity. • Understand the role of the vestibular system in posture and movement. • Know the various types of labyrinthine righting reflexes and be able to give some examples of how they may be utilized to advantage clinically. • Know the structures that constitute the basal ganglia, and learn the interconnections of the structures and the symptoms produced by lesions of the specific nuclei comprising the basal ganglia.

MOTOR SYSTEMS

When there is damage to structures of the central nervous system, varying degrees of muscular rigidity and flaccidity are observed. From a clinical point of view it is important to examine the descending influences in the central nervous system that control muscle tone and voluntary and involuntary movements, in order to understand the mechanisms that produce these conditions.

Brain Stem Influences on Spinal Reflexes

This is an appropriate place to review the information from earlier chapters about the two ways of controlling the amount of activity produced in extrafusal muscle fibers. The muscle may be stimulated to contract directly by alpha motor neurons or indirectly by means of the gamma motor system. Normally, the activity of these two pathways is organized to produce smooth, coordinated movement, but independence of function of the two systems can be demonstrated experimentally and does exist in abnormal situations.

Sir Charles Sherrington first introduced what is now considered the classic "decerebrate preparation," which is an animal in which a complete brain stem transection is done between the superior and inferior colliculi. This produces a mesencephalic animal, i.e., one in which the highest level of control of the nervous system is the midbrain, since the connections from the cerebral cortex have been cut. Such an experimental animal develops profound hypertonicity or spasticity in the antigravity muscles, which is referred to as *decerebrate rigidity*. In most quadruped animals the hypertonicity is produced in the extensor groups of muscles. In human beings, however, the hypertonicity usually occurs in the flexors in the upper extremity instead of the extensors. This may be due to the fact that man has a cervical flexure associated with the brain whereas other species do not. This flexure places the semicircular canals in man in a different orientation in space from that in lower animals, and may account for the difference.

It is interesting that the antigravity muscles of the sloth are the flexors, since his means of getting around is by swinging from limb to limb. An intercollicular section in this animal produces hypertonicity in the flexors. The increase in the muscular tone in any species is not static. It can be altered by changing the position of the head. For example, if the cervical intervertebral joints are flexed, the forelimbs or upper extremities tend to flex and the hind limbs or lower extremities tend to extend (symmetric tonic neck reflexes).

The development of hypertonicity due to intercollicular section is an example of a situation in which the alpha and gamma motor systems are not functioning in accord, and the mechanisms involved can be explained at least partially on the following basis. Part of the medullary reticular formation is inhibitory to spinal cord reflex activity. Parts of the cerebral cortex and the basal ganglia exert an excitatory influence on the medullary reticular formation, thus normally exciting inhibition. Therefore, when the connections from the cerebral cortex and basal ganglia to the medullary reticular formation are cut, as they are in the decerebrate preparation, there is no stimulus to produce medullary inhibition of spinal cord reflex activity. At the same time, other parts of the medullary and pontine reticular formation enhance spinal cord reflex activity because of a continuous afferent input from the anterior lobe of the cerebellum. These connections remain intact. The excitatory influence of those parts of the reticular formation that receive afferents from the anterior lobe of the cerebellum then act unopposed by the inhibitory portion of the reticular formation to produce muscular hypertonus in the antigravity muscles.

The evidence shows that *the facilitation of extensors occurs primarily by way of the indirect gamma route* rather than through the direct alpha route. This has been shown by two different experiments, sectioning dorsal roots and selectively anesthetizing gamma motor neurons. Either procedure eliminates the rigidity. Sectioning the dorsal roots prevents impulses from being conducted along the IA nerve fibers back to alpha motor neurons in the ventral horns, and of course anesthetizing the gamma motor neurons eliminates impulse conduction to the intrafusal fibers of the muscle spindles. If the hypertonicity had been produced by the direct alpha route neither of these procedures would have abolished it.

The following is a diagrammatic representation of the mechanisms that produce hypertonicity:

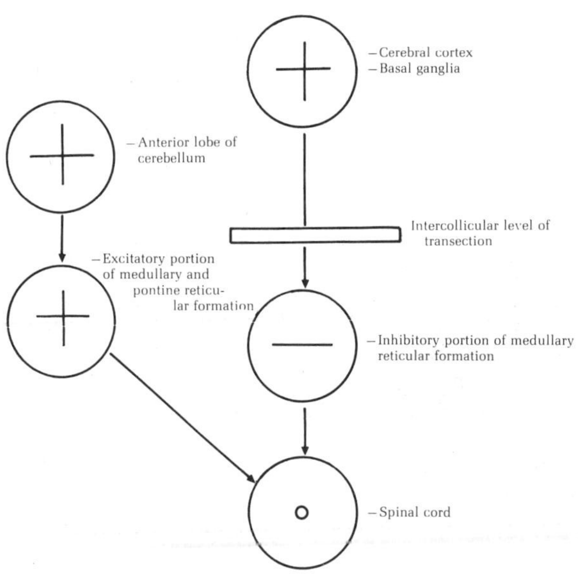

The diagram summarizes the following. The intercollicular section has eliminated the excitatory influence of the cerebral cortex and basal ganglia upon the inhibitory portion of the medullary reticular formation. Therefore, this portion of the reticular formation no longer inhibits spinal cord activity. At the same time the anterior lobe of the cerebellum stimulates the excitatory portions of the medullary and pontine reticular formation to enhance activity in the spinal cord. This enhancement of activity is now unopposed and the net effect is the production of hypertonicity.

If the anterior lobe of the cerebellum is removed in addition to an intercollicular section, the degree of hypertonicity increases. This may be explained by the fact that the lateral vestibular nucleus normally exerts an excitatory influence upon spinal cord activity by way of the vestibulospinal tracts. Although the anterior lobe of the cerebellum exerts an excitatory influence upon the reticular formation, it exerts an inhibitory influence upon the lateral vestibular nucleus. Therefore, when the anterior lobe of the cerebellum is removed, the lateral vestibular nucleus produces an unopposed excitatory influence upon the spinal cord, as followed in the illustration below. The anterior lobe of the cerebellum no longer exerts its excitatory influence upon the reticular formation or its inhibitory influence upon the lateral vestibular nucleus. In this situation the hypertonicity is due to alpha motor neuron hyperactivity. This has been shown by cutting the dorsal roots subsequent to the removal of the anterior lobe of the cerebellum, which neither abolishes nor diminishes the muscular hypertonicity.

The evidence that the influence of the lateral vestibular nucleus is excitatory is based on the fact that if one destroys that nucleus in a preparation with both an intercollicular section and removal of the anterior lobe of the cerebellum, the hypertonicity is eliminated, showing that no other center is producing the rigidity. However, if the lateral vestibular nucleus is destroyed in an animal with an intercollicular section, but with an intact cerebellum, the hypertonicity persists. This is because the anterior lobe of the cerebellum enhances activity in the excitatory portions of the reticular formation.

The mechanism by which the gamma system becomes inoperative when the anterior lobe of the cerebellum is removed is presumably the elimination of the facilitatory influence of that part of the cerebellum upon the reticular formation facilitatory regions. It must be assumed, then, that the vestibulospinal tracts have a greater influence upon alpha than upon gamma motor neurons. The switch from gamma to alpha hyperactivity is known appropriately as the

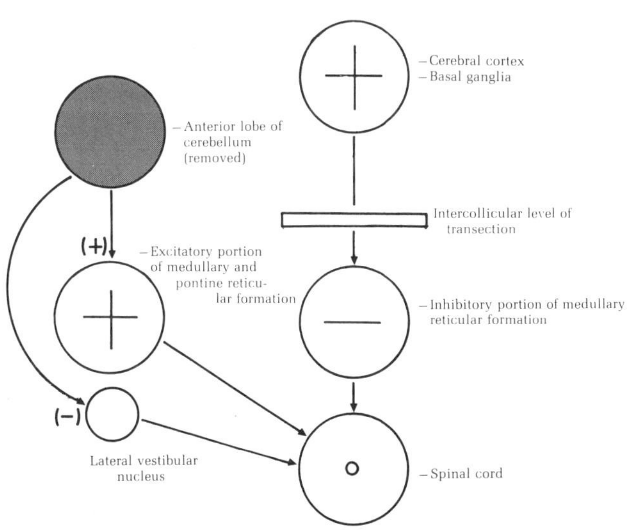

gamma–alpha switch. The point to be emphasized here is that the anterior lobe of the cerebellum plays a crucial role in the normal distribution of supraspinal influences upon alpha and gamma motor neurons. From a clinical point of view we cannot distinguish between patients with the alpha and the gamma type of hypertonicity, except that hypertonicity produced by alpha motor neurons tends to be more severe. However, the degree of rigidity present in different patients with the same lesions is variable, so that this is not a reliable criterion on which to base a decision.

Patients with injury or disease in more caudal areas of the central nervous system may also develop spasticity or hypertonicity in the musculature, which is innervated by nerves that leave the brain stem or spinal cord inferior to the level of the lesion. Patients with spinal cord injuries typically go through a period of spinal shock lasting for a period of between three and six weeks, owing to elimination of the normal background excitatory influences of the higher centers upon the spinal cord. Gradually, reflex activity returns and increases beyond normal levels so that the patient has hyperactive reflexes and spasticity that persists. The hypertonicity now reflects the absence of the normal inhibitory influences of the long descending systems upon spinal cord reflex activity.

A discussion of brain stem influences upon spinal cord activity is not complete without examination of the vestibular system, which has such an important influence upon posture and movement. The vestibular receptors are the saccule, utricle and semicircular canals, all of which are located within the petrous portion of the temporal bone. These receptors are commonly called the *labyrinths.* The saccule and utricle contain a receptor called the *macula,* which is made up of elongated sensory epithelial cells and supporting cells. Sensory hairs which extend from the sensory epithelial cells are embedded in a gelatin-like substance that covers the surface of the macula. The semicircular canals contain a similar receptor called a *crista.* The three semicircular canals, the saccule and the utricle all contain a liquid substance called *endolymph.* This is displaced in the semicircular canals when the labyrinths are stimulated. The movement of the endolymph in turn stimulates the sensory hairs of the cristae. Impulses from these receptors project to the vestibular nuclei, and some project directly to the cerebellum.

The semicircular canals are placed at right angles to each other. The anterior and posterior canals are oriented vertically and are located at an angle of about 45 degrees from the frontal and sagittal planes of the skull. The horizontal canal is placed at an angle of approximately 30 degrees inferior to the horizontal plane of the skull.

There are two types of labyrinthine reflex, referred to as labyrinthine acceleratory and labyrinthine positional reflexes. The former are elicited by passive or active movements of the head. The stimulus producing this transient type of reflex activity is a change in velocity of movement which distorts the hair cells. In the past this type of reflex activity has been attributed to stimulation of the semicircular canals, and it was believed that labyrinthine positional reflexes were elicited by the location of the maculae of the saccule and utricle in space. However, Mountcastle's review of the literature on this subject (1974) indicates that the semicircular canals and the saccule and utricle function more as a whole, and that it may be a mistake to assign specific functions to the different structures involved. The labyrinthine positional reflexes are tonic in nature so that the response lasts as long as a particular position is maintained.

One of the best examples of labyrinthine acceleratory reflexes is the normal production of nystagmus during and after rotation of the entire body. Nystagmus consists of an alternating slow and fast component of eye movement occurring in opposite directions. The movements are produced by projections from the semicircular canals to the medial vestibular nucleus, which in turn projects by way of the medial longitudinal fasciculus to the nuclei of cranial nerves III, IV and VI, which control the extraocular muscles. The nystagmus is named for the direction in which the fast component occurs. When an individual is rotated an attempt is made to keep the eyes fixed on an object, but as the rotation proceeds, this becomes impossible and the eyes quickly move in the opposite direction to gaze at a different object. This sequence is repeated over and over again. When the rotation movement ceases suddenly, the nystagmus continues, but the fast and slow components then become reversed. The nystagmus produced by rotation is due to accelerated movement; that produced by suddenly stopping the rotation is a result of deceleration. There are three main types of nystagmus — horizontal, rotatory or vertical—and the type elicited depends on how the plane of rotation relates to the semicircular canals.

The labyrinthine positional or tonic labyrinthine reflexes are illustrated best in an experimental animal which has been decerebrated and in which the tonic neck reflexes are nonfunctional. In such an animal the tone in the extensor muscles of all four extremities increases when the subject is supine and decreases when it is prone. As the body of the animal is moved into intermediate positions, varying degrees of extensor tone are produced. In the side-lying position the extensors in the extremities which are in contact with the supporting surface have increased tone in the extensors, and those muscles of the extremities of the upper side have increased tone in the flexors. These reflexes act through the vestibulospinal and reticulospinal tracts because of projections from the vestibular nuclei to the reticular formation. The tonic labyrinthine reflexes can be evoked very easily in brain-damaged children.

The role of the vestibular system in the production of motion sickness has been well established and apparently is based on the connections of the vestibular system with the cerebellum. Removal of those parts of the cerebellum to which the vestibular system projects abolishes the motion sickness.

Because of the importance of the vestibular system to movement and posture, a number of clinical tests have been developed to evaluate the integrity of this system. The most useful of these involve a *caloric* and a *rotation* test.

In the caloric test warm (112 degrees F) or cold water (68 degrees F) is introduced into the external acoustic meatus, and this normally produces nystagmus, past-pointing and turning sensations. Past-pointing is described as follows: with the eyes closed, the individual is asked to extend his upper extremity, fully flex it and then lower it in the sagittal plane. Normally, if the labyrinths are not being stimulated, he will be able to return the extremity to the original starting point. However, if the labyrinths are being stimulated it is normal not to be able to do so. The individual will return the arm further toward the direction in which he thinks he is turning. If these reactions are not produced there is a lesion in the vestibular system or in its connections with other CNS structures.

The rotation test involves rotating the individual several times with the head in a position that puts the specific semicircular canals to be tested in the plane of rotation. The same reactions should be produced as for the caloric test if the vestibular system and its connections are intact.

Abnormal function of the vestibular system has been associated with retarded development of motor skills and learning disabilities. Because of this, Rood (1956), the Bobaths (1967, 1971) and Ayers (1975) have stressed the importance of stimulation of the vestibular system in their clinical practice. Since little evidence existed to support this view, Clark, Kreutzberg and Chee (1976) set out to test this hypothesis. In one study their group exposed three preambulatory children (one normal and two with Down's syndrome) to ten sessions of semicircular canal stimulation in two weeks. The motor skills test scores were markedly improved compared with those of four control subjects.

They then studied 26 normal, preambulatory infants between three and 13 months of age to determine their level of performance on reflex and motor skills tests. Seventeen reflexes were examined. The motor skills were evaluated in five areas of increasing difficulty: prone and supine positions, sitting, creeping, standing and walking. Each infant received 16 sessions of semicircular canal stimulation over a period of four weeks. Two sessions, separated by 30 minutes, were given on each of two days of every week. A session consisted of ten spins in a rotating chair on the lap of one of the investigators in a darkened room. Each spin consisted of a rapid (one- to three-second) angular acceleration, and a one-minute period of constant velocity rotation at 16.7 revolutions per minute, followed by a sudden stop in less than one second. Further details of positioning are available in the original paper.

The performance of the infants on the reflex and motor skills tests was reassessed four days after the last day of vestibular stimulation and compared with that of infants who had not been included in the sessions. The stimulated infants scored significantly higher than the unstimulated ones on both the reflex and motor skills tests. Interestingly, the experiment included a pair of three-month-old fraternal twins. Their pretest scores were identical, but, after one of them remained in the control group and the other was exposed to vestibular stimulation, the twin in the treatment group had mastered head control and could sit independently. The twin in the control group was developing head control but had not progressed beyond motor behavior in the prone and supine positions. They were four months old when the study was completed.

The authors suggest that vestibular stimulation may be important in developing effective use of semicircular canal-controlled eye movements. The stimulation may facilitate maturation of vestibulo-ocular reflexes and provide the visual system with a more stable retinal image against which motor involvement with the environment develops more rapidly. It may also influence motor behavior through vestibulospinal reflex facilitation of spinal cord mechanisms. Studies such as this suggest that the hypothesis of the clinicians, at least with respect to development of motor skills, is correct. More positive statements may be made if follow-up studies, with such parameters as matched age and weight taken into account, produce similar results.

The vestibular system is responsible for the labyrinthine righting reflexes, which are present at birth and are most obvious in decorticate animals and brain-damaged children. In these, no matter how the body is positioned, the head has a tendency to remain in its normal position with respect to gravity as long as the body is in contact with an underlying surface. This is called the *body righting reflex acting on the head*. The *neck righting reflex* involves other parts of the body following the head into the normal position. Asymmetric stimulation of the body sometimes allows the body to right itself even though the head is tipped laterally. This is called the *body righting reflex acting on the body*.

These reflexes can be used to advantage clinically, particularly when one is working with children. For example, as the Bobaths (1967, 1971) advocate, if the goal is to get the child to move from prone or supine to sitting or standing, appropriate maneuvering of the head by the clinician can provide the sensory cues that allow the child to do so. The body righting reaction on the body provides patterns of rotation within the body axis — the hips follow the shoulders and vice versa. This type of activity is important in preparation for turning from supine to prone, sitting up from prone, side-sitting, and getting on to hands and knees in the process of standing up.

Closely related to the righting reactions are the equilibrium reactions, which are mediated by the cerebral cortex. If the center of gravity of an individual is displaced so that it is in danger of falling outside the base of support, the position of the whole body is adjusted in relation to the supporting surface in order to maintain balance. These equilibrium reactions appear at approximately six months postnatally.

It is the philosophy of the Bobaths that the righting and equilibrium reactions normally act harmoniously with each other and provide the background against which all purposeful movements and skills are performed. Their treatment procedures are based on the assumption that normal postural reflex activity can be facilitated by eliciting normal motor patterns and inhibiting patterns of abnormal reflex activity through the use of specific techniques of handling the individual. These procedures have been directed primarily toward children with cerebral palsy and are appropriately described as "neurodevelopmental treatment" because the repertoire of techniques takes into account the main aspects of the difficulties of those with cerebral palsy, i.e., the neurologic and developmental deficits.

Rood (1956) gives some very specific examples of how she utilizes the labyrinthine reflexes. A direct quote from her paper follows:

1. "In a cerebral palsied baby, the serratus for shoulder flexion may not be activated by stroking the axilla in the back-lying position because of extensor tone of the labyrinth. But if the baby is turned on its side, the ear to the ground, the top side will be flexor predominant and the serratus can be elicited immediately."

2. "Flexion predominates in the feeding pattern. A baby with increased extensor tone from irritation of the labyrinth cannot feed from a bottle in the back-lying position. This is very easily corrected. The mother's breast placement would take care of this in the normal case."

Basal Ganglia

Several of the motor systems have been discussed in earlier chapters. They include the corticospinal tracts, which represent a *direct*, somatotopically organized system by which the cerebral cortex influences the spinal cord. The corticorubrospinal system is an *indirect*, somatotopically organized pathway by which the cerebral cortex influences the spinal cord. In addition, cortical fibers project to the brain stem reticular formation and indirectly influence the spinal cord via the reticulospinal pathways, in which there is no somatotopic organization. The point to remember is that the cerebral cortex influences spinal cord activity not only directly but through a variety of projections to the brain stem, as well as through projections to a group of subcortical telencephalic nuclei called the *basal ganglia*.

The group of four nuclei comprising the basal ganglia is very important in motor function, and includes the *caudate nucleus, putamen, globus pallidus* and *amygdaloid nucleus*. Technically, the substantia nigra and subthalamic nucleus are not included as basal ganglia because the former is found primarily in the mesencephalon and the latter originates from the diencephalon, whereas the basal ganglia originate from the telencephalon. However, the functions of the substantia nigra and subthalamic nucleus are so closely related to those of the basal ganglia that they will be included in this discussion. Functionally, the amygdaloid nucleus is part of the limbic system, which

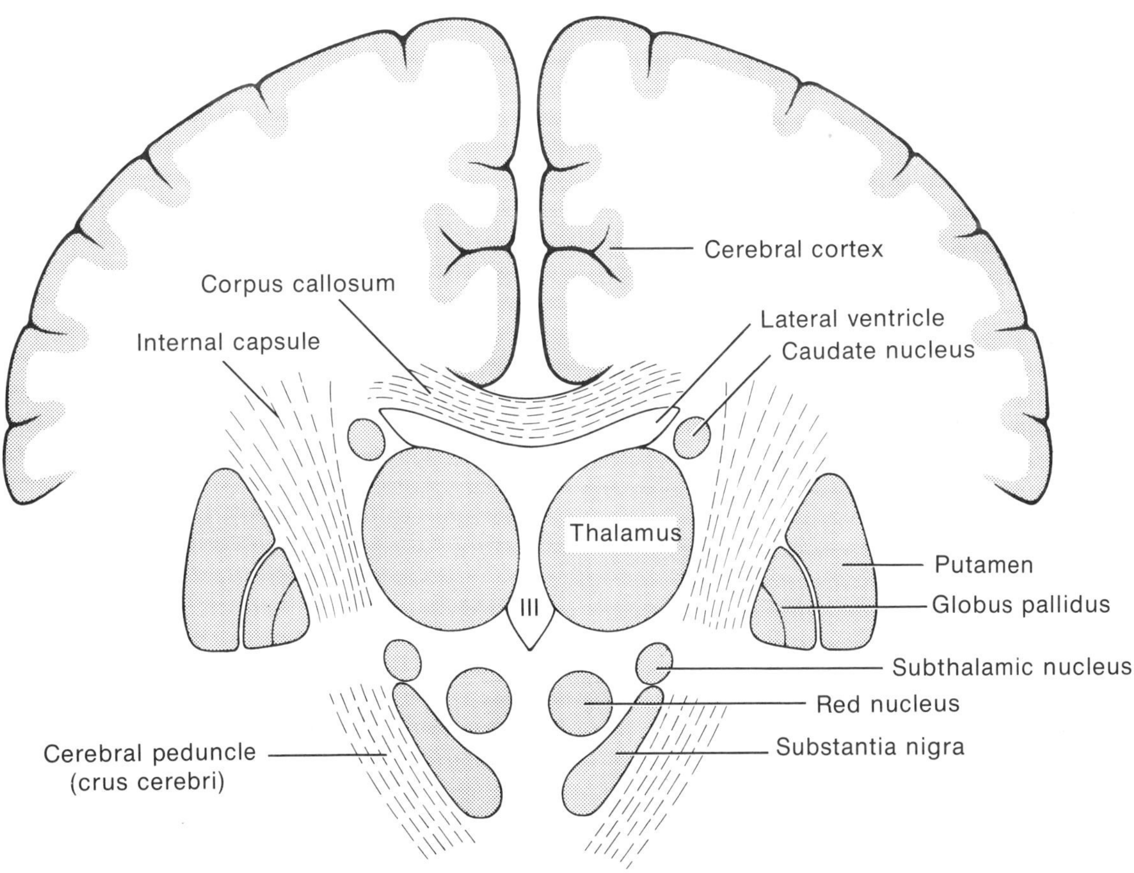

Figure 9–1. A coronal section through the thalamus and midbrain to show the basal ganglia.

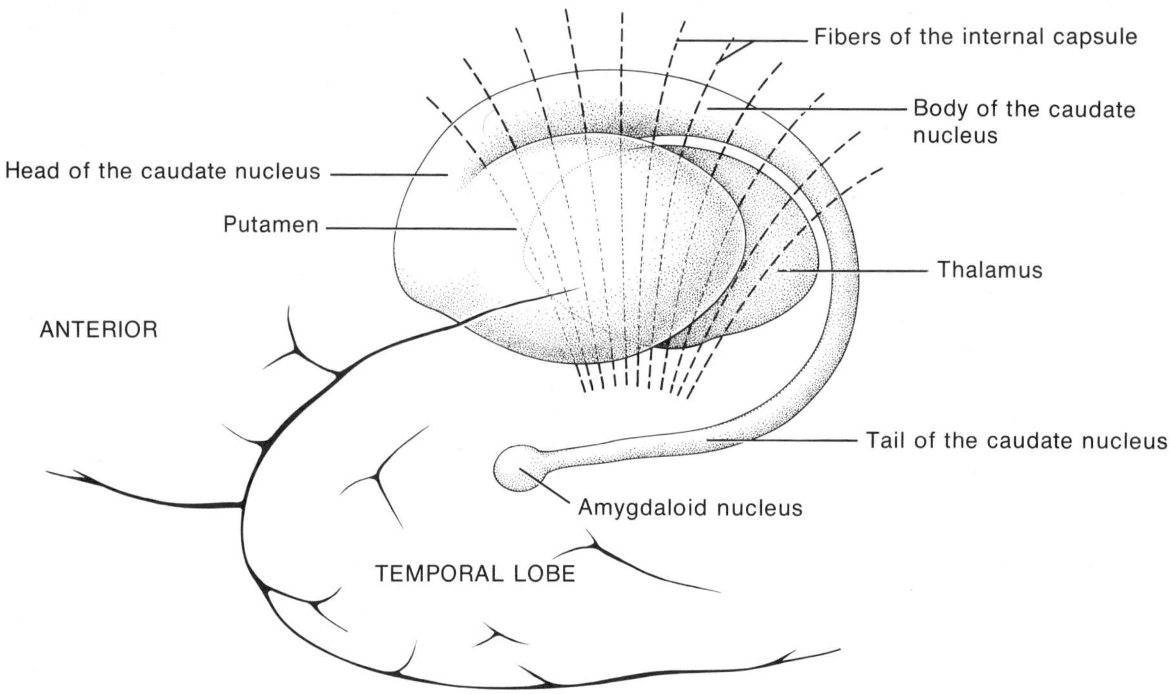

Figure 9–2. A lateral view of the putamen, caudate nucleus and amygdaloid nucleus. Notice that the head of the caudate nucleus and the putamen are continuous with each other, and the tail of the caudate nucleus is continuous with the amygdaloid nucleus. The caudate nucleus is c-shaped, following the contour of the lateral ventricle. The fibers of the internal capsule (*dashed lines*) pass lateral to the thalamus and caudate nucleus, and medial to the putamen.

will be discussed in a later chapter. The structures associated with the basal ganglia are shown in Figure 9–1, although there is a more intimate relationship between some parts of the basal ganglia than this may suggest. This can only be appreciated by a representation of the putamen, caudate nucleus and amygdaloid nucleus from a lateral view (see Fig. 9–2). The combination of the putamen and globus pallidus is called the *lentiform nucleus* and the putamen and caudate nucleus are often collectively referred to as the *striatum*.

The interconnections of the basal ganglia are quite complex, but it is necessary to know something about them if one is to understand the disorders of movement produced by their abnormal function. The striatum (putamen plus caudate nucleus) receives heavy bilateral projections from all regions of the cerebral cortex. In turn, the striatum projects to the globus pallidus and has reciprocal connections with the substantia nigra. The substantia nigra and globus pallidus both project to the reticular formation and to the ventrolateral (VL), ventroanterior (VA) and centrum medianum (CM) nuclei of the thalamus. The globus pallidus has reciprocal connections with the subthalamic nucleus. The VL, VA and CM of the thalamus, which are under the influence of the cerebellum, project back to the striatum and to the cerebral cortex. Examination of this circuitry reveals that it actually consists of a feedback loop, which in general originates in the cerebral cortex and projects to the basal ganglia, on to the thalamus and back to the cerebral cortex. This loop may be represented diagrammatically as followed on the opposite page.

The loop involves information processing by mechanisms that are not well understood. It is important to realize that the basal ganglia do not project directly to the spinal cord nor to cranial nerve nuclei. They influence the spinal cord and cranial nerve nuclei only indirectly, by their projections to the cerebral cortex and to the reticular formation, and probably are responsible for only gross types of movement.

Existing evidence strongly suggests that the globus pallidus is the efferent gateway

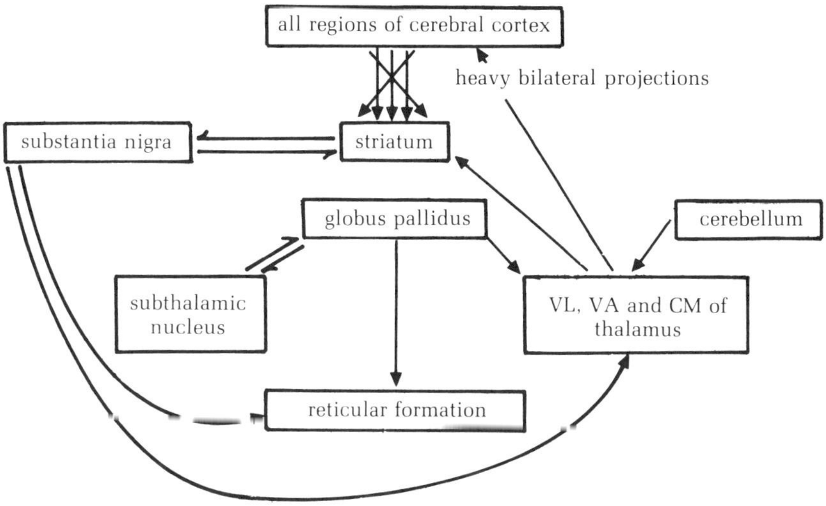

of the basal ganglia circuitry and that it exerts an excitatory influence upon structures to which it projects. In general, the nuclei that project to the globus pallidus, i.e., the caudate nucleus and subthalamic nucleus, inhibit its activity.

Attempts have been made to study the functions of each specific basal nucleus by electrical stimulation and ablation experiments. It has been found that, examined against a background of either posture or movements concurrently induced by stimulation of the cerebral cortex, stimulation of the caudate nucleus produces inhibition in the form of breaking up a sustained postural attitude or interrupting the cortically induced movement. Arrest of movement also occurs when the thalamus is stimulated. Stimulation of the caudate nucleus and putamen does not produce movement, which is consistent with the view that the striatum does not function independent of cerebral cortical influence. Rather, the striatum appears to be involved with controlling the component parts of complex movement.

LESIONS OF SPECIFIC BASAL AND ASSOCIATED NUCLEI

The basal ganglia indirectly feed back to the ipsilateral cerebral cortex, and therefore lesions of the basal ganglia are manifested on the side of the body contralateral to the lesion since the cerebral cortex controls the contralateral side of the body by way of the crossed corticospinal tracts.

Small lesions of the caudate nucleus have little effect, but large lesions produce hyperactivity involving involuntary movements known as *dyskinesias*. Two types of dyskinesia (hyperkinesias) may be produced by lesions of the caudate nucleus and putamen: *athetosis*, characterized by slow, writhing, wormlike movements, and *chorea*, a brisk, graceful series of movements. Either type is enhanced by voluntary activity, further emphasizing the fact that the striatum is concerned with inhibitory control over cortical voluntary activity. Huntington's chorea, one specific variety of dyskinesia, is an hereditary disease, the symptoms of which usually do not manifest themselves before the age of 30. Atrophy of the caudate nucleus has long been recognized as accompanying the disease, which is practically defiant of successful treatment in our current state of knowledge. Reserpine (a dopamine depleting agent) relieves the severity of the involuntary movements to some extent, but doses of up to 8 milligrams a day are required for the relief of symptoms and this amount can cause very profound depression.

We know that electrical stimulation of the globus pallidus interrupts cortically-induced movements, but the role of this nucleus is more obscure than that of the striatum. Lesions of the globus pallidus produce hypokinesias (paucity of movement), reflecting the lack of its normal excitatory influence upon the structures to which it projects. In recent years attempts to reduce extrapyramidal (all spinal pathways excluding the corticospinal tracts) symptoms such as athetosis and chorea have been made by completely destroying the globus pallidus (chemopallidectomy). This procedure has reduced the dyskinetic activity without producing any additional motor signs. Since the influence of the globus pallidus upon the structures to which it projects is excitatory, lesions of the striatum may release the globus pallidus by withdrawal of inhibitory controls upon it, to produce hyperkinesias. Subsequent destruction of the globus pallidus then logically decreases or eliminates the symptoms.

Lesions of the subthalamic nucleus produce a third type of dyskinesia, called *hemiballismus* if the lesion is unilateral and *ballismus* if it is bilateral. This is the most violent of the hyperkinesias and involves forceful, flinging, violent movements, particularly of the proximal extremities and pelvic musculature, which persist throughout every waking moment and only cease during sleep. Lesions in the subthalamus, like those in the striatum, probably release the globus pallidus and perhaps other structures from inhibitory control.

Large lesions of the substantia nigra result in almost complete loss of the gamma activating system of muscle spindles and also produce one of the most common manifestations of basal ganglia disorders, *Parkinson's disease.* Normally the projections from the substantia nigra to the striatum are rich in the transmitter dopamine, but in patients with this disease a paucity of dopamine has been found in the striatum. This produces a constellation of behavior, which includes lack of facial expression; slowed speech; stooped posture; a slow, shuffling gait that later may develop into a "festinating gait" (the patient walks faster and faster with very small steps until finally the only way he can stop himself is by running into something); a general poverty of movement; resting tremor (the fingers look as if they are "pill rolling"); and a cogwheel type of rigidity in both flexor and extensor muscle groups. Cogwheel rigidity consists of alternate contraction and relaxation as an extremity is moved passively, resulting in a very jerky type of movement.

Unlike the hyperkinesias, Parkinson's disease results in a disabling reduction in voluntary and associated movements in addition to rigidity and tremor. Although the disease was first described approximately 150 years ago, none of the mechanisms of its three major components are thoroughly understood. The severity of symptoms and the degree to which each component is manifested vary from patient to patient, suggesting that several CNS structures may be involved. It has been suggested that loss of collateral neurons from the substantia nigra relayed to the globus pallidus by way of the striatum permits hyperactivity of the pallidothalamic system, thus causing the rigidity. The tendency for hypokinesia and rigidity to occur in different proportions in different patients suggests that rigidity is not the only basis for poverty of movement, but there is no good physiologic or anatomic explanation for a selective poverty of movement in this disease.

The resting tremor involves alternating antagonistic muscular contractions that occur at a very constant rate for long periods in a given muscle group, primarily the distal musculature. Although the specific sites of damage that produce tremor are obscure, it has been found that surgical intervention in the neural loop between cortical motor areas, putamen, globus pallidus, thalamus and back to motor areas reduces tremor, rigidity and hypokinesia. Thus, one of the more attractive hypotheses to explain the production of tremor is that the reverberating circuit from the cerebral cortex back to the cerebral cortex produces an oscillation type of movement. Interruption of the circuit at any of the sites mentioned above may eliminate effectively the reverberating, oscillating type of movement that constitutes the tremor.

Good treatment by occupational and physical therapists may reduce the manifestations of Parkinson's disease. Exercise programs tailored to the individual needs of the patient can improve the stooped posture, retard the progression to general poverty of movement, improve muscle tone and assist the patient's morale.

Several drugs have been utilized for the

treatment of Parkinson's disease, with three goals in mind:

1. To increase the release of stored dopamine.
2. To decrease the activity of acetylcholine.
3. To increase the amount of dopamine in the brain.

In the past Artane, an anticholinergic agent, was the drug of choice, on the grounds that it would help to return the balance between acetylcholine and dopamine and thus restore a normal balance of excitatory and inhibitory influences. Although this drug was effective in reducing the manifestations of the disease, it produced some rather severe side-effects, which included dryness of the mouth, constipation, confusion, hallucinations, anorexia (loss of appetite), nausea and vomiting.

The discovery that amantadine, which follows in the pharmaceutical history, could benefit patients with Parkinson's disease was quite accidental. It is actually an antiviral agent, and when administered to such patients who incidentally suffered from viral infections the symptoms of Parkinson's disease diminished. It was subsequently discovered that amantadine blocks the presynaptic uptake of dopamine, thereby increasing the duration of its action. Amantadine was more effective for reduction of the symptoms of Parkinson's disease than Artane, but it produced the same side-effects in addition to disorientation, depression, nervousness and insomnia.

Something with less severe side-effects was needed and the next drug utilized was levodopa, frequently referred to as L-dopa. Levodopa is an immediate precursor to dopamine and can be incorporated into dopamine within the brain, thus increasing the dopamine level therein. The reason why dopamine itself was not the treatment of choice is that it cannot cross the blood–brain barrier, whereas levodopa can. This drug has been effective in relieving symptoms, but the biggest problem is that very high dosages are required since although levodopa can cross the blood–brain barrier only a small percentage of it does so. Levodopa is also capable of producing side-effects including nausea and vomiting, and if the required dosage is too high it may produce athetoid-like movements consisting of lip-smacking, grimacing, head-turning and involuntary movements of the limbs.

The latest drug available carries the commercial name of Sinemet, and consists of a combination of levodopa and carbidopa. Only the levodopa crosses the blood–brain barrier, but the carbidopa closely accompanies the levodopa and acts as a protective agent that prevents the destruction of the latter by enzymatic action. Under these circumstances only one-fourth of the levodopa is as effective for the relief of the symptoms of Parkinson's disease as when the levodopa is administered alone, and the side-effects, although similar to those produced by levodopa alone, are less severe.

Pyramidal vs. Extrapyramidal Systems

From a functional point of view the terms *pyramidal* and *extrapyramidal* are unsatisfactory, implying that the two systems function entirely independently, which is not the case. It has been demonstrated that all descending systems involve the cerebral cortex either directly or indirectly, and the cell bodies of both systems are interposed within the cerebral cortex. Literally, the terms are a definition of the location of the two systems as they descend in the medulla. The pyramidal system descends in the medullary pyramids and the extrapyramidal system does not. Since these expressions are currently used, it is important to know that *pyramidal system* and *the corticospinal tracts* are interchangeable terms, and that the extrapyramidal system includes all descending systems except the corticospinal tracts.

The deficits produced by lesions in the pyramidal and extrapyramidal tracts are usually complex because several fiber systems most often are involved. For example, a lesion in the internal capsule may interrupt the corticospinal and corticobulbar tracts, and corticorubral and thalamocortical fibers, as well as the cortico–striate–basal ganglia–thalamocortical loop, and this is not a complete list of the fiber systems that may be involved (see Fig. 9–3).

Selective lesions of any one descending system are extremely rare, very few naturally occurring pure corticospinal tract lesions having ever been reported in the literature. The functions of each system can only be

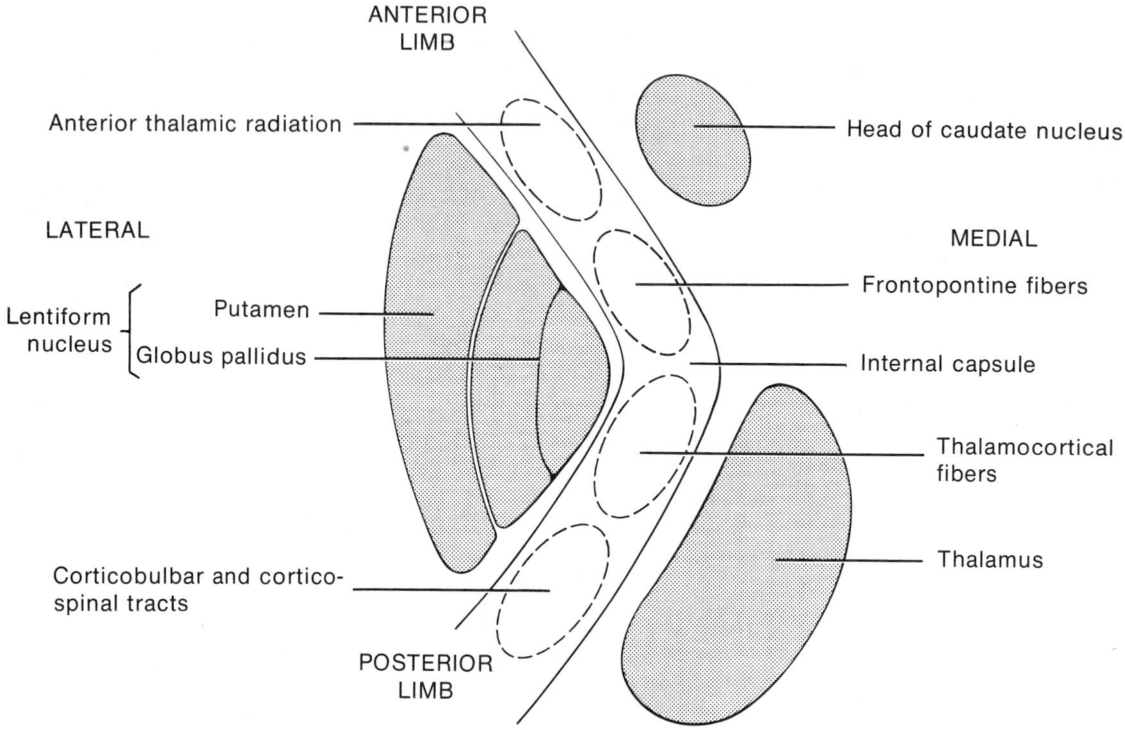

Figure 9–3. The locations of the ascending and descending systems within the internal capsule. The fibers of the extrapyramidal tracts are dispersed throughout the internal capsule. Discrete bundles of this pathway have not been traced.

analyzed by producing discrete lesions in experimental animals, and often this is difficult or impossible because of inaccessibility of tracts or structures, or because of too close an association with other structures so that damage to more than one system occurs. Therefore, the normal functions of the pyramidal and extrapyramidal systems have not been delineated clearly.

The extrapyramidal system is much older phylogenetically than the cerebral cortex. In submammalian species the diencephalon and corpus striatum are the highest sensorimotor mechanisms, the striatum being responsible for integration of motor activities and the thalamus for integrating incoming sensory information. These species are capable of only gross, postural, stereotyped kinds of movement. With the evolution of the cerebral cortex in mammals, the corpus striatum has become subservient to the cerebral cortex, but the older motor systems continue to function to produce postural adjustments, defense reactions, ambulatory activity and feeding. In other words, the older systems function in automatic types of activity, but normally these are under the control of the cerebral cortex.

REVIEW QUESTIONS

1. Explain by means of diagrams the underlying mechanisms responsible for the production of decerebrate rigidity. (This will help you to understand the basis for the varying degrees of rigidity or spasticity of the musculature in many of the patients you will see in the clinic, even though they may not be completely decerebrate.)
2. Explain the basis for the gamma–alpha switch.

3. What is responsible for the spinal shock that occurs following injury to the spinal cord?
4. Name the vestibular receptors.
5. Into which two categories do the labyrinthine reflexes fall?
6. Explain an example of a labyrinthine acceleratory reflex.
7. What position tends to produce maximum extensor tone in the musculature?
8. How would you position a patient to elicit extension in both upper and lower extremities on the right side?
9. What kinds of tests have been developed to test the integrity of the vestibular system? Explain each. What are the normal reactions to these tests?
10. What is the rationale behind the finding that vestibular stimulation improves motor skills?
11. Describe the labyrinthine righting reflexes and the equilibrium reflexes. How may they be utilized to advantage clinically?
12. Diagram the interconnections of the basal ganglia.
13. What are dyskinesias? Give specific examples of different types.
14. Name the conditions produced by lesions in specific basal nuclei.
15. What are the symptoms of Parkinson's disease?
16. Explain the goals of drug treatment for Parkinson's disease on the basis of the deficit in the neurotransmitter that causes the disease.
17. What is meant by the "extrapyramidal" system?
18. Explain why a cerebral vascular accident that involves the posterior limb of the internal capsule is so debilitating.

CHAPTER 10 • THE CEREBRAL CORTEX

OBJECTIVES

After reading this chapter you should: • Understand how the structural and functional organization of the cerebral cortex correlate with each other. • Understand the experimental methods that have been utilized to generate maps of the somatotopic representation in the cerebral cortex. • Recognize the gross divisions of the cerebral cortex (e.g., frontal, parietal, occipital and temporal lobes) and their subdivisions (e.g., superior, middle and inferior frontal gyri), and know which functions are represented in each of these divisions. • Know the symptoms that may be produced by lesions in specific areas of the cerebral cortex. • Know the function of the corpus callosum. • Know, in general, the pathology underlying epilepsy and what you might do to arrest a seizure.

THE CEREBRAL CORTEX

The cerebral cortex is more highly developed in man than in any other species, which accounts for the fact that when it is damaged the functional losses are more severe in man than are comparable lesions in other species. The large population of neurons in the cerebral cortex is responsible for the contrast in the capabilities possessed by man as compared to other species. This large population of cells allows for complex interactions within the cerebral cortex as well as with other parts of the brain. Much of the volume of the cortex is buried within the fissures; in fact it is so convoluted that approximately two-thirds of the human cerebral cortex lies within the depths of the fissures.

The cerebral cortex is of telencephalic origin and contains approximately ten billion cells, which are located mostly in six horizontal layers (see Fig. 10–1). These layers are designated by their cellular constituents, which vary greatly from one cortical area to another so that few cortical regions reveal six distinct layers. Rather, there are certain morphologic characteristics associated with specific cortical regions. For example, the somatosensory, visual and auditory cortices contain a highly developed layer 4, since afferent fibers from the thalamus appear to terminate primarily in this layer, but layers 3 and 5 are much less prominent in those areas. In the motor cortex, layer 4 is almost nonexistent, but layers 3 and 5, which contain medium- and large-sized pyramidal cells that are the origins of the descending motor fibers, are highly developed.

It can be seen, then, that structural differences can be correlated with functional differences, and this holds true for the entire cerebral cortex. These differences provide the basis for the most commonly utilized cytoarchitectonic scheme of the cortex, devised by Brodmann in 1909, who numbered the regions of the cortex according to differ-

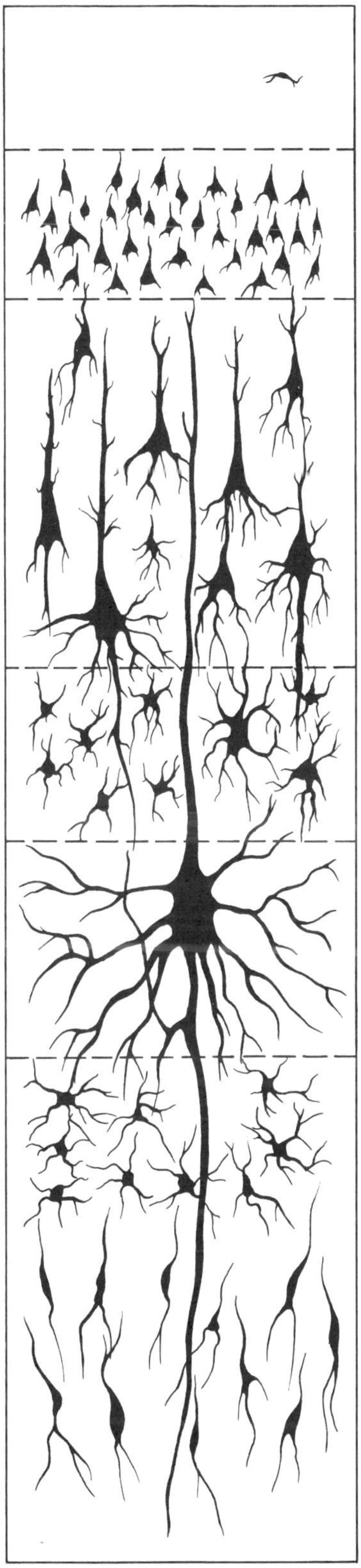

Figure 10–1. A diagrammatic representation of the six layers of the cerebral cortex.

ences in cell constituents in different areas (see Fig. 10–2).

For a time the significance of Brodmann's contribution was in question because it had not been established whether or not the morphologic differences he had demonstrated were an expression of functional differences. However, the contributions of the electrical stimulation and evoked potential methods of Woolsey and his group (1945, 1946, 1947, 1951, 1958) have shown that the major cytoarchitectonic subdivisions of the cortex are obviously related to selective activities in specific areas. The electrical stimulation techniques were utilized to map out areas of the motor cortex which are responsible for control of different areas of the body. The motor cortex was systematically electrically stimulated to induce contraction of muscles, and the somatotopic localization of parts of the body was mapped (see Fig. 10–3). Similar maps were evolved for the sensory cortex by use of the evoked potential method, which consists of stimulating sensory receptors and recording from the target points to which they project in the cerebral cortex. Such a representation of the parts of the body in the human cerebral cortex is called *an homunculus.* In both the motor and sensory cortices the face is represented laterally and the lower extremities are represented medially.

The connections of the cerebral cortex can be generalized into three categories:

1. *Projection fibers,* by which pathways interconnect the cerebral cortex with other structures. The corticospinal and dorsal column systems are examples of projection fibers.
2. *Association fibers,* which interconnect ipsilateral regions of the cerebral cortex and, in general, interconnect cortical areas with associated functions. For example, there are association fibers that connect the primary visual area (17) with the secondary visual areas (18 and 19), and there are association fibers that project from the sensory to the motor cortex.
3. *Commissural fibers,* which interconnect homotypic areas (areas which subserve functions that are the same or similar) bilaterally by way of the corpus callosum, and the anterior and posterior commissures, etc. For example, there are commissural fibers that connect the

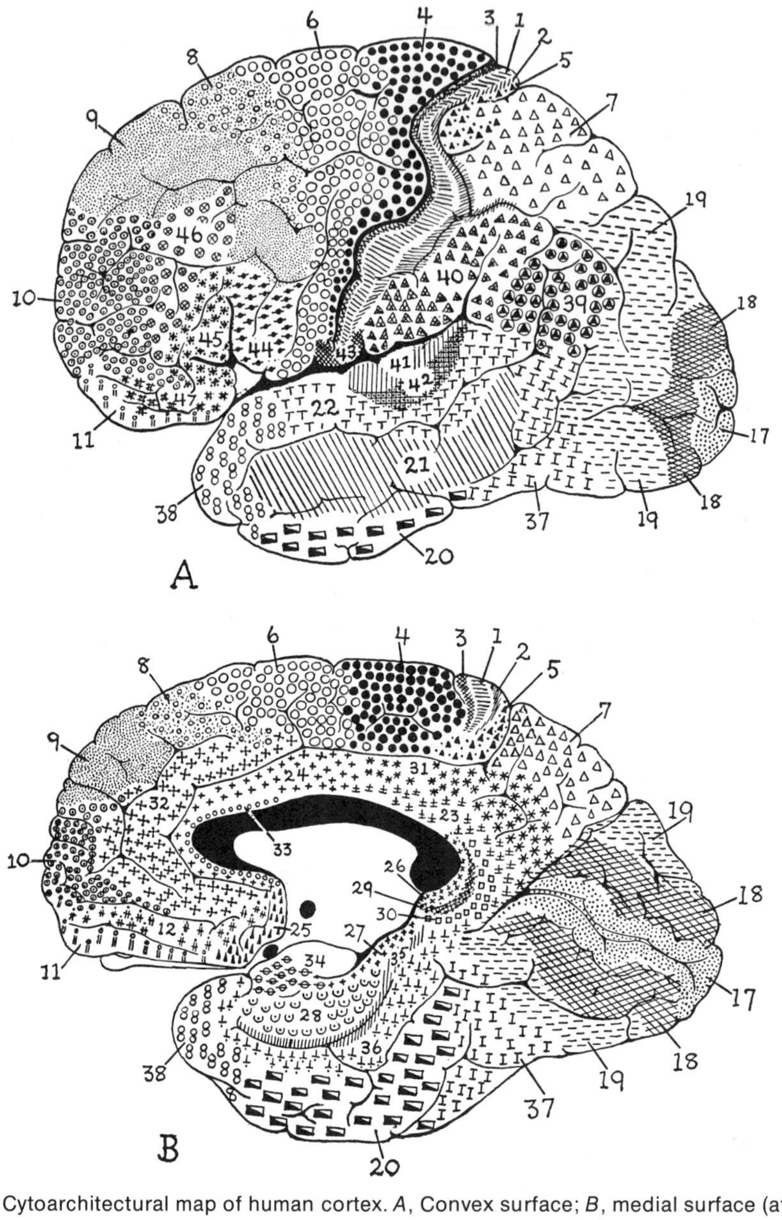

Figure 10–2. Cytoarchitectural map of human cortex. *A*, Convex surface; *B*, medial surface (after Brodmann, 1909).

right and left motor cortices and the right and left sensory cortices.

The vast majority of cortical interconnections are by way of intrinsic neurons, which constitute 75 to 90 per cent of the entire population of cortical neurons. These intrinsic neurons apparently function in processing information between its arrival and the departure of impulses controlling responses to the incoming information.

Gross Anatomy of the Cerebral Cortex

The cerebral cortex is divided into four major divisions — the frontal, parietal, occipital and temporal lobes (see Fig. 10–4*A* and *B*), separated from each other and further subdivided by fissures and sulci. The two cerebral hemispheres are separated by the longitudinal fissure, which is bounded inferiorly by the massive corpus callosum.

The frontal lobes extend from the most rostral (frontal) pole of the cerebral cortex to the central sulcus. They contain the motor areas of the brain, the prefrontal (association) areas and the area of Broca, which is functionally related to speech and will be discussed in some detail later in this chapter.

The parietal lobes extend posteriorly from the central sulcus to the parieto-occipital sulcus, and laterally and inferiorly to the lateral or Sylvian sulcus. The parietal lobes contain the somatosensory areas of the brain and large expanses of association cortex.

The main function associated with the occipital lobe is the reception and perception of visual stimuli, the primary receptive area of which is located on the banks of the calcarine fissure.

The temporal lobe subserves a variety of functions, including conscious perception and interpretation (Wernicke's area) of auditory stimulation, olfaction and memory, and has numerous connections with the limbic system (*to be discussed later*), which functions in emotional and autonomic responses to the environment.

A very old portion of the cerebral cortex, from a phylogenetic point of view, can be seen only when the temporal and frontal lobes are separated at the Sylvian fissure. This is called the *insula*. The function of this very old portion of the cerebral cortex has not been clearly determined.

When the cerebral cortex is observed from its medial aspect (Fig. 10–4*B*), a number of gyri and sulci can be identified, some of which have definite functions assigned to them. The calcarine fissure can be seen best from this view (vision); the paracentral lob-

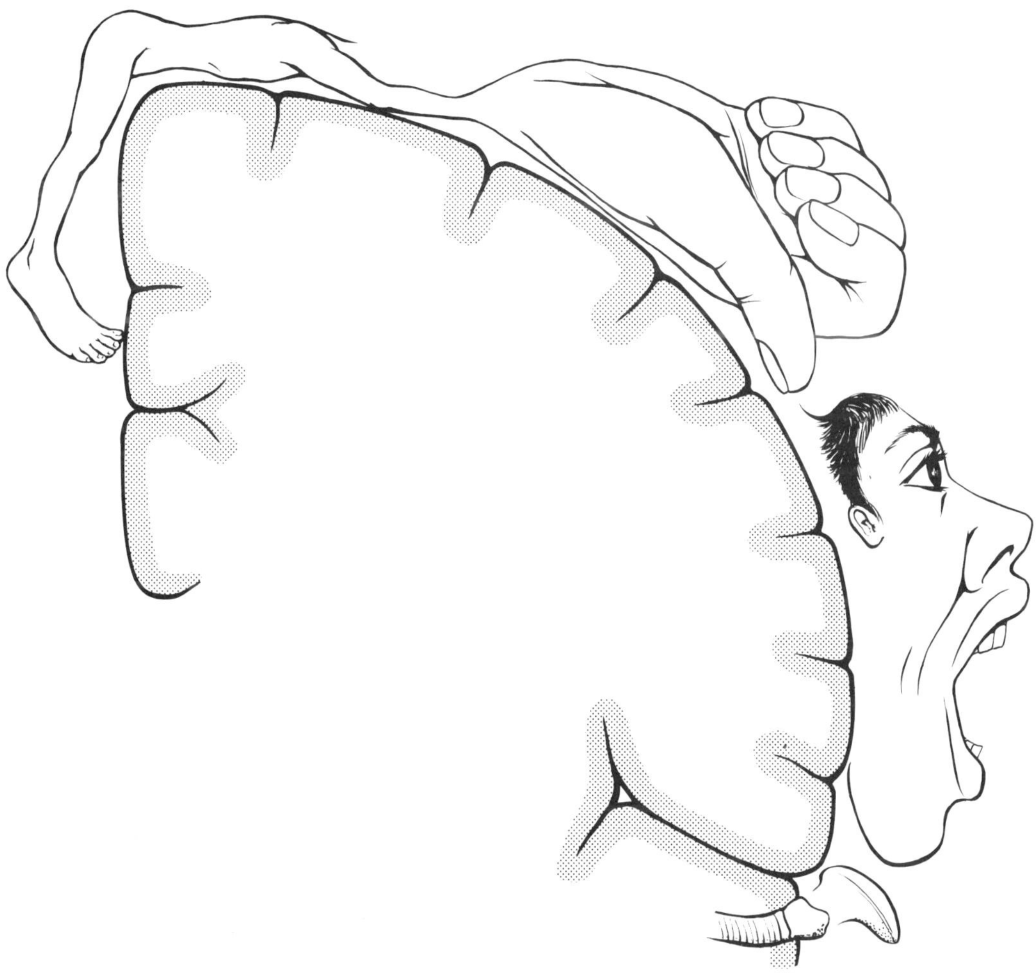

Figure 10–3. The motor homunculus of the human brain.

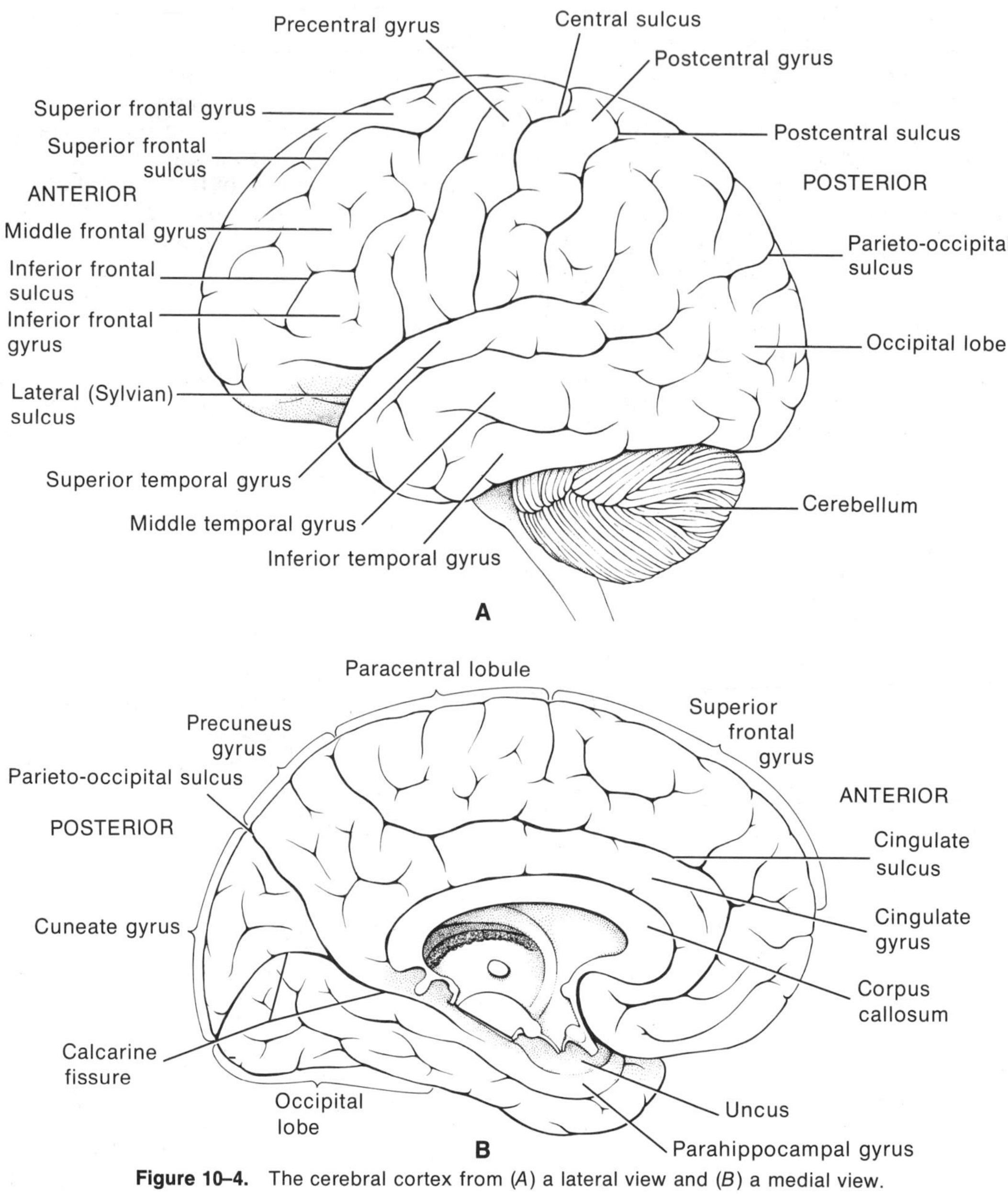

Figure 10–4. The cerebral cortex from (*A*) a lateral view and (*B*) a medial view.

ule contains the cerebral representation of the areas of the body innervated by the sacral segments of the spinal cord, the cingulate gyrus is associated with the limbic system; the uncus receives information from the olfactory system; and structures within the parahippocampal gyrus function in memory and autonomic and emotional responses by way of connections with the limbic system.

The Motor Cortex

Many maps of cortical representation of muscles and movements have been developed by electrically stimulating specific areas of the cortex and observing the responses. One of the major findings from all this work is that there is considerable overlap of function between areas, and this should be kept in mind as we generalize in the following discussion.

Area 4 (of Brodmann), which is just anterior to the central sulcus, tends to provide more control over the distal musculature, and area 6, just anterior to area 4, provides more control over the musculature of the trunk and proximal extremities. Areas 4 and 6 together comprise the primary motor area (MI), which contains a complete representation of the contralateral side of the body. Woolsey and his associates have discovered that there is also a secondary motor cortex or motor association cortex (MII) on the medial surface of the frontal lobe, just rostral to area 6. The somatotopic organization is such that the face is represented anteriorly and the hindlimb posteriorly. There is more overlap of the control of individual muscles in MII, and instead of containing a complete representation of the contralateral side of the body, MII contains a complete bilateral representation of the skeletal musculature. Electrical stimulation of MII elicits gross, postural types of movement, whereas electrical stimulation of MI elicits finer, more discrete types of movement.

Recent work has provided evidence that there are also motor areas in the *postcentral gyrus* that coincide with sensory areas I and II. Each of these areas also has a complete motor representation of the body. The evidence for the existence of these motor areas has been provided by removing the entire precentral gyrus and then electrically stimulating the sensory areas. Motor responses have been elicited in such preparations, but the pathways utilized to do so remain obscure.

Experiments in monkeys have shown that lesions in the cortical motor areas produce characteristic deficits. When MI is destroyed, a contralateral hypotonic paresis (paralysis) is produced. There is not a complete paralysis, but the movements are slower and not well coordinated. Bilateral destruction of MII is necessary to produce any symptoms, which include some spasticity, but little paralysis. Concomitant destruction of MI and MII produces a combination of symptoms. Initially there is hypotonia of the musculature, later followed by hypertonia. The latter persists and is accompanied by a severe paresis, which develops immediately after the lesion is made and persists in company with the hypertonia.

Pure lesions of the corticospinal tracts can be produced only at the level of the medullary pyramids, where their course is very superficial. The result is contralateral hypotonic paresis, which is more severe than that produced by destruction of MI. This may be interpreted to mean that the fibers of origin of the corticospinal tracts must be located in areas other than MI, and of course we know this to be true. The fact that selective destruction of the corticospinal tracts produces hypotonic paralysis serves to emphasize that the spasticity which results from upper motor neuron lesions is due to damage to the extrapyramidal pathways and is *not* due to damage to the corticospinal tracts alone.

The Somatosensory Cortex

The somatosensory cortex has also been mapped by Woolsey and his associates by the evoked potential method. The primary somatosensory area (SI) is located in areas 3, 1 and 2 of the postcentral gyrus. The overlap is similar to that in MI, and there is complete contralateral representation except for bilateral representation of the intra- and perioral structures. SI receives information primarily from the dorsal column system, but also receives some from the anterolateral system. More specifically, area 3 obtains information primarily from cutaneous receptors with small receptive fields that project from the contralateral side of the body; areas 1 and 2 receive most of their impulses from joints as well as other deep structures, and all three areas receive impulses from a few pain and temperature receptors.

The secondary somatosensory area (SII) is located on the parietal cortex within the banks of the Sylvian fissure. It contains a complete somatotopically organized bilateral representation of the body with the face represented rostrally and the hindlimb caudally. Its sensory characteristics closely resemble those of the anterolateral system, which is predominantly represented in SII; that is, it receives most impulses from cutaneous receptors with large receptive fields (consistent with the conveyance of the modality of diffuse touch in the anterolateral system) from both sides of the body. It receives from more nociceptive (unpleasant sensations) receptors than SI and is entirely lacking in information from the joint receptors. Temperature has yet to be investigated.

There is also some sensory representation in motor area 4 which is still considered as part of SI. It has somatotopic organization and bilateral representation. The most important projections to this area are from muscles, so that it presumably is involved with the integration of motor functions. The pathways by which these fibers reach the cerebral cortex are unknown, but apparently they do not pass through the cerebellum or the sensory cortex.

In humans, lesions in SI are manifested by a contralateral impairment of function that involves loss of appreciation of the spatial characteristics of a stimulus. There is difficulty with precise localization of a stimulus, loss of two-point discrimination and loss of the sense of body position and movement. Some functions are generally preserved, such as recognition of having been touched, of painful sensations and of temperature changes. All these may require more intense stimulation than normal to reach consciousness. The preserved functions are probably mediated through subcortical structures such as the thalamus or by an intact SII.

Ablation of SII alone produces relatively minor disturbances in sensation.

The Visual Cortex

The primary visual cortex is located on the banks of the calcarine fissure in the occipital lobe and is designated as area 17. This is the termination point for the last order neurons of the visual system which project from the lateral geniculate nucleus of the thalamus to the cerebral cortex (geniculocalcarine fibers). The production of homonymous hemianopia by lesions of the optic tract posterior to the optic chiasm has been dealt with in the discussion of the optic nerve. This deficit in one-half of the visual field may also be produced by a hemorrhage or occlusion of the posterior cerebral artery, or by the presence of a tumor or trauma that completely destroys area 17 on one side. A left-sided lesion will manifest itself by complete loss of vision in the right visual field, and vice versa.

Areas 18 and 19 comprise the secondary visual areas, which are interconnected with area 17. This latter projects to both of the secondary areas on the ipsilateral and contralateral sides of the brain by way of the splenium of the corpus callosum. The secondary visual centers do not receive direct projections from the lateral geniculate nucleus.

The Auditory Cortex

The auditory cortex consists of Brodmann's areas 41 and 42, which are hidden in the transverse temporal gyri just medial to the superior temporal gyrus. The last order neurons of the auditory system project from the medial geniculate nucleus of the thalamus, through the internal capsule, to terminate in those areas (geniculotemporal fibers). It should be recalled that auditory impulses are distributed bilaterally in the auditory cortex. Therefore, a unilateral lesion of the auditory cortex produces a partial bilateral deafness that may not be recognized clinically. The loss on the side contralateral to the lesion is more profound, indicating that although the fibers of the auditory system are both crossed and uncrossed the number of crossed fibers in the system outnumbers the uncrossed component.

Speech

The cerebral cortex as it relates to speech is of particular interest to clinicians. Speech involves two processes — *articulation,* which requires coordination of the muscles responsible for control of speech, and *symbolism,* or formulation of what one wants to say. Articulation is a purely mechanical event, but symbolism involves the synthesis of intangible elements into ideas. Lesions in the precentral (motor) gyrus of the cerebral cortex cause difficulty with articulation owing to lack of control of the appropriate musculature. Difficulty with symbolism is due primarily to lesions of Broca's area (Fig. 10–5) of oral representation in the inferior frontal lobe of the *left* cerebral hemisphere. The evidence to date indicates that Broca's area is not related to cerebral dominance, so that it is located in the left hemisphere in the

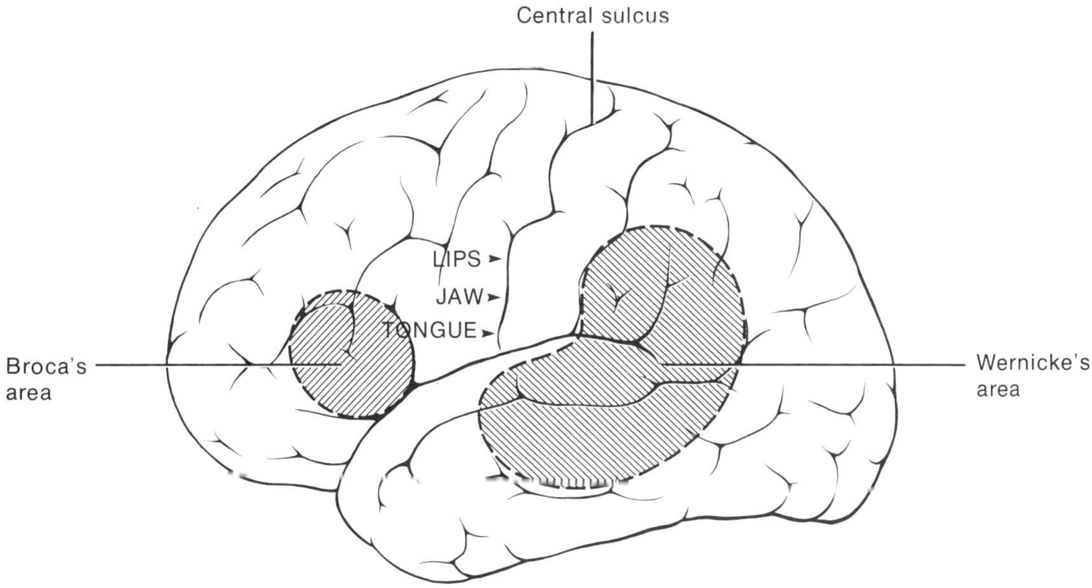

Figure 10–5. The locations of Broca's and Wernicke's areas in the human brain.

vast majority of persons, regardless of whether an individual is right- or left-handed. If Broca's area is removed the result is what is known as *expressive aphasia* or *dysphasia* (aphasia = complete lack of speech; dysphasia = difficulty with speech).

Another area, Wernicke's, which overlaps the auditory cortex in the temporal lobe, also plays an important part in speech (Fig. 10–5). If Wernicke's area is destroyed or damaged, the ability to recognize or interpret words is lost. This is called *receptive aphasia*. The two kinds of aphasia or dysphasia are frequently encountered in the clinic, particularly in association with cerebral vascular accidents that occur in the left cerebral hemispheres, since both Broca's and Wernicke's areas are located on the left side in most people. It is interesting that patients who cannot express themselves in any other way usually are capable of swearing even when they have no intention of doing so and expect to say something altogether different. Strangely, even those who have never sworn may have this difficulty if they become aphasic or dysphasic. It is important for the clinician to understand that this is a completely involuntary reaction to the environment in most cases. It does not indicate anger and should certainly not be taken as a personal affront.

One may go into the room of an aphasic person and say "hi." Very quickly and on a reflex basis the patient answers "hi," but he cannot initiate the conversation. He has to hear the word first and then he can respond. These patients can also sing and in the context of a familiar tune they can sing the right words as the tune progresses. This is a way to have fun with patients as you are working with them because they realize they are saying the right words and it tends to boost their morale. Unfortunately there seems to be no therapeutic value to the singing because, at least in the author's experience, there has been no carry over into improved speech. The fact that patients are capable of responding in these ways presumably means that some functions of memory and reflex activity related to speech are located in the right cerebral hemisphere. The fact that speech therapy may meet with some success in aphasic and dysphasic patients probably is due to either some return of function of the damaged left side of the brain, or the ability of the right side of the brain to take over some of this function, or both.

The Association Cortex

The association cortex includes all areas of the cerebral cortex without specific functions assigned to them. In general, the higher the position of the species on the phylogenetic scale, the larger is its association cortex. These parts of the neocortex have evolved to the greatest extent in primates and therefore must be responsible for those capabilities that characterize human behavior in terms of speech, thought, memory, etc. However, it is precisely these areas that are most difficult to analyze in terms of input, output and intrinsic organization. Because relatively little is known about the association cortex, we will not spend a great deal of time on it except to cite some interesting experiments that afford some insight into the function of some areas.

In the early 1940s a procedure called *prefrontal lobotomy* (disconnection of the anterior portions of the frontal lobes) was extremely popular. Approximately 50,000 of these radical surgical procedures were carried out for relief of intractable pain and in profoundly psychotic patients. This is considered a low point in neurosurgery because subsequently it has been found that simply cutting the connections to the rostral portion of the frontal lobe by a surgical approach through the nasal passages accomplishes the same result. This procedure does not actually relieve the pain, but the patients do not seem to care that the pain exists. They experience a feeling of euphoria (a false sensation of well-being). This tells us that the prefrontal areas have something to do with the patient's affective behavior, i.e., his emotional response to the environment. In addition, contusions to the prefrontal area result in the loss of the three "T"s — tact, tenacity and tenseness — and can also cause impairment of intellectual capabilities.

When the temporal lobe is removed (*temporal lobectomy*) the individual may have a tendency toward hypersexuality, but is otherwise very placid except for a few mild symptoms. The most disabling manifestation of the removal is that the patient cannot learn anything, because recent memory is a function of the medial portion of the temporal lobe. Contusions of this lobe may result in hallucinations and delusions, transient irritability, and depression. Some patients also display withdrawal, anxiety, paranoia, insecurity, religious fanaticism and paroxysmal outbursts of temper with abusiveness. Between these outbursts the individual is good-natured, but the characteristic of temporal lobe contusion is agitated aggression.

One clinical manifestation characteristic of a lesion in a specific area of the cerebral cortex other than those customarily attributed to the principal motor and sensory areas is *apraxia*. This consists of the inability to perform certain tasks which the patient has been doing all his life and which he takes for granted, such as getting out of the bathtub, removing his shoes and so on. These deficits may occur without any signs of paralysis or sensory loss and may reflect a localized abnormality in the nondominant hemisphere.

There are a number of different types of *agnosia*, which means inability to recognize; Carpenter (1976) describes three:

1. *Tactile agnosia* — failure to recognize objects by means of cutaneous and proprioceptive sensibilities when both are normal in the part of the body involved. This is particularly associated with lesions in the left cerebral hemisphere, and it is not clear whether the deficit is due to inability to interpret tactile information or whether there is an inability to synthesize the information from the different cutaneous and joint receptors from which the impulses originate.
2. *Visual agnosia* — failure to recognize objects when there is no impairment of vision and there is normal intellectual capacity. This deficit has been attributed to lesions in the visual association areas.
3. *Auditory agnosia* — inability to recognize what is heard when there is no impairment in hearing. Lesions in area 22 of the superior temporal gyrus of the dominant side are implicated in this deficit, particularly when the damage is bilateral.

The function of the corpus callosum was originally thought to be that of keeping the cerebral hemispheres from sagging. We know that this is not true through some interesting experiments designed to define the role of the corpus callosum. The function of this great mass of commissural fibers is to connect areas of the two cerebral hemispheres that have the same or a similar function. The following experiments have helped to elucidate this function.

In animals in which the corpus callosum

and the optic chiasm have been completely severed along the midline in the sagittal plane, there remains the ability to see only the ipsilateral side with one side of the cerebral cortex as long as one eye is covered or closed. If the animal is taught a discrimination task with one eye covered, and the eye with which he has seen the cues to learn is then covered, he cannot perform the task because the normal pathways by which the information would have been transmitted to the contralateral cerebral cortex have been destroyed.

If only the optic chiasm is severed in the midline the animal learns the activity bilaterally with only one eye open. He can then perform the activity with either eye open because there has been transfer of input to the contralateral cerebral cortex by way of the corpus callosum.

If only the corpus callosum is severed and the optic system is intact, the animal still learns a task bilaterally with only one eye open because there is visual stimulation of both cerebral hemispheres via the crossed optic fibers.

If an animal is trained first and then both the corpus callosum and optic chiasm are severed, there is no effect on learning because the task has been taught by the information already transferred and learned by both sides of the cerebral cortex.

The corpus callosum has been severed in some individuals to prevent the spread of epileptic seizures from one cerebral hemisphere to the other. These are referred to as "split brain" patients. Interestingly, such individuals have very little disability, and are difficult to recognize as long as they have an intact visual system to receive visual cues from both eyes. Their sensory surroundings are thus conveyed to both cerebral cortices by way of the visual system and they can respond normally. Their difficulties arise if for some reason they are deprived of vision in one eye.

Many of you may be encountering epileptic patients in clinical practice, and it may be beneficial to know something about the condition and what you may do to ward off a seizure. These occur as a result of pathologic focal discharges at a specific area of the brain, due to some factor that upsets the environment of the cells. The pathologic factor may be in the form of scar tissue from earlier trauma, abnormal blood flow, a chemical imbalance, etc. The seizure itself involves what is known as a *recruitment phenomenon*, i.e., cells adjacent to the initial focal point become involved and the seizure spreads. It may begin with a twitching of the thumb and then spread to the hand, proceed to the arm, and so on. One can map out the cortical areas involved just by watching the progress of the involvement.

From a therapeutic point of view, some things may be done to ward off a seizure if there is some warning that one may be imminent. If the area surrounding the focal point of the seizure can be put into functional use, the seizure sometimes can be warded off. This is called *occlusion*, in which two processes are competing for the participation of the same cell. If the cell can be recruited into doing something useful, the rhythmic seizures may be prevented. Verbal commands that distract the patient may also be helpful. If the seizures are audiogenic in nature (brought on by stimulation of the auditory system), music or some kind of noise other than the type that induces the seizure may prevent it. Any time you can prevent a full-blown epileptic seizure you are doing the patient a real favor because the more often a seizure occurs, the stronger the circuitry involved grows, and the seizures tend to become more intense.

There are some interesting sidelights concerning the training of patients in motor activities. Amputees with artificial limbs (prostheses) are now being trained to use cortical signals to move parts. Another interesting phenomenon is that one can rehearse movements just by thinking about them, but the movements must have been learned first. This has been shown by comparing two groups of athletes, one of which practiced by doing the movements and the other by thinking about them. There was very little if any difference in the postexperimental performance. If this can work with normal individuals it may work with patients as well. However, it is important to realize that there is a difference between learning active and passive movements. A patient cannot be taught how active movement feels by taking him through a passive range of movement.

There is now evidence that in monkeys the sensory modalities of light touch or skin pressure and/or passive joint movements project to the primary motor areas of the cerebral cortex. This means that there is a feedback loop between the motor cortex and the periphery, which may play an important role in tactile exploration. In addition, if this loop exists in man, and there is no reason to believe that it does not, the neurophysiologic basis on which Margaret Rood's brushing techniques are founded is strengthened. If the skin is lightly brushed over the muscle in which a contraction is desired, the impulses elicited may take a direct route to the cells in the more superficial layers (II and III) of the motor cortex. These cells in turn synapse with neurons in layer V where some of the cells of origin of the corticospinal tracts are located. The effects produced are excitatory to neurons within a restricted region and inhibitory to neurons in a wider area. The net effect may be contraction of the muscle underlying the stimulated skin and inhibition of the adjacent musculature. Presumably this feedback loop involves the dorsal column and corticospinal systems, but many more elements may be involved.

REVIEW QUESTIONS

1. In which areas of the cerebral cortex is layer IV especially well developed? Layers III and V? What is the functional significance of the variability in development of these layers in different areas?
2. What experimental methods have been utilized to map the somatotopic representation of the body in the motor and sensory areas of the cerebral cortex? Explain each method.
3. What is meant by:
   a. cortical projection fibers?
   b. cortical association fibers?
   c. cortical commissural fibers?
4. In both the motor and sensory cortices, which areas of the body are represented medially and which laterally? Which areas are represented in the paracentral lobule on the medial surface of the cerebral cortex?
5. Compare the results of stimulation of cortical areas MI and MII.
6. What are the symptoms of lesions in cortical area MI? MII?
7. In what way does a pure corticospinal tract lesion differ from an upper motor neuron lesion?
8. Compare cortical areas SI and SII in terms of:
   a. areas of the body represented (which side)?
   b. tracts that terminate in these areas.
   c. types of receptors represented in each.
9. What are the symptoms of lesions in cortical area SI? SII?
10. What are the two processes involved in speech? Lesions in which areas will interfere with each of these processes?
11. What is meant by receptive aphasia? Which area functions in understanding the spoken word? Where is this area located?
12. What is meant by expressive aphasia? A lesion in which area will produce this disability?

13. What is the function of the corpus callosum?
14. What are some of the pathologic factors that may produce epileptic seizures? Name some actions you might take to prevent a seizure if there are signs that one is imminent.
15. What is apraxia? Agnosia?
16. From the information available to you to date, consider all the interconnections at suprasegmental levels by which incoming sensory information may influence motor output.

CHAPTER 11 • THE THALAMUS

OBJECTIVES

After reading this chapter you should: • Understand which nuclei comprise the thalamus. • Be able to diagram a generalized scheme of the interconnections of the specific thalamic nuclei. • Be familiar with the symptoms that may accompany the thalamic syndrome. • Understand how the perception of pain may be modified by various kinds of influences. • Know the peripheral receptors and central pathways by which pain perception is transmitted and interpreted by the central nervous system. • Be able to explain the "gate theory" of pain. • Be familiar with some of the treatment techniques and surgical procedures utilized for the alleviation of pain, and whenever possible explain the underlying basis for the success of the procedure under discussion.

THE THALAMUS

The word thalamus means inner chamber, which is quite appropriate considering that the thalami lie deeply hidden under the convolutions of the very massive cerebral cortex. The third ventricle separates the two walnut-shaped thalami, which are often partly connected by a bundle of fibers called the *massa intermedia,* which spans the third ventricle.

The thalamus is subdivided into a number of nuclear groups, each of which is characterized by specific afferent connections and by efferent fibers that link it to a particular area of the cerebral cortex. The simplest way of dealing with the relationships of the nuclear groups is by means of diagrammatic representations. Figure 11–1 shows a frontal view of the thalamus at approximately the midlength of the third ventricle. The thalamus is seen to be subdivided by the *internal medullary lamina*, which is a dense layer of myelinated fibers within which lie a number of cell groups called *intralaminar nuclei.* In general, the ventral nuclei are located ventrolateral to the internal medullary lamina; a group of lateral nuclei lies dorsolaterally and the medial dorsal nuclear mass is located medially. The specific nuclei within these general groupings are more easily visualized in a lateral view of the thalamus as illustrated in Figure 11–2.

The interconnections of the thalamus have been the subject of very extensive research so that a great deal of detail is available. The discussion here will be limited to the major connections that will be of most value to those who will be involved in clinical situations. Those interested in learning more detail regarding the thalamus are urged to read Carpenter's *Human Neuroanatomy,* Chapter 15 (1976).

In general, the ventral nuclei receive afferent fibers from the dorsal column system, from the anterolateral and trigeminothalamic tracts (from the principal sensory and

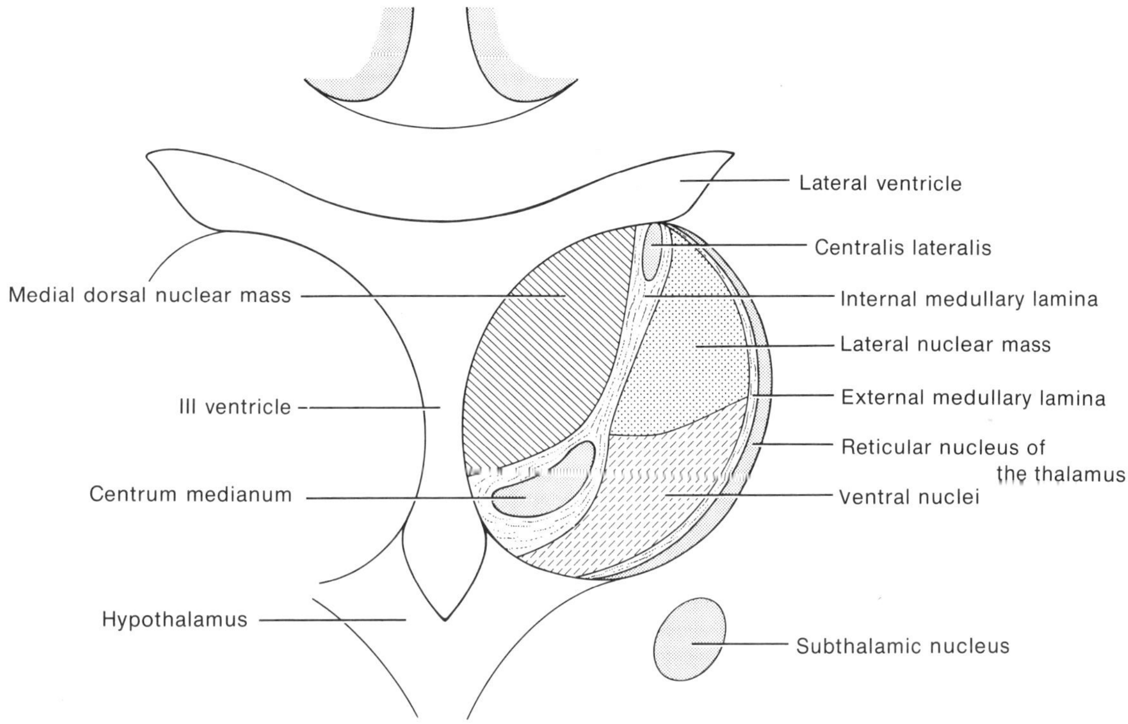

Figure 11–1. A frontal view of the thalamus at approximately the midlength of the third ventricle.

spinal nuclei of the trigeminal nerve), from the neocerebellum by way of the superior cerebellar peduncles, and from the globus pallidus, substantia nigra and nucleus solitarius (taste).

Ventrolateral and Ventral Anterior Nuclei

More specifically, *afferent* fibers project to the ventrolateral and ventral anterior nu-

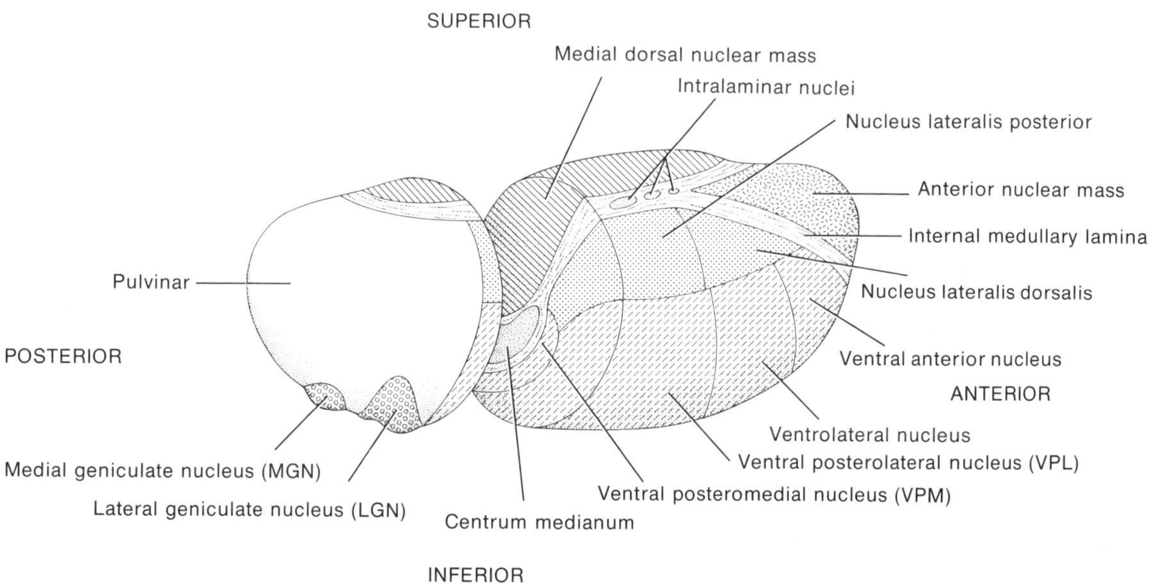

Figure 11–2. A lateral view of the thalamus. The reticular nucleus of the thalamus and the external medullary lamina have been removed.

clei from the neocerebellum, globus pallidus, substantia nigra and cerebral cortex. *Efferent* fibers from these nuclei in turn project to the precentral (motor) cortex, the orbitofrontal cortex and the striatum. It seems worth re-emphasizing here that these projections to the cerebral cortex via the ventrolateral and ventral anterior nuclei of the thalamus indicate clearly that the cerebellum, globus pallidus and substantia nigra are involved in modulating motor activity. These nuclei are somatotopically organized with the face represented medially, the lower extremity laterally, and the upper extremity and trunk in an intermediate position.

Ventrobasal (Ventroposterior) Nucleus

The ventral posterolateral and ventral posteromedial nuclei collectively are called the *ventrobasal nucleus* or *complex*, which has been mentioned several times in connection with the ascending pathways of the dorsal column and anterolateral systems.

Several systems synapse in the ventrobasal complex en route to the cerebral cortex. These afferent systems project to the ventrobasal complex from the dorsal column system, anterolateral tracts, trigeminal system and nucleus solitarius. Areas 3, 1 and 2 of the somatosensory cortex also project to this complex so that the connections with the cortex are reciprocal, since the efferent projections from the ventrobasal complex project to those areas in the postcentral (sensory) cortex.

Recall that the somatotopic organization in the ventrobasal complex is such that the face is represented medially and the feet laterally. The fibers rearrange themselves en route to the cerebral cortex so that the face is ultimately represented laterally and the feet medially in the cerebral cortex.

The modality of taste, conveyed by fibers from the nucleus solitarius to the ventrobasal complex, projects finally to the cerebral cortex, but its area of termination has not been well defined.

Medial and Lateral Geniculate Nuclei

The medial and lateral geniculate nuclei comprise the *metathalamus*, which functions in the special senses of vision and hearing.

The *medial geniculate nucleus* receives information from the auditory receptors of the cochlea by way of the inferior colliculus, and provides a relay station for these impulses to project to the auditory, motor and sensory cortices, with which it has reciprocal connections.

The *lateral geniculate nucleus* receives visual impulses from the retinal ganglion cells and provides a direct relay station for visual impulses to reach the visual cortex, and indirect pathways to reach the motor and sensory cortices.

Anterior Thalamic Nuclei (Mass)

The anterior thalamic mass includes the anterior dorsal, anterior medial and anterior ventral nuclei. This group of nuclei receives afferent fibers from the mamillary bodies by way of the mamillothalamic tracts. The mamillary bodies in turn are in receipt of information from the hippocampus via the fornix, the midbrain and other hypothalamic areas. The anterior thalamic nuclei also receive fibers directly from the fornix and connect reciprocally with the cingulate cortex. These connections with the cingulate cortex comprise part of the limbic system, which is concerned with basic emotional drives and memory mechanisms; it will be dealt with in more detail in a later chapter.

Medial Dorsal Thalamic Nucleus

The medial dorsal thalamic mass has reached enormous proportions in man and has the most precise projections of all the thalamic nuclei. It receives afferent fibers from the olfactory (piriform) cortex, which includes the uncus and amygdaloid nucleus, and projects efferent fibers to the orbitofrontal cortex (the area just superior to the orbits) via the anterior limb of the internal capsule. These connections are reciprocal and are the ones cut during prefrontal lobotomy. A cerebral vascular accident in this area produces euphoria (a false feeling of well-being) just as does prefrontal lobotomy.

The interconnections of the remaining thalamic nuclei have not been as well defined as those just discussed, but a few facts are worth noting.

Nucleus lateralis dorsalis, nucleus lateralis posterior and the pulvinar may receive only intrathalamic and widespread cortical fibers, including sensory, motor, visual and association areas. Relatively recent evidence also suggests that there are projections from the tectum to the pulvinar. Efferents from these nuclei project primarily to the cingulate gyrus and to the parietal lobe, principally to association areas involved with processing and interpreting information received by the primary sensory areas of the cortex. The function of these fibers is incompletely understood, although we do know that a lesion in the association cortex disturbs the ability to interpret sensory input. There is some evidence that the part of the pulvinar which receives projections from the tectum may in turn project to parts of the visual cortex.

Within the internal medullary lamina lie a group of nonspecific nuclei called *intralaminar nuclei*, of which the largest is the centrum medianum (CM). This nucleus receives afferents from the globus pallidus and from the reticular formation, and in turn projects to widespread areas of the cerebral cortex as well as to the striatum. When the widespread projections to the cerebral cortex are stimulated, diffuse cortical arousal is produced. Another intralaminar nucleus is the centralis lateralis (CL). Its connections are very poorly understood, although it is known to be important in pain mechanisms. Other nuclei include the parafascicular, paracentral and central lateral nuclei, of which the parafascicular is the most important. It receives information from the cerebellum, spinal cord, reticular formation, motor cortex and basal ganglia, and in turn projects to the striatum and to the cerebral cortex (as does the centrum medianum).

The reticular nucleus of the thalamus consists of a thin sheet of cells that surrounds the ventral and lateral aspects of the thalamus. It separates the thalamus from the internal capsule so that all fibers interconnecting the thalamus and cerebral cortex must pass through the reticular nucleus, but its function has not been well defined.

This is a very brief account of the morphology and function of the thalamus, which is a very complex structure; we have mentioned only those points that complete the picture of the interconnections between the cerebral cortex and the subcortical structures dealt with in this book. The important generalization to remember about the thalamus is that it is an important way-station for all pathways en route to the cortex, with the exception of the olfactory system. Therefore, the cerebral cortex depends almost entirely on the thalamus for receipt of sensory information. However, it is emphasized that the thalamus is not simply a relay station. There is now evidence to show that neurons which originate in the cerebral cortex are capable of inhibiting activity in the thalamus. These projections from the cerebral cortex suggest that the thalamus is capable of refining or concentrating information that ultimately reaches the cortex.

It is very difficult to learn all the interconnections of the specific thalamic nuclei as they have been presented here. A generalized scheme such as the one diagrammatically presented below may be worth remembering.

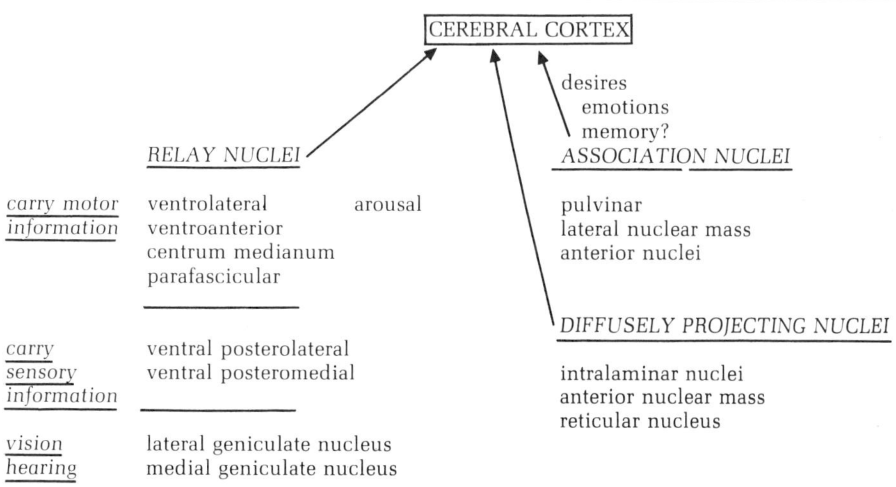

The cerebral cortex is actually an outgrowth or continuation of lower brain centers, especially of the thalamus. Therefore, although this is not shown in the above diagram, for each area of the cerebral cortex there is a corresponding and connecting area of the thalamus. Thus, activation of a minute portion of the thalamus activates the corresponding and much larger portion of the cerebral cortex, and the evidence to date shows that, for each projection of the thalamus to the cerebral cortex, there is a reciprocal projection from the cerebral cortex to the thalamus.

Pain

Pain is a sensation encountered on a daily basis by every clinician in practice. Since all sensations of pain are associated with systems that pass to or through the thalamus, this seems an appropriate place to increase one's understanding of pain and some of the therapeutic approaches to its alleviation.

Since the detection of pain persists after complete destruction of the sensory areas of the cerebral cortex bilaterally, it is believed that the thalamus is capable of functioning in some conscious awareness of pain. This is an exception to the notion that in most cases sensory information must reach the cerebral cortex to be consciously appreciated. When the cortical sensory areas are removed one cannot accurately localize the pain sensation, but nevertheless there is recognition of the existence of pain.

The function of the thalamus in the recognition and transmission of pain sensibility is reflected in a condition most often produced by hemorrhage or occlusion of the posterior cerebral artery, which supplies the blood to the thalamus. Destruction of parts or all of the thalamus by such cerebral vascular accidents may result in what is called the *thalamic syndrome.* With a complete lesion of the thalamus sensation is almost completely lost on the entire contralateral side of the body, including the face, trunk and limbs. All sensations are severely affected, but especially the deeper ones such as position sense and vibration. In addition, there may be central sensations in part of or the entire contralateral side of the body which are deep, spasmodic and excruciatingly painful. The patient may be hypersensitive to painful stimuli and may overreact. This type of spasmodic pain does not always accompany lesions of the thalamus, but when it does it is very agonizing and tends to be resistant to medication.

The most characteristic sensory changes that accompany total or partial thalamic lesions are the tendencies for the patient to overreact to stimuli and to experience the sensation produced for long periods after the stimulus has been removed. If the internal capsule is involved in the same lesion that has produced the thalamic damage there may be an accompanying contralateral hemiparesis or hemiplegia.

The classic or traditional view of spinal cord pain mechanisms may be generalized by the diagram below.

The perception of pain presumably occurs when impulses that ascend in the anterolateral system activate the thalamic ventral posterolateral nucleus or cortical neurons, or both. The character of pain actually has so many dimensions that this simple traditional concept is not really adequate to explain it. It not only involves the discriminative capacity to identify the

---

pain perception	somatosensory cortex ↑ ventral posterolateral nucleus of the thalamus
	↑
pain pathway	anterolateral system ↑ pain fibers (free nerve endings)

onset, duration, location, intensity and physical characteristics of the stimulus, but also includes several functions: the motivational (what are the patient's motivations?); affective (the state of mind the individual is in and the influence of his past experiences); and cognitive (awareness and recognition of the situation). These functions influence the patient's own private response to painful stimuli, and the response is usually aversive behavior, i.e., a tendency to avoid the noxious stimulus.

In addition, pain is profoundly modified by attention, emotions, suggestion and pathologic conditions of the central and peripheral nervous system that can increase or decrease the intensity of the pain. A good example of the role attention may play in the experience of pain is the frequency of telephone calls the general practitioner receives in the late night hours from patients who have been uncomfortable all day. The events of the day have provided a distraction from the discomfort, but at night the distractions are absent and patients have ample opportunity to concentrate on the discomfort, which becomes unbearable to the point at which they must consult their physician at once.

We are well aware of the peripheral mechanisms involved with pain. It is mediated by free nerve endings provided by small type III and C nerve fibers that enter the dorsal horns of the spinal cord. Subsequently the central nervous system must provide for both spatiotemporal discriminative and motivational–affective functions. Normally, then, the noxious stimulus to the body surface is quickly located in time and space, and the mechanisms leading to aversive behavior that is often accompanied by autonomic and emotional responses are activated quickly. Continuing experimental and clinical observations are providing some insight into the neural mechanisms underlying the discriminative and motivational dimensions of pain. Kenneth Casey (1973) has diagrammed some of the major relevant CNS pathways involved and the following is a modification of his work.

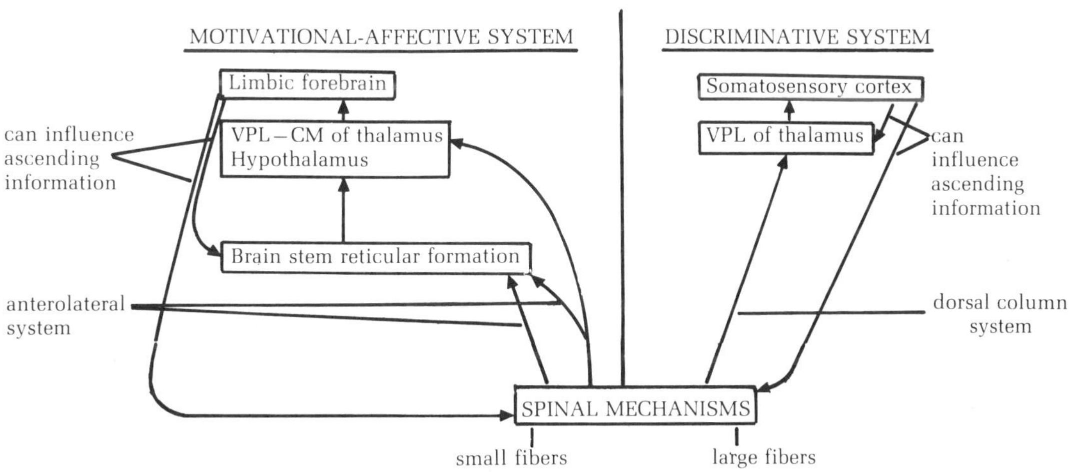

VPL = ventral posterolateral nucleus
CM = centrum medianum nucleus

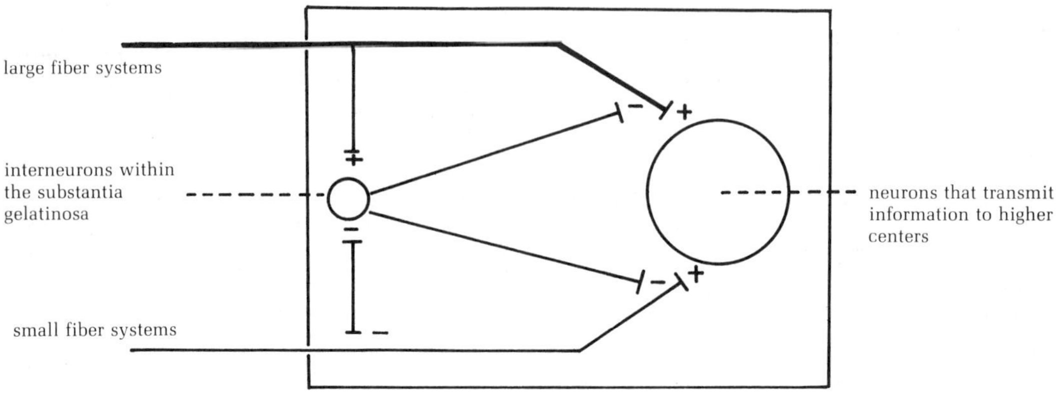

We are now very familiar with the discriminative system, and it should be recognized that the anterolateral system may contribute some information to that system by way of its projections to the ventral posterolateral nucleus of the thalamus.

The diagram shows that in the motivational–affective system the anterolateral tracts project freely to the reticular formation and to the thalamus, and then to the limbic forebrain, which functions in emotional responses. Therefore, these projections may represent the ascending system which provides a neural basis for the aversive, motivational dimension of pain.

With this background information we can now consider the *gate theory of pain control* as presented by Melzack and Wall (1965). We know that both large- and small-diameter peripheral nerve fibers enter the dorsal horn of the spinal cord, where their terminals form synaptic contacts with various neurons in the dorsal spinal gray matter. Here, large-diameter nerve fibers enhance activity in a population of spinal neurons, which in turn depress synaptic transmission which has been produced by stimulation of cutaneous receptors subserved by nerve fibers of both large and small diameter. Nerve fibers of small diameter lack the ability to excite the inhibitory interneurons, and in fact may facilitate synaptic transmission. The activity of the large and small fiber systems may be represented diagrammatically as shown above.

These differences in the influences of the large- and small-diameter fibers at the spinal level prompted Melzack and Wall to postulate the existence of the gate control mechanism in the dorsal spinal gray matter. Finally, it is proposed that the entire gating mechanism shown above is modulated by impulses that descend from cortical and subcortical supraspinal neurons. These control neurons are initially activated by the large, rapidly conducting fibers of the dorsal column system.

There is much current debate regarding the gate control hypothesis. It is not universally accepted because the complexity of synaptic arrangements in the spinal gray matter defies decisive anatomic evidence for or against the hypothesis. In addition, some neurophysiologic experiments have not supported certain details of the theory. What is of most importance is the general agreement that *the large diameter cutaneous fibers are predominantly effective in inhibiting spinal sensory input from both large and small fibers.* Therefore, the basic elements of the proposed gate control mechanism are present and provide a mechanism by which the excitation of the anterolateral system by sensations of pain can be modulated at the spinal level.

The role of the large-diameter fibers in inhibition may be exemplified in the case of peripheral neuropathies (lesions of peripheral nerves) in which it is thought that there may be destruction of the nerves of large diameter. The loss of their normal inhibitory control may lead to a pathologic increase in spinal synaptic input by way of the small-diameter fibers, which in turn leads to a decrease in the threshold for pain; thus, the patient experiences intense sensations of pain with minimal amounts of stimulation. One must be cautious about making dogmatic statements regarding selective damage to the large-diameter fibers in the neuropathies, however, because so far this is merely a hypothetical conclusion which requires the confirmation of additional experiments and careful clinical observation.

Recently the literature has been bombarded with papers that deal with *acupuncture analgesia*. The gate control mechanism is often referred to as the neurophysiologic basis for the success of this procedure. However, there does not seem to be any reliable experimental evidence to support its role in acupuncture. In fact, the successful therapeutic use of this treatment method has not been explained in terms of any solid neurophysiologic basis.

Pain does not automatically follow presumably noxious stimuli for reasons that now can be understood. Its perception or lack of perception is strongly influenced by complex spinal cord interactions and by complex cerebral cortical functions, such as fear and anxiety, which tend to intensify the perception of pain. Attention and hypnosis can minimize this perception. If an individual is distracted by having his attention drawn to other things he will tend to forget about his discomfort, and hypnosis is a means by which he can be induced to ignore the presence of pain.

In summary, then, we may say that nerve impulses that are conducted by small-diameter, slow conducting nerve fibers are essential for the detection of the sensation of pain. These nerve fibers synapse with neurons in the dorsal spinal gray matter, where they activate the anterolateral system. This system projects to the reticular formation, hypothalamus, thalamic nuclei and limbic forebrain, which subserves the motivational–affective dimensions of pain. Impulses in the large-diameter, rapidly conducting somatosensory nerve fibers ascend in the dorsal column system to activate the ventral posterolateral nucleus of the thalamus and cerebral cortical neurons, providing the spatiotemporal discriminative capability for pain. These two parallel systems together constitute the neural basis for somatic pain.

In addition, pain sensation and perception can be modified by CNS activity. At the spinal cord level, large-diameter fibers can modulate synaptic transmission from somatic nerve fibers to spinal cord cells. Impulses descending from cerebral and other supraspinal structures also can act at spinal, brain stem and thalamic levels to influence the activity in the ascending pathways. This provides a means by which higher integrative and psychologic functions can affect pain sensation and the means by which the patient may respond to pain.

The foregoing facts provide the basis for some of the treatment techniques presently being utilized for alleviation of chronic pain. One of these involves implanting stimulating electrodes into the dorsal column system. Some success has been documented by use of this method as well as by electrical stimulation in the periaqueductal (around the cerebral aqueduct) gray matter within the midbrain. Although the gate theory may have been responsible for the initial trials of such methods for the therapeutic relief of pain, more recent evidence indicates that another mechanism is behind their success. It is thought that stimulation of various areas of the CNS produces an analgesic effect by causing the release of endorphin substances that are present normally in the brain and pituitary gland. The endorphins mimic the analgesic effects of opiates such as morphine. A direct connection between the periaqueductal gray area and spinal neurons has been demonstrated by injecting tritiated leucine into that area, and observing that it was transported down the spinal cord to the region of the incoming pain fibers in Lissauer's tract. This finding puts the use of these electrical stimulation techniques on a fairly firm physiologic basis.

Some other quite radical surgical procedures for the relief of pain include section of the anterolateral tracts in the cervical region. This procedure is effective only for pain that occurs below the level of the cervical region; in some cases the relief from pain is only temporary because, if the anterolateral system is sectioned only on one side, the uncrossed fibers of the system may continue to transmit the pain impulses to higher centers. For pain that persists in the cervical and head regions, stereotactic destruction of the thalamic nuclei that transmit pain is sometimes done; however, this is a major surgical procedure usually reserved for patients who suffer from a terminal disease.

Transcutaneous electrical nerve stimulation is a method now often used in the clinic. It involves administration of electrical stimulation to the skin in the painful area. If the pain is located in the extremities, and no relief is achieved with the electrodes placed in the painful area, the electrodes may be moved to a more proximal area over the nerves that supply the involved area. The gate control theory is presumably the basis for the success of this method. Apparently the electrical stimulation activates large peripheral nerve fibers, which subsequently inhibit the small fibers that transmit the pain impulses. There is a very low percentage of success with this method, but when such a therapeutic tool is available it is worth the attempt because it may prevent the patient from becoming addicted to such pain relievers as drugs and alcohol, and may eliminate the need for the radical surgery required for implantation of stimulating electrodes in the brain or spinal cord.

REVIEW QUESTIONS

1. List the afferent and efferent connections of the following thalamic nuclei:
   a. ventrolateral.
   b. ventrobasal (VPM and VPL).
   c. medial geniculate.
   d. lateral geniculate.
2. Is the thalamus thought of primarily as a relay station, or does it have greater functional significance? Explain.
3. Explain the somatotopic organization in the ventral nuclei of the thalamus.
4. Reproduce the diagram of the generalized scheme of the interconnections of the specific thalamic nuclei.
5. Which symptoms may be associated with the thalamic syndrome?
6. Which functions may influence a patient's response to pain?
7. Which ascending system is responsible for the discriminative perception of pain? For the motivational–affective aspects of pain?
8. Diagram and explain the "gate theory" of pain.
9. Explain why electrical stimulation of various areas of the central nervous system may produce an analgesic effect.
10. What is transcutaneous electrical nerve stimulation? What is thought to be the neurophysiologic basis for its success?
11. Of the methods for the alleviation of pain included in this discussion, which would you prefer to see tried first? Why?

CHAPTER 12 • THE HYPO-THALAMUS

OBJECTIVES

After reading this chapter you should: • Understand the importance of the influence of the hypothalamus on every aspect of the body and, in general, the means by which this influence is exerted. • Know the differences in origin, the pathways and general functions of the sympathetic and parasympathetic nervous systems. • Understand the importance of the limbic system.

THE HYPOTHALAMUS

The hypothalamus is very old phylogenetically and is of diencephalic origin. It lies inferior to the ill-defined hypothalamic sulcus and extends from the preoptic area, which is just anterior to the optic chiasm, to the midbrain tegmentum. It comprises the ventral floor of the third ventricle (see Fig. 12–1). The hypothalamus contains several nuclear groups in addition to the pituitary gland. The optic chiasm is morphologically but not functionally included in the hypothalamus, since its sole function is conveyance of visual impulses from the retina. Of the nuclear groups the mamillary bodies and the paraventricular and supraoptic nuclei are the most prominent, not because of their size but because they contain large, deeply staining cells. More is known about the connections of these nuclear groups than about other nuclear groups of the hypothalamus, and they will be the only ones considered here.

For many years the hypothalamus was neglected so that very little was known of its function, but in the last 35 years intensive research has provided evidence that it exerts an influence upon almost every aspect of function of the body, either directly or indirectly by a variety of connections. Because of this widespread influence the hypothalamus is often called the *head ganglion* of the autonomic and endocrine systems. It is directly involved in the control of respiratory, cardiovascular and thermoregulatory mechanisms, feeding and drinking behavior, sexual activity and reproduction, as well as the affective status of the individual, which includes drive, motivation and emotion.

All behavior occurs against a background of visceral and endocrine activity, which is in large part coordinated by the hypothalamus by way of connections with the brain stem reticular formation, the autonomic nervous system, the limbic system and the pituitary gland.

In general, *afferent* fibers project to the hypothalamus from olfactory regions, the midline thalamic nuclei, the brain stem reticular formation, the retina, the frontal lobe of the cerebral cortex and structures of the limbic system (hippocampal formation, amygdaloid complex and cingulate gyrus of the cortex).

Efferent projections of the hypothalamus include fibers that terminate in the hippo-

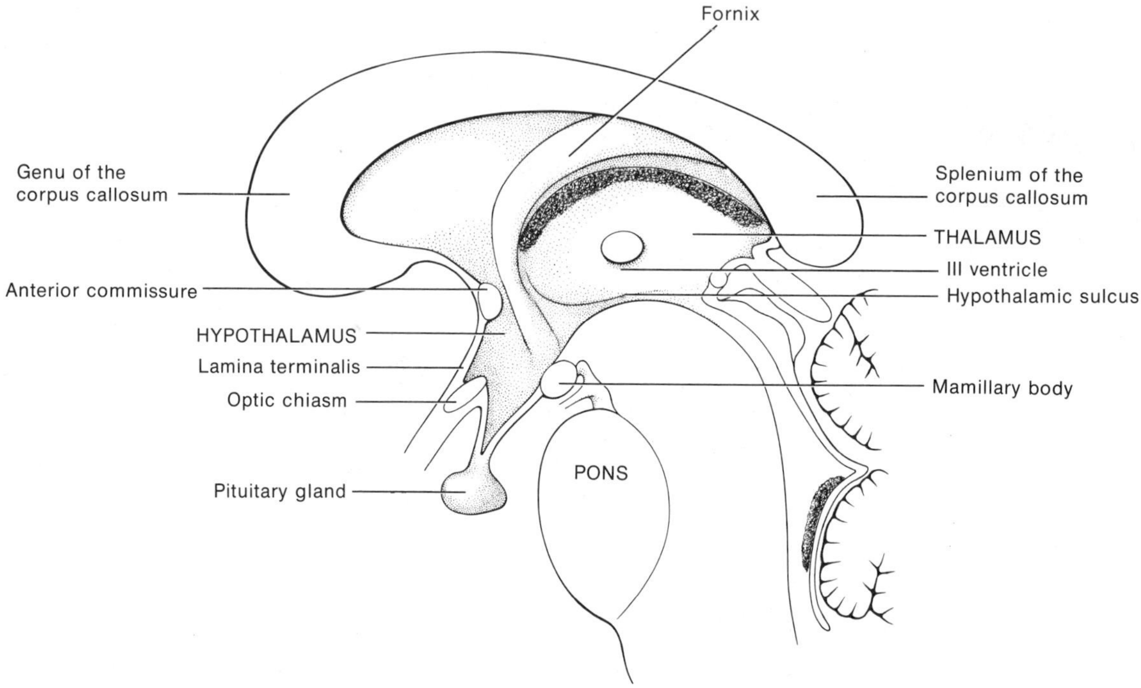

Figure 12–1. The hypothalamus and related structures.

campal formation, the amygdaloid complex, the midbrain directly and by way of the thalamus, the reticular formation and the posterior pituitary gland. Those fibers that project to the anterior thalamic nuclei originate in the mamillary bodies, which in turn receive projections from the hippocampus via the fornix. The anterior thalamic nuclei project to the frontal cortex and limbic portions of the cortex where they function to influence emotional states. The projections to the reticular formation apparently supply brain stem parasympathetic nuclei and also have relay connections with spinal sympathetic preganglionic neurons in the intermediolateral horns. Projections to the posterior pituitary gland (neurohypophysis) originate in the supraoptic nucleus and operate in the control of water balance in the body. There is also a neurohumeral link between the hypothalamus and the anterior pituitary gland, but this is via messengers carried in a portal circulatory connection rather than a direct neuronal connection.

It has been established that the hypothalamus is the chief subcortical center for regulation of both sympathetic and parasympathetic activities. Although few functions have been established for some hypothalamic nuclei we can make some general statements about them. Stimulation of anterior and medial hypothalamic areas produces a decrease in heart rate and an increase in tone and motility of the alimentary canals as well as vasodilatation and salivation through vagal and sacral parasympathetic neurons. Stimulation of the lateral and posterior hypothalamus produces activity in the sympathetic system that results in increased specific metabolic processes in certain organs and tissues which are characteristic of emotional stress, combat or flight.

The posterior lobe of the pituitary gland or neurohypophysis has its embryonic origin in the hypophysis and is considered part of it. The remainder of the pituitary gland, the adenohypophysis or anterior lobe originates as an outgrowth from the buccal cavity, and during development wraps itself around the tip of the neurohypophysis. The latter is under direct neural control of the hypothalamus, but the adenohypophysis is linked to the hypothalamus by the portal circulation mentioned previously. This portal circulatory system transmits neurohumors from the hypothalamus to the adenohypophysis. The perikaryons of the cells of the nuclei synthesize hormones which are packaged in the Golgi apparatus. These neurosecretions pass down the axons by axoplasmic flow to the neurohypophysis where they are released into the blood stream. The principal hormone produced by the supraoptic nucleus is called *antidiuretic hormone* (ADH), and that produced by the paraventricular nucleus is called *oxytocin*. ADH functions in the control of water balance and oxytocin stimulates activity of the smooth muscles of the uterus and mammary glands.

The adenohypophysis is stimulated to secrete hormones by the central nervous system through the hypothalamus. A hypothalamic–hypophyseal portal system is necessary for normal function of the anterior lobe, and it is a reasonable deduction that some substance is added to or removed from the blood as it passes through the hypothalamus, which either stimulates or inhibits the secretion of adenohypophyseal hormones. A number of hormones are secreted by the adenohypophysis, including gonadotropin, adrenocorticotropin and thyrotrophic hormone. These hormones will not be discussed in any detail here except to say that they function in the regulation of growth, basal metabolism rate, composition of body fat and sexual development.

Two areas of the hypothalamus have an important function in the regulation of body temperature. The anterior hypothalamus is sensitive to increases in temperature, and when stimulated it produces sweating and vasodilatation of cutaneous blood vessels so that excessive heat may be eliminated. The posterior hypothalamus is stimulated by decreases in temperature and responds by producing shivering and constriction of blood vessels for conservation of heat.

THE AUTONOMIC NERVOUS SYSTEM

The autonomic nervous system includes both sympathetic and parasympathetic systems, and consists of neural mechanisms involved with effectors that regulate the internal processes of the body by means of reflex responses that are not under voluntary control. The afferent pathways in the somatic and autonomic systems are very similar in that the neuronal cell bodies of both systems are located in the dorsal root ganglia, or in peripheral sensory ganglia associated with cranial nerves, but the efferent pathways are quite different. Somatic motor neurons make direct synaptic contact with their effectors, whereas autonomic motor pathways relay or synapse within a system of peripheral ganglia. Thus, the motor pathway consists of a preganglionic and a postganglionic neuron.

The division of the autonomic nervous system into sympathetic and parasympathetic portions is based on the work of Langley, who found that their anatomic features were different and that drugs affected the process of transmission differently in the two systems. *Sympathetic* preganglionic fibers are derived exclusively from the thoracic and upper lumbar segments of the spinal cord. These preganglionic fibers synapse with postganglionic fibers either in the sympathetic chain ganglia or in more peripherally located ganglia, such as the celiac, superior and inferior mesenteric ganglia. These peripherally located ganglia are referred to collectively as *prevertebral* or *preaortic* ganglia. *Parasympathetic* preganglionic fibers originate in the nuclei of several of the cranial nerve nuclei and from the motor roots of sacral nerves 2, 3 and 4. The preganglionic fibers of the parasympathetic system synapse with postganglionic fibers close to or within the structures that the postganglionic fibers innervate.

All preganglionic fibers are cholinergic (they utilize acetylcholine as a transmitter), and postganglionic fibers are either adrenergic (sympathetic nervous system) and utilize norepinephrine as an effector agent or are cholinergic (parasympathetic system) and employ acetylcholine as the final active agent.

Sympathetic System

The sympathetic chain ganglia, in which many of the sympathetic preganglionic fibers synapse, are interlinked by longitudinal fibers producing a fiber system that extends from the base of the cranium to the coccyx along the anterolateral aspect of the vertebral column. Figure 12–2 shows that the preganglionic fibers originate in the intermediolateral horn of the spinal cord, and after coursing through the ventral roots and mixed spinal nerves they gain access to the

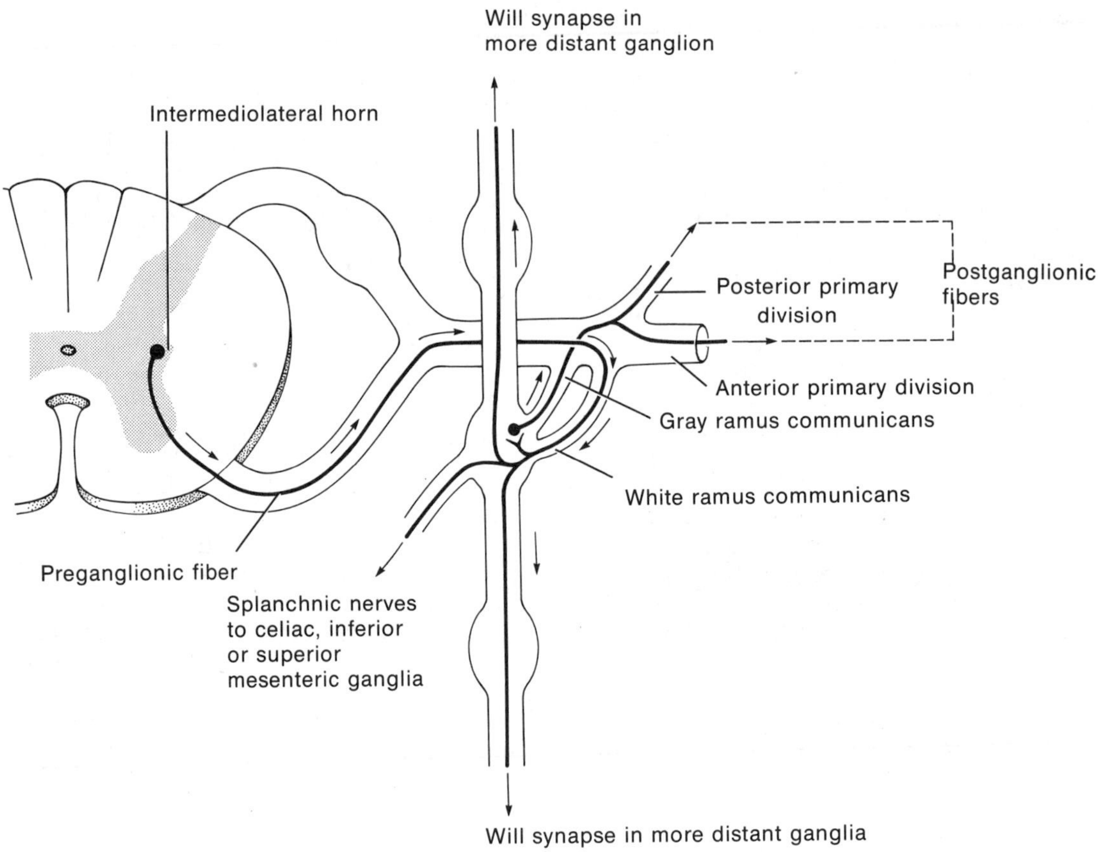

Figure 12–2. The origin and routes taken by pre- and postganglionic fibers of the sympathetic nervous system.

sympathetic chain ganglia by way of the white rami communicantes. Preganglionic fibers are myelinated, and since myelin is white in the living state these fibers make up the white rami. Within the ganglia the preganglionic fibers may synapse with postganglionic neurons at the level at which they emerge from the spinal cord; they may ascend or descend to synapse in more distant chain ganglia; or they may course through the sympathetic chain ganglia en route to the prevertebral ganglia.

Those fibers that project to the prevertebral ganglia without synapsing make up the greater, lesser and least splanchnic nerves. The preganglionic sympathetic fibers that comprise the splanchnic nerves synapse with postganglionic sympathetic neurons within the prevertebral ganglia. The postganglionic fibers then distribute to abdominal viscera. The postganglionic sympathetic fibers that originate within the sympathetic chain ganglia project back into the spinal nerves by way of the gray rami communicantes. After entering the spinal nerve they may distribute by way of either the posterior or the anterior primary divisions.

Postganglionic fibers are unmyelinated and therefore are not white; they thus make up the gray rami communicantes. Connections with the sympathetic chain in the cervical region and regions inferior to upper lumbar spinal segments are exclusively by way of gray rami, since no myelinated sympathetic preganglionic fibers enter the chain in these areas. Preganglionic fibers of the sympathetic system originate only from spinal segments T1 to L3, so that the cervical and sacral segments provide no sympathetic outflow even though their motor nerves contain postganglionic fibers from the sympathetic chain. Figures 12–3 *A* and *B* illustrate an example of how the preganglionic fibers may course into these areas.

There are fewer chain ganglia in the cervical region than elsewhere, there being only the superior, middle, intermediate and in-

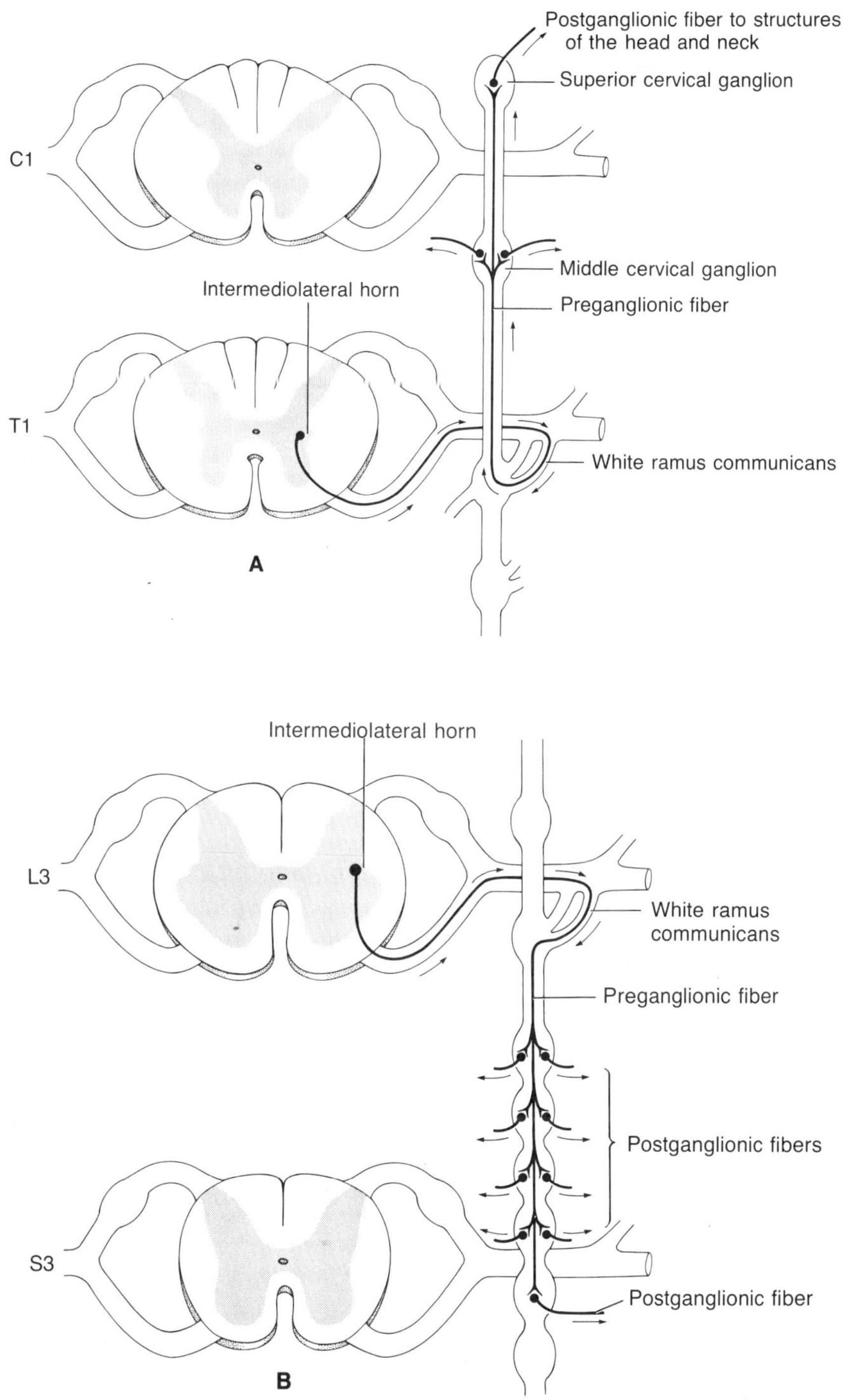

Figure 12–3. An illustration to show how preganglionic fibers extend into (*A*) the cervical areas and (*B*) areas inferior to the upper lumbar segments to synapse with postganglionic sympathetic fibers in those areas.

ferior cervical ganglia. Often the middle and intermediate ganglia are absent, and usually the inferior ganglion is fused with the first thoracic ganglion. In this case the two fused ganglia are called the *stellate ganglion.*

Postganglionic sympathetic fibers that supply the vascular smooth muscle, sweat glands and piloerector muscles may reach these structures by one of two routes. They may go from the chain ganglion back into the motor distribution of a spinal nerve to reach their destination or they may travel along the walls of arteries. For example, postganglionic sympathetic fibers that innervate the upper extremities are derived from the middle cervical ganglion and the stellate ganglion, and distribute to their effectors by way of the brachial plexus. The lower extremities receive their postganglionic sympathetic fibers from the lumbar and sacral ganglia and distribute through the lumbosacral plexus. The sympathetic postganglionic fibers that supply the head and neck course along the carotid arteries from their origin in the superior cervical ganglion.

The preganglionic fibers that supply the upper extremities originate at spinal levels T1 and T2, and those that supply the lower extremities originate at lumbar levels.

The splanchnic nerves originate in spinal segments T4 to T11 and may be contributed to by some small branches from lumbar roots. As stated earlier, the splanchnic nerves contain preganglionic fibers that terminate in the prevertebral ganglia which are located in close association with the large arteries that supply the digestive tract. The postganglionic fibers from these ganglia supply all of the abdominal viscera.

The preganglionic fibers that supply the head and neck originate in the first and second thoracic segments of the spinal cord, and after synapsing in the superior cervical ganglion the postganglionic fibers supply all the structures of the head and neck that receive sympathetic innervation. They produce secretion from the sweat glands, contraction of the piloerector muscles and constriction of the blood vessels. Fibers that project to the salivary, lacrimal and buccal glands produce secretory activity. The blood vessels of the brain receive vasoconstrictor fibers and the eye receives fibers that produce dilatation of the iris. (Recall that constriction of the iris is produced by the oculomotor nerve with the parasympathetic cells of origin located in the Edinger-Westphal nucleus.) Lesions of the superior cervical ganglion result in lack of perspiration, inability to contract the piloerector muscles and dilatation of the blood vessels of the head and neck. In addition there is lack of glandular secretory activity and constriction of the iris. Pupillary constriction of one eye, loss of sweating on one side of the face and drooping of the eyelid, associated with a lesion in the sympathetic nervous system, is known clinically as *Horner's syndrome.*

The thoracic viscera are supplied by preganglionic fibers from spinal segments T2 to T4. These fibers synapse in the stellate or cervical ganglia, after which the postganglionic fibers distribute to the heart and lungs. Those postganglionic fibers that innervate the heart produce cardiac acceleration as well as dilatation of the coronary blood vessels. Those fibers that innervate the lungs produce dilatation of the bronchi and constriction of the pulmonary vessels.

The abdominal viscera receive their innervation through postganglionic fibers that originate in the prevertebral ganglia. The sympathetic innervation of the stomach and intestines produces constriction of the blood vessels, inhibition of peristalsis and contraction of the sphincter muscles, all of which causes retention of the contents of the digestive system. Sympathetic fibers that project to the urinary bladder are inhibitory, but those to the sphincter of the bladder cause the sphincter to contract, which also causes retention of its contents.

Parasympathetic System

The parasympathetic outflow originates from cranial nerves III, VII, IX and X and from sacral spinal segments 2, 3 and 4. The pathway of innervation is also a two-neuron one, but in contrast to the sympathetic system the ganglia where synapses occur are located close to or within the effector organs.

The functions of cranial nerves III, VII and IX were discussed in Chapter 7. The vagus nerve contains the vast majority of fibers that contribute to the parasympathetic system. Its motor root sends efferent fibers to most of the thoracic and abdominal viscera. Parasympathetic fibers produce cardiac deceleration and constriction of the coronary arteries, constriction of the bronchi, augmentation of peristalsis and inhibition of the sphincters, thus enhancing emptying of the digestive tract. The vagus nerve also stimulates secretion by the stomach and pancreas and produces dilatation of small blood vessels.

Innervation by the vagus nerve extends only as far inferiorly as the junction of the transverse and descending colons. The abdominal and pelvic viscera inferior to that point are innervated by sacral segments 2, 3 and 4. Structures innervated by these spinal segments are parts of the large intestine, the rectum, the urinary bladder, the uterus and the external genitalia.

From the foregoing it is clear that the influences of the sympathetic and parasympathetic systems are generally opposed to each other, providing organs that are supplied by both with a double control of function. It is interesting that the parasympathetic system is directed with greater precision to its effector organs than is the sympathetic system. The parasympathetic fibers are preganglionic until they are very close to the organ to be innervated, so that their effect is quite precise. On the other hand, the preganglionic sympathetic fibers synapse with many postganglionic fibers which are located at long distances from the organs to be innervated, so that one preganglionic fiber may produce effects over a large area. This morphologic dichotomy fits well with the concept that the parasympathetic system functions to maintain homeostasis in the internal milieu, whereas the sympathetic system is activated in emergency situations characterized by widespread responses, including sweating, piloerection, constriction of blood vessels, dilatation of the iris, cardiac acceleration and dilatation of the bronchi.

Reflex activity of the autonomic nervous system is dependent on afferent input from both the somatic and visceral systems. For example, somatic afferent fibers convey sensation of pain from nerve endings in the skin, which may produce a number of visceral responses, including dilatation of the pupils, constriction of the peripheral blood vessels, and so on. More often, however, afferent impulses originate within the viscera, in which case the afferent fibers conveying the impulses course uninterrupted to the dorsal roots by way of splanchnic or spinal nerves through the sympathetic ganglia and the preganglionic trunks (white rami communicantes). Here, some fibers terminate in the dorsal horn of the spinal gray matter. Their distribution may be diffuse, but ultimately, after polysynaptic contacts are made with cells in the intermediolateral horn, efferent sympathetic fibers emerge to provide the efferent link of the reflex arc (see Fig. 12–4). The ascending pathways to higher centers remain rather obscure, but it is known that they terminate in the posterior thalamic nuclei and posterior hypothalamus. Afferent autonomic stimuli produce very diffuse responses, exemplified by the fact that stretching of the intestines produces dilatation of the pupils.

Visceral afferents are also known to be constituents of cranial nerves III, VII, IX, X and XI. From the discussion in Chapter 7 it is known that these afferent fibers have their cell bodies in ganglia similar to dorsal root ganglia of the spinal cord. An example of how a cranial autonomic reflex arc works is that of impulses traveling centrally via the glossopharyngeal nerve when the carotid sinus is stimulated. These fibers terminate in the dorsal motor nucleus of the vagus nerve, and the efferent link is provided by the fibers of the vagus nerve, which produce cardiac deceleration and a decrease in blood pressure. Some clinicians have utilized this reflex successfully to reduce blood pressure in individuals who suffer from hypertension. The method utilized is to put the patient in an inverted (head down) position, which increases pressure in the carotid sinus, thus stimulating the carotid sinus reflex. This method of treatment must be used with caution, however, and should not be employed in those individuals in whom the carotid sinus is not functioning normally.

The autonomic and somatic systems do not function independently from each other but rather interact very extensively, so that if one is in a state of parasympathetic dominance the muscles tend to be relaxed, and if one is in a state of sympathetic dominance the muscles tend to be tense. There are a number of ways by which the state of autonomic dominance can be shifted along the spectrum between the two extreme states.

A

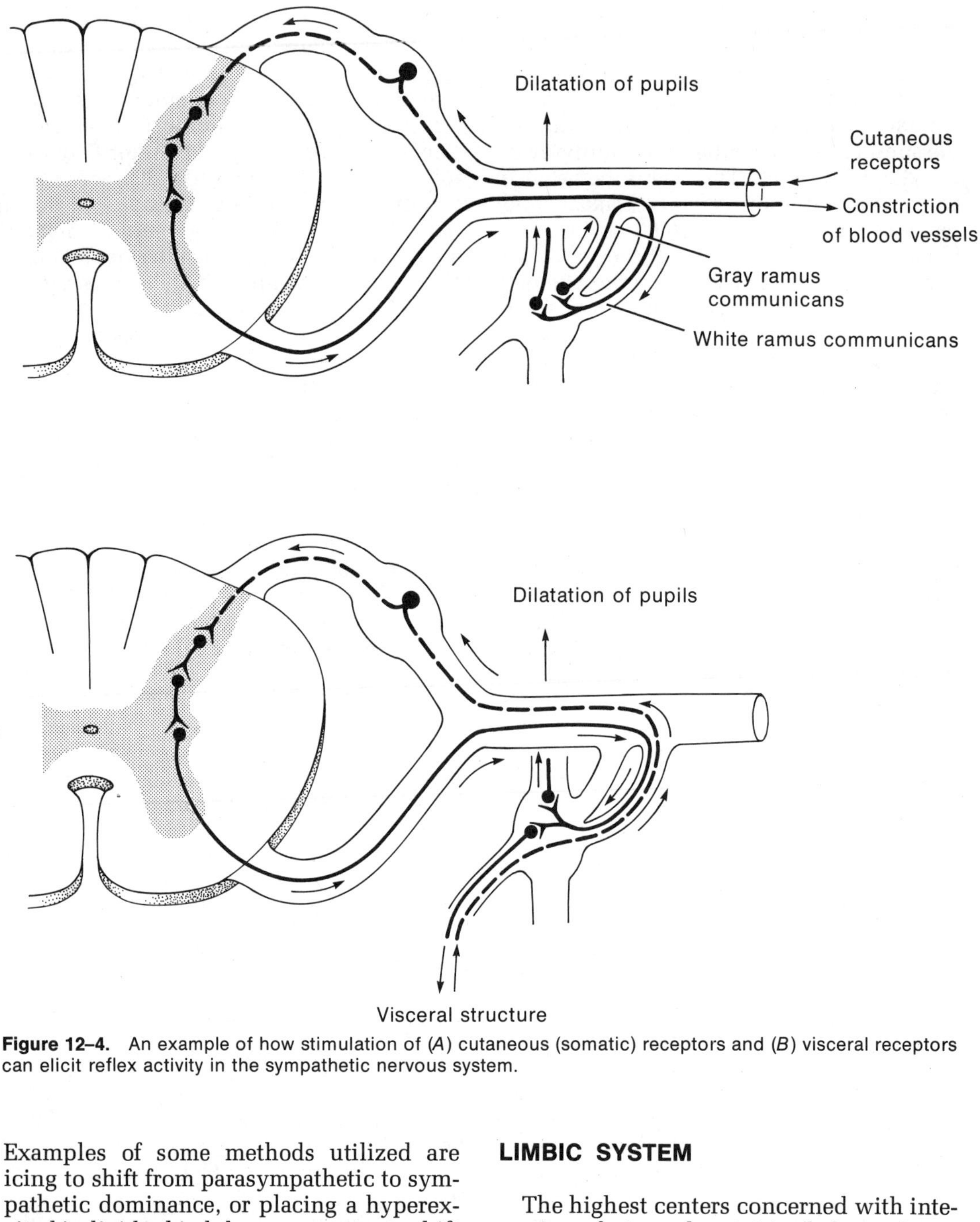

B

Figure 12–4. An example of how stimulation of (*A*) cutaneous (somatic) receptors and (*B*) visceral receptors can elicit reflex activity in the sympathetic nervous system.

Examples of some methods utilized are icing to shift from parasympathetic to sympathetic dominance, or placing a hyperexcited individual in luke-warm water to shift from a sympathetic dominant state further toward the parasympathetic end of the spectrum. It should be remembered, however, that any method used to stimulate the autonomic nervous system to elicit either responses of a systemic nature or specific somatic responses must be carefully and judiciously administered in order to avoid rebound effects or overstimulation.

LIMBIC SYSTEM

The highest centers concerned with integration of visceral activities belong almost exclusively to the limbic system, which is sometimes called the *visceral brain.* This system is associated with the emotional aspects of behavior. It includes the hippocampus and its connections, the piriform lobe, the cingulate gyrus, the insula, the septal nuclei (located within and anterior to the septum pellucidum) and the amygdaloid complex.

The interconnections of the limbic system are highly complex and only incompletely worked out. Knowledge of these complex interconnections is of very little clinical value in most instances, and therefore only a few will be briefly mentioned here. The hippocampus and septal region connect massively with the hypothalamic nuclei, primarily by way of the fornix. The hypothalamus also receives fibers from the olfactory system, the head of the caudate nucleus, the piriform cortex and the amygdaloid complex. The caudate nucleus receives from the cingulate gyrus and intralaminar nuclei of the thalamus, and the reticular formation receives fibers from the hippocampus and cingulate gyrus. Since the reticular formation is able to influence large areas of the cerebral cortex by way of various nonspecific thalamic nuclei, this is no doubt a very important means by which the autonomic nervous system exerts such a widespread influence upon the nervous system.

REVIEW QUESTIONS

1. The hypothalamus is directly involved in the control of which functions?
2. In general, through which connections does the hypothalamus exert such widespread influences?
3. Through which very important brain stem structure does the hypothalamus regulate the activity of the sympathetic and parasympathetic systems?
4. In what ways are autonomic neuronal pathways the same as somatic neuronal pathways, and in what ways do they differ?
5. State the origin and describe the pathways by which the sympathetic innervation reaches the head and neck, the upper and lower extremities, and the thoracic and abdominal viscera.
6. What are the sites of origin of the parasympathetic system? The sympathetic system?
7. In general, how do the sympathetic and parasympathetic systems differ in function? How may this be explained on a morphologic basis?
8. Diagram the routes by which afferent impulses may produce an effector response through the sympathetic nervous system.
9. What structures are included in the limbic system? Why is it important?
10. Select an ascending or descending pathway of the nervous system and discuss its anatomic connections thoroughly and logically, the types of information it carries, how the information is conveyed to other parts of the nervous system as the pathway ascends or descends, and how it might affect other ascending or descending systems. The pathway selected must be described or diagrammed completely; e.g., if the dorsal column is selected, begin with the receptors involved with that system.

CHAPTER 13 • CEREBRAL CIRCULATION AND CEREBROSPINAL FLUID

OBJECTIVES

After reading this chapter you should: • Be familiar with the most common causes of cerebral vascular accidents. • Know the origins and distribution of the blood supply of the spinal cord. • Know the consequences when the blood supply to the spinal cord is cut off. • Know the origins of the blood supply to the brain and be familiar with the vessels that enter into the make-up of the circle of Willis. • Know which structures receive their blood supply from the : a. anterior cerebral artery; b. middle cerebral artery; c. posterior cerebral artery. • Know the consequences of occlusion or hemorrhage of the: a. anterior cerebral artery; b. middle cerebral artery; c. posterior cerebral artery. • Be able to diagram the route of venous drainage from the brain. • Know the functions of cerebrospinal fluid • Know the origin and direction of flow of the cerebrospinal fluid and the means by which it gets back into the general circulation. • Know the causes of hydrocephalus. • Be familiar with some of the diagnostic laboratory examinations utilized to localize damage to the CNS.

INTRODUCTION

The brain has one of the highest metabolic rates of any structure in the body. Although it comprises only approximately 2 per cent of total body weight, it consumes about 20 per cent of the oxygen utilized by the entire body. Since there is almost no glucose or oxygen stored in the brain, its metabolism depends almost entirely on aerobic mechanisms that demand adequate flow of oxygenated blood. In fact, the brain is so very dependent on adequate blood flow that if it is deprived of its circulation consciousness can be maintained for less than ten seconds.

It is extremely worthwhile to understand the blood supply to the brain and spinal cord because of the frequently occurring cerebral vascular accidents and spinal cord injuries seen in a significant percentage of the patient population in most health care facilities.

The most common causes of deprivation of adequate blood supply to the brain (cerebral vascular accident) are:

1. *Arteriosclerosis* (atherosclerosis), which may lead to closure of the arteries if a *thrombus* forms or becomes attached to the arterial lumen.
2. *Embolisms,* which are potential obstructions that move in the blood stream until they become lodged in a narrowed area. An embolism may consist of a blood clot, air, fat, or pieces of tumors.
3. *Hemorrhage,* which is due to pathologic changes in the cerebral blood vessels.

The most common type of cerebral vascular accident involves vascular deprivation only in local areas. Those areas deprived of their blood supply degenerate so that there may be loss of function of the specific area involved.

CIRCULATION OF THE SPINAL CORD

The blood supply of the spinal cord is furnished primarily by the *vertebral arteries* and *radicular arteries*, which are branches of the deep cervical, intercostal, lumbar and sacral arteries. The radicular arteries enter the vertebral column along with the spinal nerves by way of the intervertebral foramina. They then divide into anterior and posterior radicular arteries, which contribute to both the *anterior* and *posterior spinal arteries*. The anterior and posterior spinal arteries in the cervical region are formed primarily by the vertebral arteries. The latter originate from the subclavian arteries bilaterally. They then ascend to the sixth cervical vertebra where they enter the foramen transversarium of that vertebra. They continue to ascend in the foramina transversaria of the upper cervical vertebra and enter the posterior cranial fossa via the foramen magnum.

The vertebral arteries unite to form the basilar artery, which lies in the basilar sulcus of the pons, but each vertebral artery also gives off two branches along the anterolateral surface of the medulla. These branches provide for the two descending posterior spinal arteries, one on either side of the cord, and the two anterior spinal arteries. The initial two anterior spinal arteries unite at the level of the medullary pyramids to form a single descending anterior spinal artery, which lies in the median longitudinal fissure. The posterior spinal arteries supply the posterior horns and posterior funiculi of the spinal cord, and the anterior spinal artery supplies the lateral and ventral horns and funiculi (see Fig. 13–1). If the blood supply is deprived in certain areas of the spinal cord, the symptoms will be those of a spinal cord lesion, since deprivation of the blood supply leads to necrosis of spinal cord tissue. The venous drainage has a distribution similar to that of the arteries. It consists of *anterior* and *posterior radicular veins*.

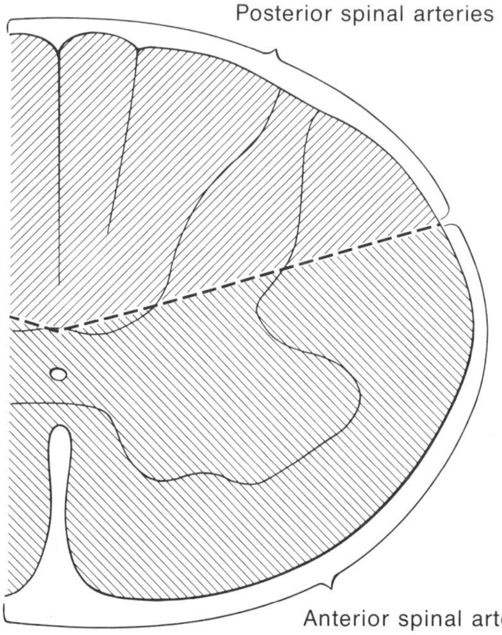

Figure 13–1. A cross-section of the spinal cord showing the areas of distribution of the anterior and posterior spinal arteries.

CIRCULATION OF THE BRAIN

The origin of the blood supply of the brain is entirely from the *vertebral* and *internal carotid arteries*. The two vertebral arteries unite to form the *basilar artery*. The latter then bifurcates to form the posterior cerebral arteries. The internal carotid arteries continue as the middle cerebral arteries after giving off the anterior cerebral arteries. The arterial configuration known as the *circle of Willis* (Fig. 13–2) consists of the anterior, middle and posterior cerebral arteries, the anterior communicating artery, which forms an anastomosis between the two anterior cerebral arteries, and the two posterior communicating arteries. The posterior communicating arteries connect the middle and posterior cerebral arteries in some cases, and in other cases connect the internal carotid and posterior cerebral arteries.

Although the circulation of the two cerebral hemispheres is connected by the anterior and posterior communicating arteries, it is important to understand that functionally these anastomoses usually are very inadequate: i.e., if there is a massive occlusion of one of the major blood vessels in one hemisphere, there is not adequate

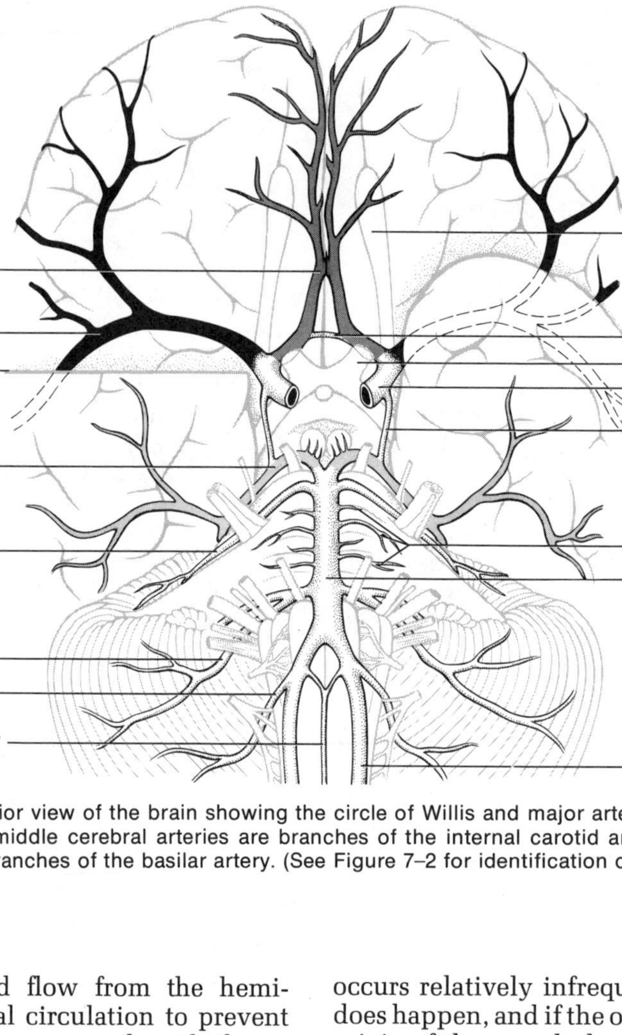

Figure 13–2. An inferior view of the brain showing the circle of Willis and major arteries of the brain. Note that the anterior and middle cerebral arteries are branches of the internal carotid artery and the posterior cerebral arteries are branches of the basilar artery. (See Figure 7–2 for identification of the cranial nerves.)

crossover of blood flow from the hemisphere with normal circulation to prevent subsequent brain damage on the side that is deprived of its circulation. This is the reason for the severity of symptoms following most cerebral vascular accidents.

The three main vessels that branch from the circle of Willis are the anterior, middle and posterior cerebral arteries.

Anterior Cerebral Artery

This supplies the medial surface of the cerebral cortex as far posteriorly as the precuneus gyrus, the rostrum of the corpus callosum, the inferior part of the head of the caudate nucleus, the septum pellucidum and septal nuclei, the anterior portions of the putamen and globus pallidus, and part of the anterior limb of the internal capsule (see Fig. 13–3).

Occlusion of the anterior cerebral artery occurs relatively infrequently, but when it does happen, and if the occlusion is near the origin of the vessel, the ensuing symptoms may include severe hemiplegia (particularly involving the contralateral lower extremity), some sensory loss over the contralateral lower extremity, personality changes and urinary incontinence.

Middle Cerebral Artery

This courses through the Sylvian fissure and supplies almost the entire lateral surface of the cerebral cortex, which includes motor, sensory, auditory and association cortices and those areas that function in speech (see Fig. 13–4). Within the Sylvian fissure the very important *lenticulostriate arteries* branch off from the middle cerebral artery and penetrate the insular cortex to supply most of the putamen, all of the caudate nucleus except for the inferior portion

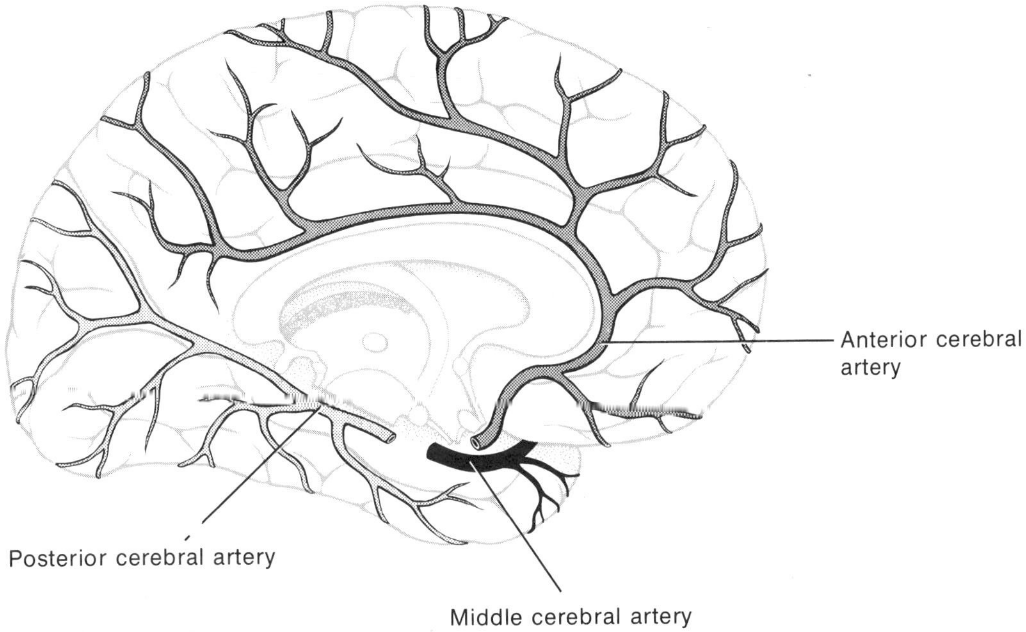

Figure 13–3. The medial aspect of the brain showing part of the distribution of the anterior, middle and posterior cerebral arteries.

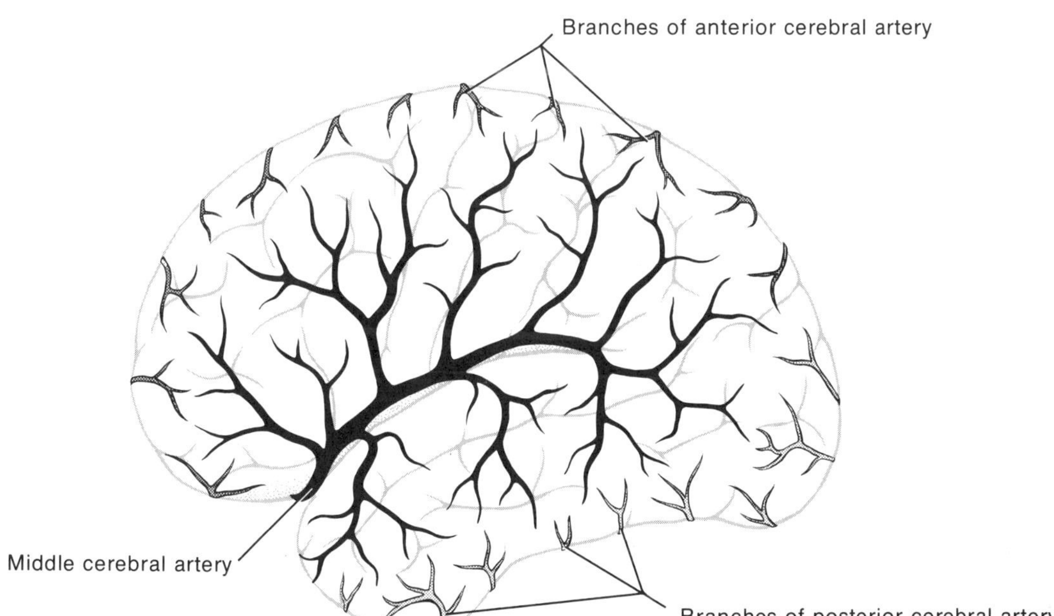

Figure 13–4. The lateral aspect of the brain showing the blood supply of the cerebral cortex. The Sylvian fissure has been opened slightly to show the course of the middle cerebral artery.

of the head, the posterolateral portion of the globus pallidus, and the posterior portion of the anterior limb and part of the posterior limb of the internal capsule.

The middle cerebral artery is the most common site of vascular occlusion. If the occlusion occurs close to its origin the symptoms are severe and very disabling if not fatal. The contralateral hemiplegia or hemiparesis that results involves the upper extremity and face most severely. In addition to supplying many of the nerve cells of origin of the corticospinal and extrapyramidal tracts, the middle cerebral artery also supplies cells of origin of the corticobulbar pathways, hence the resulting weakness of the face and other structures innervated by the cranial nerves. Patients with cerebral vascular accidents should always be evaluated very carefully for damage of cortical fibers that project to the cranial nerves. There may be a contralateral sensory loss in the same areas in which the motor deficits occur. If the lesion is in the left hemisphere there may be both motor and sensory disturbances of speech, since these areas are located in the superior temporal lobe and the inferior frontal gyrus. If the lesion is in the right hemisphere the patient is likely to be dyspraxic or apraxic, and may not even recognize the existence of the left side of the body. Homonymous hemianopia very frequently accompanies the rest of these symptoms.

One of the most common localized sites of occlusion of the middle cerebral artery is in the lenticulostriate branches that supply the internal capsule and parts of the basal ganglia. This lesion produces the typical contralateral spastic hemiplegia or hemiparesis so often seen clinically. The disability is the result of damage to the ascending and descending systems located in the internal capsule.

The severity of symptoms that result from cerebral occlusion always depends on the location of the lesion. If it is near the origin of one of the major vessels, large areas of the body may be severely involved, whereas if the lesion restricts itself to a small local branch, or occurs in an intermediate position, it may go unnoticed or may result in a monoplegia (involvement of just one extremity). In general, the nearer the occlusion is to the origin of a vessel, the more severe will be the symptoms, since more extensive areas of the brain are damaged.

Occlusion of the internal carotid artery most frequently occurs at the level at which the common carotid artery bifurcates to form the internal and external carotid arteries. The symptoms of internal carotid artery occlusion are very similar to those of middle cerebral artery occlusion combined with anterior cerebral artery occlusion, unless the anterior communicating artery becomes functional.

Posterior Cerebral Artery

This is derived from the vertebral-basilar arterial system and supplies almost all of the medulla, pons, midbrain and cerebellum along with the cerebellar arteries that are derived from the basilar artery. In addition it supplies the medial, inferior and posterior surface of the occipital lobe, including the primary visual cortex, the posterior portion of the posterior limb of the internal capsule, the inferior surface of the temporal lobe, the thalamus, hypothalamus and infundibulum, and the choroid plexus of the principal portion of the lateral and third ventricles.

The results of occlusion of the posterior cerebral artery tend to be quite variable because there are several anastomotic branches between it and the middle cerebral artery, but the occurrence of these anastomotic branches varies from individual to individual. The symptoms that may be produced are homonymous hemianopia and the "thalamic syndrome," which may include contralateral hemianesthesia, hemichorea and "central pains." The hemianesthesia may be complete, involving all modalities, or it may be partial, depending on the extent of the damage to the thalamus, but sensation is never normal. Central pains are sometimes present following posterior cerebral artery occlusion. This type of pain is referred to as *thalamic pain* because it is caused by damage to the thalamus.

Thalamic pain is characterized as a deep, lancinating and boring pain which is felt in the soft tissues and bone. This type is difficult to tolerate and unfortunately is not usually relieved by treatment with analgesics or by surgical intervention. There is a considerable suicide rate among those who

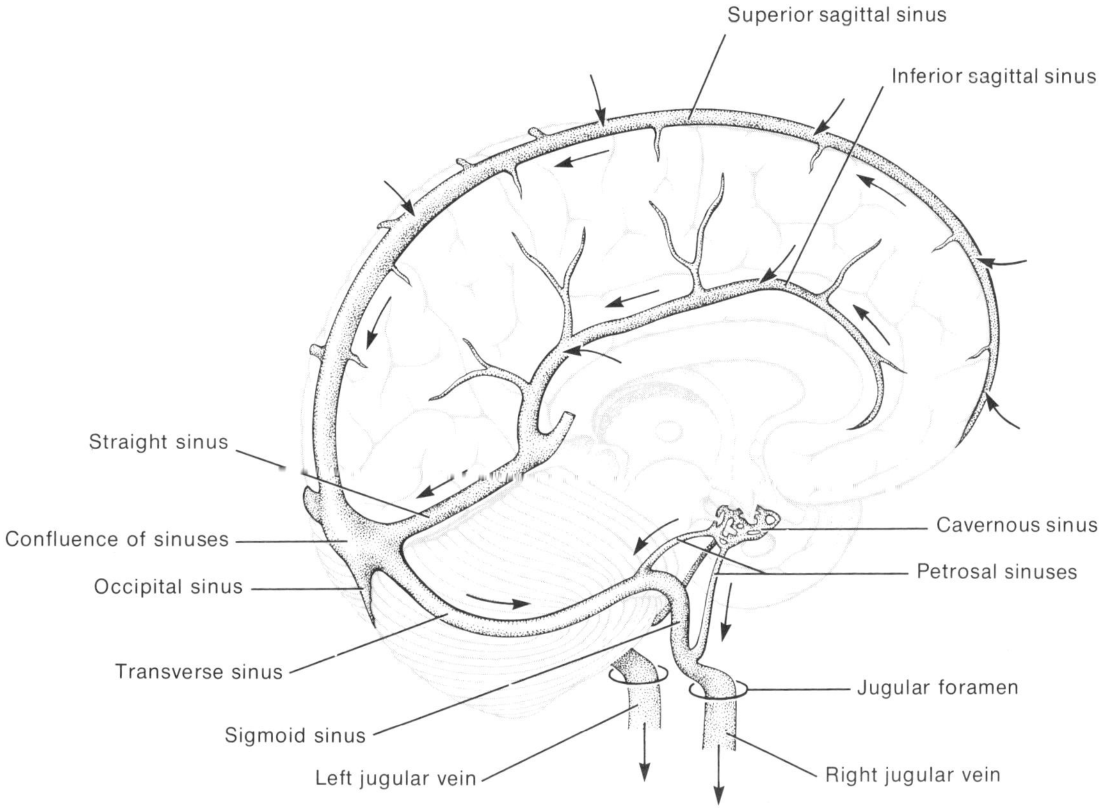

Figure 13–5. A diagrammatic representation of the venous drainage of the brain from a postero-medial view.

suffer from this syndrome. Another characteristic of thalamic lesions is that these patients have a tendency to overrespond to stimuli and to feel their effects long after the stimuli have ceased. The choreic movements, when present, are flinging and violent in nature, but can be controlled by the administration of chlorpromazine. Other symptoms that may accompany posterior cerebral artery occlusion are a contralateral hemiparesis due to involvement of the internal capsule, and abnormal autonomic function if the hypothalamus is damaged.

Cerebral Venous System

Superficially, the cerebral veins follow the courses of the arteries fairly closely, but their courses diverge centrally as the veins drain into dural sinuses, so-called because they are formed by splitting of the dural sheath. The veins may empty into the superior or inferior sagittal sinus or into the cavernous sinuses. The superior sagittal sinus drains directly into the transverse sinuses, whereas the inferior sagittal sinus drains into the straight sinus, which then drains into the transverse sinuses. The point at which the superior sagittal, straight and transverse sinuses converge is called the confluence of the sinuses. The transverse sinuses are continuous with the sigmoid sinuses, which return the blood to the general circulation by way of the internal jugular veins that originate at the jugular foramina. The cavernous sinuses drain by way of the petrosal sinuses into the sigmoid sinuses, after which the route of the venous blood is the same as that of the other sinuses (see Fig. 13–5).

CEREBROSPINAL FLUID

The cerebrospinal fluid (CSF) is located in the ventricular system of the brain, the subarachnoid spaces of the brain and spinal cord, and the central canal of the spinal cord. In man these spaces contain approximately 125 ml of CSF of which there is an appreciable turnover, since 45 to 130 ml of new CSF is produced per day.

The functions of CSF are to provide: (1) a protective layer to cushion the central nervous system; (2) a fluid pathway for chemical substances to be transported to and from the CNS; and (3) a pathway by which neural metabolites may return to the venous system.

The chroid plexus of all of the ventricles elaborate CSF and secrete it into the ventricles. The general direction of flow is from the lateral to the third ventricle and then to the fourth ventricle via the cerebral aqueduct. From the fourth ventricle it reaches the subarachnoid spaces of the brain and spinal cord by way of the medially located foramen of Magendie and the two laterally located foramina of Luschka. There is also a slight upward current of CSF from the spinal central canal. This fluid is probably derived from the ependymal lining of the central canal. The circulating fluid is passively returned to the venous system by passage through the arachnoid villi, which are located primarily in the venous lacunae of the superior sagittal sinus. It is then returned to the general circulation by the same route by which the venous blood is returned into the internal jugular vein.

If the flow of CSF is blocked somewhere in the ventricular system, or if for some reason it is not absorbed, hydrocephalus is produced. This is discussed in Chapter 5.

The CSF is clear to somewhat yellowish and slightly viscous. It contains small quantities of inorganic salts, primarily potassium chloride and sodium chloride, in addition to small amounts of dextrose and traces of proteins. Normally, it contains very few cells. Very frequently lumbar puncture, and less frequently puncture into the cisterna magna (cisterna cerebellomedullaris), is done to measure the pressure of and to obtain CSF from the subarachnoid space for diagnostic purposes. The preferred location for lumbar puncture is between the third and fourth lumbar vertebrae. Cistern punctures are done between the first and second cervical vertebrae.

Normally, CSF pressure is between 100 and 200 mm. Pressures recorded outside these limits are abnormally high or abnormally low. Increased pressure may be observed in patients with brain tumors, subdural hematoma, brain abscesses or cysts, infection, head injury, cerebral hemorrhage or occlusion, subarachnoid hemorrhage and metabolic encephalopathies. The pressure also may increase in conjunction with hydrocephalus and benign intracranial hypertension. Decreased pressure may be caused by dehydration or spinal cord tumors that may block the flow in the subarachnoid spaces.

The cell content of CSF increases in a great number of abnormal conditions. In general, if more than six white cells or any red cells are present it is of pathologic significance. Alterations in protein and sugar content may also be present in a number of pathologic conditions. The reader is referred to Alpers and Mancall's "Essentials of the Neurological Examination," 1973, pp. 129–135, for more detailed information regarding abnormalities that may be detected by examination of CSF.

Laboratory Examinations

The evaluation of CNS deficits will be discussed in Chapter 15, but it seems appropriate here to mention some of the diagnostic laboratory examinations currently used to determine the sites of cerebral vascular accidents.

Electroencephalography is sometimes utilized to locate the site of a cerebral lesion. Electrical activity of groups of cortical neurons is recorded by the application of scalp electrodes. The electrical potentials are amplified, recorded and analyzed for abnormalities. The electrodes are moved from site to site, and abnormal electrical activity occurs when they are placed over the site of the lesion. The closer the lesion is to the surface of the cerebral cortex, the more reliably can it be localized.

Cerebral arteriography may be employed to evaluate a number of vascular diseases. It involves direct injection of a radiopaque substance into the vertebral or carotid arteries or into the aortic arch or brachial vessels. The substance then circulates through the blood vessels of the brain, during which time serial radiographs are taken. From these information may be obtained regarding structural abnormalities of vessels, alterations in positions of vessels and alterations in blood flow patterns.

Radioisotope (scintillation) brain scan-

ning is one of the methods of choice presently used to diagnose intracranial lesions. A number of different isotopes have been utilized. They are injected and the brain is then scanned for areas in which the concentration of isotope is increased. Hematomas, tumors and vascular malformations may all be demonstrated by this safe diagnostic technique.

Another relatively new method is called *echoencephalography*. This is a safe technique that uses ultrasound, which produces echoes that rebound from the deep structures of the brain. The echoes are recorded and their characteristics can determine the location of cranial contents (i.e., shifts away from the midline), and sometimes the thickness of hematomas can be determined.

Computerized Axial Tomography (CAT scanning) is in current widespread use and has replaced some of the older procedures such as pneumoencephalography. CAT scans are a form of computerized x-ray densitometry, which has many advantages. The biggest disadvantage is the great expense of the x-ray equipment and computer instrumentation required to process the results (Patten, 1977).

REVIEW QUESTIONS

1. What are the most common causes of cerebral vascular accidents?
2. Which arteries supply the spinal cord?
3. Which parts of the spinal cord are supplied by:
   a. the anterior spinal artery?
   b. the posterior spinal arteries?
4. In general, what symptoms may occur if the blood supply to part of the spinal cord is occluded?
5. From which arteries is the entire blood supply of the brain derived?
6. Diagram and label completely the arterial configuration of the circle of Willis.
7. Name the structures that receive their blood supply from:
   a. the anterior cerebral artery.
   b. the middle cerebral artery.
   c. the posterior cerebral artery.
8. What symptoms may occur if there is occlusion of:
   a. the anterior cerebral artery?
   b. the middle cerebral artery?
   c. the posterior cerebral artery?
   d. the internal carotid artery?
9. Diagram and label completely the venous drainage of the brain.
10. What are the functions of cerebrospinal fluid?
11. From what structures is CSF derived?
12. Explain the direction of flow of CSF from its origin to its return into the general circulation.
13. What is hydrocephalus? What causes it?
14. What are some of the laboratory examinations by which CNS deficits may be localized? Briefly explain each one.

CHAPTER 14 • DEGENERATION AND REGENERATION OF NERVES SUBSEQUENT TO TRAUMA

OBJECTIVES

After reading this chapter you should: • Understand that when nerve cell perikaria are destroyed they are not replaced. • Know that regeneration *may* occur when axons have been damaged without damage to the perikaria. • Know the difference in potential for regeneration of nerves in the central versus the peripheral nervous system • Understand wallerian degeneration. • Understand retrograde degeneration. • Be able to describe the changes that occur during chromatolysis. • Be aware of the factors essential for successful regrowth of axons to their appropriate end organs. • Know the rate of regeneration in the peripheral nervous system. • Know some of the causes of CNS lesions. • Be aware of some of the available electrodiagnostic tests that determine the integrity of peripheral nerves.

DEGENERATION AND REGENERATION

In the mammalian brain, essentially all nerve cells are produced by the time the individual is born. No new cells are produced subsequent to that time. If the perikaryon of a nerve cell is destroyed, the entire nerve cell is lost permanently and cannot be replaced. The nerve cell body and its processes are destroyed because the *Nissl substance*, which produces protein for the maintenance of the whole cell, is located primarily in the cell body. However, if axons have been interrupted without damage to the cell bodies, regeneration of the peripheral segment of the axon may occur.

In order to understand the recovery of function that might be expected subsequent to peripheral nerve injuries and CNS lesions, it is important to have first some understanding of both the degeneration and the regeneration process.

In the peripheral nervous system new functional connections can be made by regenerating axons, but in the central nervous system new functional connections generally are not made. Once a central pathway is cut, it cannot be reestablished. For example, when the ascending and/or descending pathways are damaged by a spinal cord injury, the damaged axons do not make functional connections with their appropriate target cells.

When a peripheral or central axon is cut, the portion of the axon which is distal to the damage degenerates. This is called *wallerian degeneration*, named after Waller, who formulated the law that "when an axon is divided, the part that is separated from its perikaryon undergoes degeneration," i.e., an axon cannot survive without its perikaryon.

The rate of degeneration is faster in the peripheral than in the central nervous system. In the peripheral nervous system degeneration of axons begins within 24 hours and is well advanced five or six days later. In the central nervous system degeneration does not begin until about three days after a lesion occurs and is not well advanced until seven to 14 days afterwards.

Myelin degeneration roughly follows the same time course as axon degeneration, but begins within two minutes after injury. However, the debris from degenerating myelin persists in the area longer than that of axons, especially in the CNS.

The degenerating axons and myelin of the peripheral segments are removed by the phagocytic activity of invading macrophages and Schwann cells in the peripheral nervous system, and primarily by microglia in the central nervous system.

In the peripheral nervous system, after being freed of the degenerating myelin, the Schwann cells divide and line themselves up in continuous rows within the persistent original endoneurial sheath, if the Schwann cell basal lamina and endoneurium is left intact. These rows of Schwann cells are called *bands of Büngner* and function as mechanical guidelines for regenerating axonal sprouts.

Degenerative changes also occur proximal to the site of injury, but these changes are extremely variable. Degeneration *proximal* to the site of injury is called *retrograde* degeneration. Some cell bodies show no change at all, but others degenerate and die within a few days. Most commonly the changes that occur are somewhere between these two extremes and include: (1) swelling of the perikaryon; (2) peripheral displacement of the nucleus; and (3) dispersion of Nissl substance. This triad of modification is referred to as *chromatolysis*. Figure 14–1 shows a comparison between a normal and a chromatolytic nerve cell.

Chromatolysis has been found to occur in dorsal root ganglion cells, some motor cells of cranial nerves, and in general in the larger cells of the CNS, and usually is most marked seven to 14 days following a lesion. Degeneration of the proximal segment of the axon for a length of approximately one or two nodes of Ranvier is also a part of the retrograde degenerative process. This process may be reversible, and the cell may return to a completely normal state, or it may lead to cell death. The changes that comprise chromatolysis appear to be related to the formation of new protein for the purpose of repair-

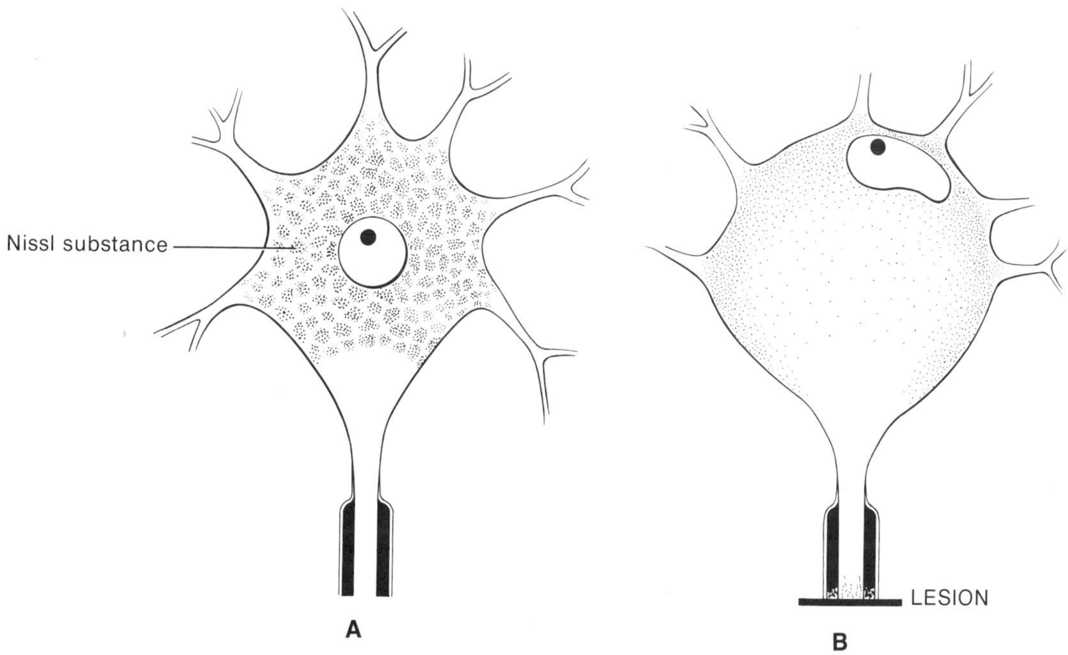

Figure 14–1. *A,* A normal nerve cell body. *B,* A chromatolytic cell body, which is swelled, has a peripherally placed nucleus and dispersed Nissl substance.

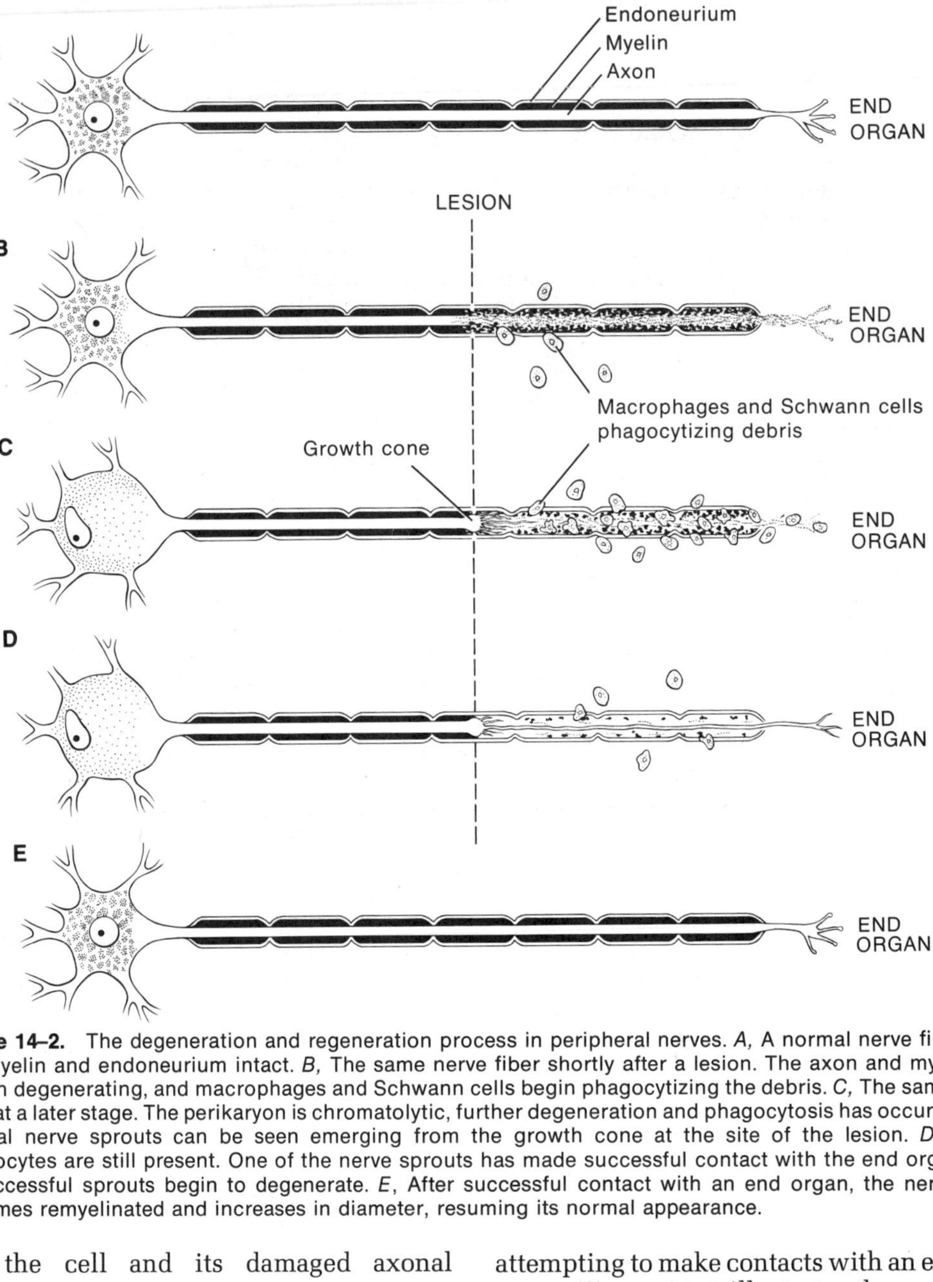

Figure 14–2. The degeneration and regeneration process in peripheral nerves. *A,* A normal nerve fiber with the myelin and endoneurium intact. *B,* The same nerve fiber shortly after a lesion. The axon and myelin are shown degenerating, and macrophages and Schwann cells begin phagocytizing the debris. *C,* The same nerve fiber at a later stage. The perikaryon is chromatolytic, further degeneration and phagocytosis has occurred, and several nerve sprouts can be seen emerging from the growth cone at the site of the lesion. *D,* A few phagocytes are still present. One of the nerve sprouts has made successful contact with the end organ. The unsuccessful sprouts begin to degenerate. *E,* After successful contact with an end organ, the nerve fiber becomes remyelinated and increases in diameter, resuming its normal appearance.

ing the cell and its damaged axonal process.

If the perikaryon does not die as a result of retrograde degeneration, the axon remains intact proximal to the lesion except for the previously mentioned degeneration along the length of one or two nodes of Ranvier. The proximal segment of the axon can then form axonal sprouts at the cut ends of the nerve fiber.

Regeneration may begin as early as three hours after injury, at which time the tips of the axonal stumps enlarge to form *growth cones*. These send out from 10 to 40 exploratory pseudopodia which make their way along the mechanical guidelines in the bands of Büngner in the area and distally, attempting to make contacts with an effector organ. Figure 14–2 illustrates the regeneration process.

Successful growth of the nerve sprouts back to their effector organs is dependent on:

1. The pathways offered by the remaining peripheral degenerating nerve stump. If the epineurium is not intact there is very likely to be formation of a neuroma. In addition, bands of Büngner must be laid down by the Schwann cells for good regeneration to proceed. For these two reasons, suture of the epineurium may be necessary if the nerve trunk has been completely severed.
2. The amount of scar tissue at the site of the

lesion. If dense scar tissue has been produced, it may be impossible for the axon sprouts to cross it to enter the bands of Büngner.

3. Successful contact with an end organ.

If conditions allow the axon to enter Büngner's bands, successful regneration with restoration of function will generally occur. The fact that each regenerating axon can produce many new sprouts increases the chance of making successful contacts with end organs, but only those branches that make successful contact with end organs become remyelinated and survive. Therefore, although there is a great overproduction of axon sprouts during the early stages of regeneration, the number becomes greatly reduced, since the first axon within an endoneurial sheath to make a successful connection is the only one to survive. The successful axon becomes remyelinated only after it connects with an end organ, which brings up one of the most interesting questions in neuroscience: why is it that remyelinization does not occur until an axon makes a successful contact with an end organ? What turns on the myelin production switch?

In general, in the mammalian peripheral nervous system, motor axons reinnervate motor organs and sensory peripheral processes reinnervate sensory organs. Cross-connections of motor nerves to sensory organs and vice versa are not formed. For example, cutaneous nerves do not reinnervate muscles nor do alpha or gamma motor neurons reinnervate pacinian corpuscles. However, there appears to be very little specificity beyond this: a peripheral alpha motor neuron, in general, will innervate any muscle and the muscle will then function according to its new connections with the CNS. The first regenerating nerve to reach a muscle reinnervates it, whether it is the appropriate one or not, which may lead to complications. For example, if a nerve previously innervated a flexor muscle, and upon reinnervation that nerve establishes connections with an extensor muscle, one must think flexion in order to get that muscle to do extension.

Generally one new motor end plate will be formed on each extrafusal muscle fiber as in the normal situation. Hyperneurotization usually does not occur either normally or upon reinnervation.

The rate of regeneration in the peripheral nervous system varies from 1 to 4 mm per day, although most clinicial histories of recovery indicate that 1 mm per day is more accurate. This is important to keep in mind when working with patients with peripheral nerve injuries in order to estimate roughly the time within which it is reasonable to expect some return of function. One must also allow some additional time for the regenerating axons to cross the scar tissue and to make functional connections after they reach their target organs.

Diagnostic Tests

Several diagnostic tests are available for testing the function of peripheral nerves.

THE REACTION OF DEGENERATION

The procedure consists of initially attempting to stimulate the peripheral nerve in which damage is suspected with alternating current. If the nerve is functioning normally all the muscles which are innervated by the nerve distal to the point of stimulation will respond with a tetanic contraction. A normally functioning nerve which is stimulated with direct current will respond by producing a brisk twitch in each muscle that it innervates distal to the point of stimulation. Both or either of these responses indicates that there is no reaction of degeneration.

A *partial reaction of degeneration* is indicated by a diminished response to both types of electrical stimulation in all muscles innervated by the nerve distal to the point of stimulation. If each of the muscles is stimulated directly, the response to alternating current is diminished and it may require higher-than-normal intensities to produce any response. The response to direct current will be diminished and may be slower than the normal brisk twitch. A partial reaction of degeneration may be present immediately after the nerve is damaged before degeneration of the peripheral stump is complete, during the reinnervation process before it is complete and when the damage to the nerve is only partial.

A *total* or *full reaction of degeneration* is present when there is no response in the muscle when the nerve trunk is stimulated by either alternating or direct current. When the muscle is stimulated directly, there is no response to alternating current and only a slow, sluggish, wormlike response to direct current. The total reaction of degeneration occurs 14 to 21 days after a peripheral nerve has been completely severed. It indicates that there is loss of excitability of the nerve and this state may persist for a period of several weeks to several years.

If there is an *absolute reaction of degeneration*, neither the nerve nor the muscle will respond to either alternating or direct current. This indicates loss of excitability of both the nerve and the muscle. The absolute reaction does not occur until several years after the injury when the contractile muscle tissue has been replaced by fibrous connective tissue.

STRENGTH-DURATION CURVES

This procedure employs determination of a value called *rheobase*, which according to Brown and Meng is defined as the intensity of an electrical impulse of infinite duration required to evoke a threshold response in a muscle. Three hundred milliseconds is usually long enough to be considered infinite. The duration of the electrical impulse then is gradually decreased and the intensity of stimulation necessary to produce a threshold response is established for each duration. The intensity of stimulation required for a threshold response at 15 durations between 300 and 0.1 milliseconds is usually adequate for a determination of the integrity of the nerve supply to a muscle. The test is complete when a threshold response to the shortest duration is attained or when the stimulation is too painful for the patient at any given duration. The results may be interpreted as follows:

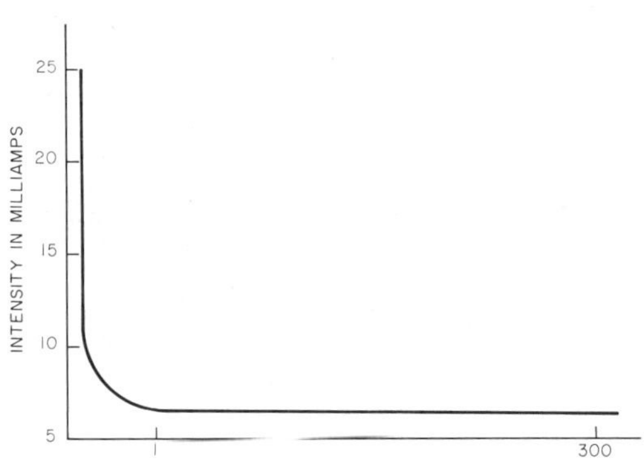

The above flat, continuous curve indicates a normally innervated muscle. There is very little, if any, increase in the intensity required to produce a minimal muscle contraction until the impulse duration is below 1 millisecond.

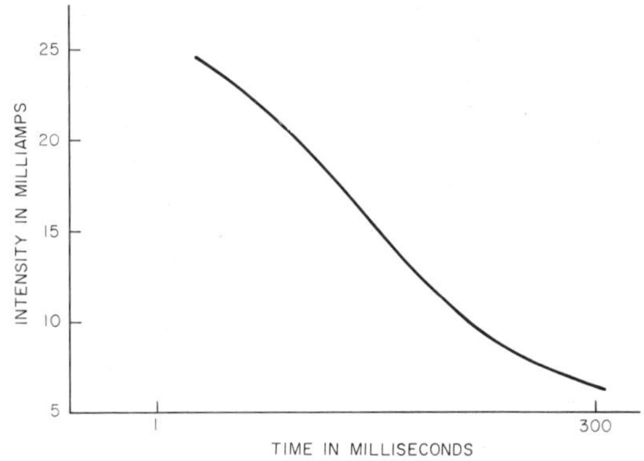

This steep, continuous curve is shifted to the right and a rapid increase in intensity is required as the duration decreases to produce a minimal muscle contraction (threshold response). The patient's intolerance of the high intensities required to produce a reaction at shorter duration usually limits the testing that can be done at shorter durations. This type of curve indicates denervated muscle tissue.

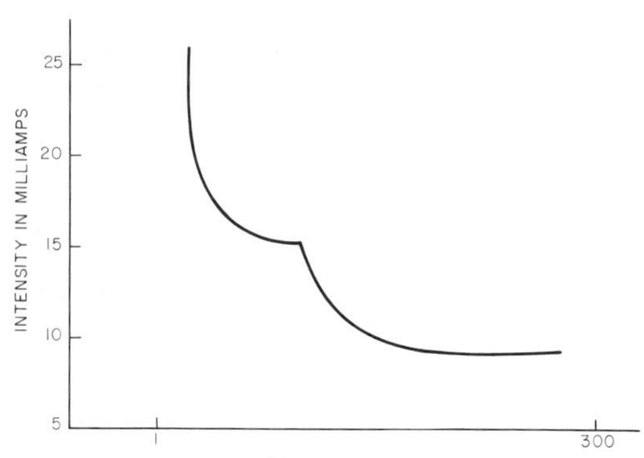

This discontinuous curve, which tends to be positioned between the normal and denervated, indicates that the muscle is partially denervated. It may mean that there has been a partial injury or that the nerve is degenerating or regenerating. "The significance of this curve can be determined only in relation to the time of injury, by comparison with previous or subsequent tests, in conjunction with other medical and neurological findings" (Brown and Meng, 1974).

DETERMINATION OF CHRONAXY

Chronaxy is defined as the minimum duration that an electrical current of twice the intensity of rheobase must have in order to evoke a muscular contraction. "Some feel that this measure follows most consistently the process of degeneration and reinnervation" (Brown and Meng, 1974).

To administer this test the point of optimal response must first be located and rheobase must be established. The intensity of the electrical current should then be set at a value twice that of rheobase. The impulse duration is then increased slowly from 0 until a threshold response identical to the rheobase response is obtained.

The chronaxy of normally innervated muscle is below 1 millisecond and may approach 0.1 millisecond. *Degeneration* is indicated when serial chronaxy measurements show a gradual *increase*. *Denervation* is indicated when chronaxy is in excess of 15 milliseconds. *Regeneration* of a nerve is reflected by a gradual *decrease* in chronaxy and voluntary motion may be present before the value of chronaxy reaches normal. An *increase* in chronaxy from 1 to 15 milliseconds may be indicative of a partial lesion.

Other classic electrodiagnostic tests include the strength-rise curve and lambda ratio tests.

More recent additions to the diagnostic armamentarium for the determination of the integrity of peripheral nerves include *electromyography*, which records the electrical activity generated during muscle contraction; and *nerve conduction velocity* studies that, as the name implies, measure the velocity at which impulses are conducted along a nerve trunk. *Biofeedback* works on the same principle as the electromyograph. In addition to recording the electrical activity produced by contracting muscles, this instrument may be used to reeducate weak muscles.

The details of administration and interpretation of the above tests may be found in "Fundamentals of Electrotherapy (Course Guide)" by Brown and Meng, 1974.

In the mammalian CNS axonal regeneration is abortive in the vast majority of cases. There is no return of function when axons are completely severed from connections with their cell bodies. The reasons for failure of functional return are unclear, but some of the possible explanations are:

1. Too much glial scarring produced by astrocytic processes occurs so that the axonal sprouts cannot grow across the area that has been injured.
2. There may be differences in Schwann cells and oligodendroglial cells. It is not known whether the latter are capable of laying down mechanical guidelines similar to Büngner's bands for the axons to follow during regeneration.
3. Other axons may take over the synaptic contacts previously occupied by the degenerating axons so that when (if) they do regenerate they cannot make functional contacts.
4. Allergic factors, since Feringa et al have found that immunosuppressive agents have produced some physiologic regeneration in the long descending tracts of the adult rat spinal cord.

We do know that axonal regeneration in the CNS is most successful when vascular damage and scarring are minimal or absent, but even under these conditions there is no significant functional return. However, it is important to understand that when axons become demyelinated without interruption of the axons themselves, regeneration of myelin can occur in both the peripheral and central nervous systems. This accounts for the remissions and exacerbations characteristic of demyelinating diseases, an example of which is multiple sclerosis. Degeneration of myelin in this disease accounts for the periods of exacerbation; regeneration of myelin accounts for the periods of remission.

Some of the major causes of CNS lesions are:

1. Mechanical, such as forceps injuries at birth, or trauma later in life.
2. Anoxia or asphyxiation during birth.
3. Viruses, which may selectively affect sensory fibers; others selectively affect motor neurons.
4. Chemicals and heavy metals such as lead, copper, cadmium, etc.
5. Heredity, e.g., some types of muscular dystrophy, Huntington's chorea, etc.
6. Vascular trauma or abnormalities.

REVIEW QUESTIONS

1. Explain why nerve cells cannot regenerate if the perikaryon is destroyed.
2. What is wallerian degeneration?
3. Describe the process of peripheral nerve regeneration.
4. Explain the changes that may occur during retrograde degeneration.
5. Upon what factors does successful growth of nerve sprouts back to their effector organs depend?
6. When do regenerated neurons become remyelinated?
7. Do sensory neurons reinnervate motor organs or motor neurons reinnervate sensory organs? Do regenerating axons always reinnervate the same structure that they innervated before being damaged?
8. What is the rate of regeneration of peripheral nerves?
9. Does regeneration in the central nervous system usually lead to functional recovery? Give some reasons for your answer.
10. What are some of the electrodiagnostic tests used for testing the integrity of peripheral nerves?
11. When myelin has been destroyed either in the central or peripheral nervous system can it regenerate?
12. What are some of the major causes of CNS lesions?

CHAPTER 15 • EVALUATION OF CENTRAL NERVOUS SYSTEM LESIONS

OBJECTIVES

After reading this chapter you should: • Be familiar with the names of some of the evaluative scales and procedures that have been developed for infants. • Be familiar with the sequence of normal growth and development. • Be able to use the glossary of reflexes and reactions to enhance your understanding of CNS function. • Know, in general, what types of symptoms may be produced by CNS deficits. • Know how to test for function of the cranial nerves. • Recognize the importance of determining the state of the patient's autonomic nervous system.

INTRODUCTION

This chapter is not intended to encompass the complete neurologic examination, but rather to provide reference to the literature that describes the details of evaluation of infants and adults, to give information about the approximate timing and sequence of normal infant development, to discuss generally the symptoms that may be produced by CNS lesions and to describe a few of the basic procedures by which we can determine the integrity of the CNS. Lesions of the CNS may be hereditary, they may occur at birth, or they may appear at any time during the life span of an individual.

EVALUATION OF THE NEONATE

The major causes of lesions at birth may be mechanical factors such as trauma produced by the use of forceps, or may be anoxia or asphyxiation as the result of twisting of the umbilical cord or induced by long labor. To reduce the possibility of anoxia or asphyxiation, long labors should be avoided, and cesarian section is the method of choice if parturition does not proceed at a reasonable rate.

A number of evaluative scales and procedures have been developed for neonates and infants. Among these are the Brazelton Neonatal Behavioral Assessment Scale (Brazelton, 1973), the Milani-Comparetti Developmental Scale (Milani-Comparetti and Gidoni, 1967), Doudlah's Motor Development Checklist (Doudlah, 1976) and the Denver Developmental Screening Test (Frankenburg and Dodds, 1969).

The Brazelton scale assesses the performance of newborn babies in response to manipulations intended to recapitulate everyday life situations in a condensed form to give a profile of behavior. This type of assessment requires a great deal of practice and skill. Excellent illustrative films are available through EDC Distribution Center, 39 Chapel Street, Newton, MA 02160.

The Milani-Comparetti scale correlates reflexes with spontaneous movement and maturation of body control, and is widely used by occupational and physical therapists, nurses and personnel in well-baby clinics. It has the advantage of being easy to administer, but the disadvantages are that the procedure is not standardized and is not useful for children with severe disabilities.

Doudlah's checklist ignores the concept of age-related motor milestones in favor of looking at phases of activity. She believes in observing spontaneous movement rather than manipulating the children to perform specific tasks. Her phases and transitions consist of movement in place, rolling, movement through space in a quadrupedal position, being upright in space and movement through space in the upright position. Films of these phases of development are available through Anna Doudlah, Perceptual-Motor Research Section, Central Wisconsin Center, 317 Knutson Drive, Madison, WI 53704.

The Denver test is a simple, task-oriented screening tool with which to discover disabilities in children. It has several distinct advantages. It is simple to administer so that it can be done by lay people; it has been standardized with 1000 children in Denver, Colorado; it can be utilized in a variety of settings; and, realistically, an age range is given at which specific capabilities should develop rather than a single specific time for the determination of normality. In addition, this test has a correlation rate of over 90 per cent when compared with other motor developmental tests. The disadvantages are that the test is task-oriented rather than based on observation of spontaneous behavior; it cannot be used for treatment planning; it does not consider the quality of movement; and no inter-rater reliability norms have been established.

To aid in the detection of CNS dysfunction, the following chart provides information regarding the *approximate* times at which specific voluntary and reflex functions should normally appear and disappear during development. The chart is followed by a glossary which describes reflexes and reactions that appear during development.

Text continued on page 188

NORMAL GROWTH AND DEVELOPMENT CHART

Chronologic Age	General Motor Development	Postural Reflexes	Hand Function, Dressing and Feeding	Speech and Language	Vision
1 month	*Supine*—back rounded; flexion and lateral rotation attitudes predominate. Head to one side; hands fisted. Never kicks into full extension. *Prone*—head bobs reflexly but is usually turned to one side. Flexion predominates. *In ventral suspension*—the whole body conforms to gravity. *PTS**—head lags completely *Sitting*—head erects momentarily; spine is uniformly curved. *Standing*—reflex stepping; little support.	Responds to pain with diffuse movements, crying, flexor withdrawal. ATNR**—strong in some children, fleeting in others. Moro reflex is present. There is violent neck righting. Retrusion tongue reflex is present, as are hand and foot grasp reflexes. No equilibrium reactions are present.	Puts one hand to mouth; hands clench on contact; thumb is nonfunctional. Hand can be pried open to hold an object, but only fleetingly.	Mouth functions in breathing, sucking, swallowing crying, choking and vomiting. Child listens passively to sounds and has a rather impassive face.	Vision tends to lag behind touch, smell and hearing at birth and is not well developed at 1 month. Infant follows a dangling object only to the midline.
2 months	*Supine*—legs exhibit more extension and reciprocal kicking. *In ventral suspension*—head extends to the neutral position. *Sitting*—head bobs to the erect position more frequently.	Labyrinthine head righting is present. Reflex stepping disappears. No equilibrium reactions are present.	Holds a toy briefly if placed in hand. Grasp is accomplished in the pronated position. Fingers on ulnar side are the strongest.	Smiles socially and has an alert expression. Makes single vowel sounds such as "ah," "ɔh," "un."	Eyes begin to follow an object past the midline. Infant can hold an object without looking at it.
3 months	Head is held in the midline more frequently in all positions. Hands are closed loosely. *Prone*—gets up on forearms; head is fully extended. Hips are more extended, but knees are still flexed. *Standing*—takes weight briefly; may lift one foot.	Moro and ATNR are weak. Labyrinthine head righting is further developed. *In ventral suspension*—head lifts above plane of body horizontally. No equilibrium reactions are present.	Holds toy and looks at it briefly. Pulls at clothes (automatically).	Coos, chuckles, makes social vocal responses.	Range of vision is now through 180 degrees. Eyes follow a moving object for short distances. Color vision develops at 3–5 months.

*PTS—pull to sitting.
**ATNR—asymmetric tonic neck reflex.

NORMAL GROWTH AND DEVELOPMENT CHART *(Continued)*

Chronologic Age	General Motor Development	Postural Reflexes	Hand Function, Dressing and Feeding	Speech and Language	Vision
4 months	*Supine*—symmetric postures predominate. *Prone*—legs are well extended. The child often props up on forearms with one elbow extended, and tends to tip over because equilibrium reactions are not yet present. The first roll to supine is accomplished in this manner. *PTS*—head lags only slightly. *Sitting*—head is erect but set forward in relationship to the trunk.	Moro and ATNR are seen only occasionally and should disappear completely by 6 months. Grasp reflex disappears. Downward parachute reaction appears at 4–5 months. Landau reaction appears now.	Fingers are more often extended. Hands may engage near face. Child approaches toy with hands and may take it to mouth. Is mostly bidextrous. Pulls clothing over face.	Anticipates feeding by opening mouth for a nipple. Biting and sucking can be inhibited. Sucks fingers or fist. Laughs aloud and expresses excitement by rapid breathing, squealing and grunts.	Arms are activated by sight of a toy. Child prefers midline head position for best all-around vision.
5 months	*Prone*—draws up knees trying to crawl; makes swimming-like movements.	Landau response becomes stronger. Knees now extended. Labyrinthine and optical reflexes are strong. Prone equilibrium is positive.	Pats a bottle. Puts object to mouth but still cannot grasp it. Scratches and rakes.		
6 months	*Supine*—lifts head and legs high. Pulls from supine to prone voluntarily. *PTS*—lifts head and legs to assist actively. *Sitting*—sits on chair with erect trunk and sits briefly on floor using hands for support. *Standing*—bears almost full weight when held in standing.	Parachute in sitting appears. May see STNR* from 6–8 months.	Has palmar grasp in pronation. Grasps foot in supine and plays with toes. Holds arms out to be picked up. Can pick up a 1-inch cube. Sits propped for 30 minutes. *Teething*—incisor teeth appear at 6 months + or − two months	Turns head toward sounds.	Eyes and hands come into joint action. Eyes "pathfind" intently for hands.
7 months	*Supine*—infant does not like this position for long. *Prone*—can reach up for a toy; tries to pivot. *Sitting*—sits erect alone for brief periods. *Standing*—bounces actively.	Landau reaction is now full-blown. Body righting reaction acting on the body is present. Forward parachute is present. Supine equilibrium is positive. At 7–9 months child can localize pain stimuli and deliberately withdraw the stimulated part.	Still quite bidexterous. Transfers objects from hand to hand and mouths objects. Grasps in half-supination with more of a radial grip but still not with fingertips. Pats a mirror, bangs objects on a table and can feed self a biscuit.	Says "da-da;" babbles at toys; imitates sounds of others; produces more consonant sounds. Can transfer food in mouth with tongue. Real chewing begins. Can recognize strangers.	

*STNR—symmetric tonic neck reflex.

8 months	*Prone*—trunk pivoting begins. At this point the legs do not contribute much. *Sitting*—sits erect for approximately one minute, but is unsteady.	Sitting equilibrium is positive.	Has inferior scissors grasp. Reaches for toys out of reach. Bites and chews toys. Likes to play "peek-a-boo."	
9 months	*Supine*—stops kicking and holds legs more still. *Sitting*—sits alone for ten minutes. Can lean forward and return to erect sitting. Goes from sitting to prone and crawls on hands and knees. Often crawls backward. *Standing*—pulls to stand; holds railing, taking full weight, but cannot get down.	Foot grasp gone. Backward parachute in sitting appears between 9 and 11 months. Positive all-fours equilibrium reaction appears between 9 and 12 months.	Holds bottle with hands and feet. Prehends pellets with a scissor grasp. Has radial digital grasp.	Eats crackers. Munches rather than sucks. Responds to name and "no, no."
10 months	*Supine*—tolerates this position only while asleep. Sits up immediately on awakening. *Sitting*—sits indefinitely with good control. *Standing*—can pull up to a railing and lower self. Supports entire weight when hands are held.		Has inferior pincer grasp. Approaches objects with extended index finger and pokes at things. Picks up crumbs or pellets and can put two cubes together. Can now release objects.	Plays patty-cake and waves bye-bye. Can say one word besides "ma-ma" and "da-da." Babbles and smiles in a mirror.
11 months	*Sitting*—pivots. *Standing*—takes steps at a railing, but does not cruise yet.		Drinks milk from a cup which is held for him. Puts cube in cup. Likes activities that involve putting objects into containers. Is gaining in wrist extension.	
12 months	Plantigrade creeping is present. Cruises at a railing; walks with hands held and may stand alone momentarily.	Responds to pain at 12–15 months. Attempts to push painful stimulus away with hands. Eyes respond to painful stimulus. STNR may be seen in form of Landau response. See-saw is present. Standing equilibrium is positive in a few children.	Hits two objects together. Grasps with almost adult facility, but still releases with too much extension (especially small objects). Tries cube tower, but fails. Releases ball after demonstration. Cooperates in dressing. Can dangle a ring by a string. Eating is messy.	Reacts to music and some words and sentences. Can say two words besides "ma-ma" and "da-da." Watches adult facial expressions. Gives away toy on request.

NORMAL GROWTH AND DEVELOPMENT CHART *(Continued)*

Chronologic Age	General Motor Development	Postural Reflexes	Hand Function, Dressing and Feeding	Speech and Language	Vision
13 months	Gradual change from creeping to two-hand walking to one-hand walking. Some children walk alone with high guard.	Body righting changes. Child does not turn all the way to prone in order to sit up.	Grasps two 1-inch cubes in one hand. Scribbles in imitation.	Imitates adult speech, copying the melody and dynamics of speech, but can say only three to four words; comprehends a few objects by name.	
15 months	Bipedal walking develops; creeping is discarded soon. Child gets into standing alone. Walks a few steps, starts, stops, falls down. Many walk with medium guard by this time. Creeps up stairs.	Standing equilibrium should be positive.	Builds two-cube tower.	Uses jargon but can say four to five words, including names. Pats pictures in book and helps turn pages; begins to recognize pictures. Shows toys to others. Says "ta-ta" upon receipt of objects. Points or vocalizes wants; indicates wet pants.	
18 months	Walks, seldom falls, arms at sides. Walks fast but wobbles. Runs stiffly and flat-footed without moving knees much. Walks up stairs with one hand held. Seats self in small chair, climbs into adult chair. Walks against ball, but cannot kick it.	Landau response often inhibited. All equilibrium reactions are quite reliable.	Hands are really free for the first time now that walking is stable. Hurls ball; puts pellets into a bottle; carries and lugs dolls; scribbles spontaneously or on request; makes vertical strokes. Feeds self but not without spilling. Likes pots and pans, magazines, blocks and push-pull toys. Builds a three-cube tower. *Teething*—has all deciduous teeth (they are at least visible by 18 + or − three months).	Begins to master symbols. Looks selectively at pictures; names ball. Can say approximately ten words. Indicates wants by pointing. Understands simple sentences.	
21 months	Squats in play. Kicks large ball. Walks up stairs holding railing. Walks down stairs with one hand held.		Handles cup well, but spills if too full. Throws cup away when finished. Builds a five- to six-cube tower.	Can say approximately 20 words.	

24 months (2 years)	Runs fairly well without falling and may prefer running to walking. Ankles and knees are more flexible. Climbs stairs alone, one step at a time.	Neck righting present in 11 out of 19 children. Half of the children rise in transitional form.	Pulls on socks; pulls up pants. Makes horizontal strokes. Can imitate a circle, but cannot initiate it. Also imitates a "V." Likes crayons, clay and building towers. Begins to turn spoon over in mouth (supination).	Uses simple expressions. Uses "I, me, you." Discards jargon and can say three-word sentences. Calls self by name usually. Understands about 50 words. Verbalizes toilet needs consistently.	
30 months	Can walk on tiptoes. Jumps with both feet. Tries to stand on one foot but cannot.		Holds crayon in fingers rather than in fist.		
36 months (3 years)	Runs well. Rides tricycle and likes climbing on low planks, boxes and jungle gyms. Can stand on one foot only a moment. Goes *up* stairs alternating feet. Jumps down from the bottom step.		Builds a nine- to ten-cube tower; copies a circle well. Feeds self well and can put on shoes and unbutton clothes. *Teething* – deciduous teeth are all the way in.	Names drawings. Can tell own sex. Uses phrases and can form simple sentences. Refers to self by pronoun form. Speech still limited to concrete situations, but is building sentences rapidly. Asks rhetorical questions. Begins dramatic play. Knows some rhymes and songs. Understands taking turns and obeys two prepositional commands.	
42 months	Can stand on one foot for two seconds. Goes *down* stairs alternating feet.	Gets up from supine with only partial rotation (transitional form).	Likes pounding activities.		
48 months (4 years)	Does broad jump. Likes hopping, skipping and jumping.	At age 4 to 5 years *neck righting* is usually seen and then is inhibited. *Body righting* – five of 17 rise like adults, seven in transition, five in a primitive manner.	Throws ball overhand. Can copy a square and a cross. Draws a man with two parts added. Washes face and hands. Brushes teeth and laces shoes.	Counts three objects; names one or more colors; knows front from back of clothes. Obeys five prepositional commands.	
5 years	Skips, alternating feet. Jumps rope; walks a chalk line; stands on one foot more than eight seconds. May use roller skates.	Neck righting is now inhibited; child gets up like an adult.	Draws a good man. Copies a triangle and prints a few letters. Dresses and undresses alone.	Counts to ten. Knows four colors and names penny, nickel and dime. Asks meanings of words.	Vision – 20/30.
6 years	Stands on each foot alternately with eyes closed. After age 6, all basic motor skills have been acquired (primarily through maturation). Further motor learning involves superimposition of advanced skills on the basic patterns.		Has acquired an advanced throwing pattern. Copies a diamond. Puts clothes on drawings of a man. Ties shoelaces. Hand preference is now stable.	Knows morning from afternoon and right from left	Vision 20/20 by age 7.

GLOSSARY OF REFLEXES AND REACTIONS*

Amphibian Reaction

Receptors: joint and cutaneous.
Stimulus: subject prone, lift one hip off support and exert unequal pressure.
Response: flexion of the ipsilateral lower extremity.
Therapeutic use: facilitation of lower extremity flexion, as in crawling and creeping patterns.

Babinski Reflex

Receptors: cutaneous.
Stimulus: stroking of the lateral aspect of the plantar surface of the foot.
Response: extension of the metacarpophalangeal joint of the great toe; abduction of the four lateral toes.
Age of normal occurrence: 0 to 12 months.
Therapeutic use: developmental and/or neurologic testing. Its retention suggests an upper motor neuron lesion.

Crossed Extension Reflex

Receptors: cutaneous.
Stimulus: nociceptive, a painful stimulus to the sole of the foot.
Response: flexion (withdrawal) of the stimulated extremity; extension and adduction of the contralateral extremity. The response outlasts the stimulus.
Area of integration: spinal cord.
Purpose: protection of the threatened side; maintenance of posture on the contralateral side.
Therapeutic use: neurologic testing.

Equilibrium Reactions (Tilting)

Receptors: semicircular canals.
Stimulus: slow shifting of the base of support or slow displacement of the body in space.
Response: lateral flexion of the spine toward the elevated side of the support (abduction of the extremities on the elevated side and parachute reactions in the depressed extremities will also be seen).
Area of integration: midbrain.
Purpose: to keep the center of gravity over the base of support.
Age of normal appearance: prone – 5 months.
supine – 7 months.
sitting – 8 months.
all-fours – 8 months.
standing – 12 months.
Therapeutic use: developmental testing; as a treatment procedure to improve balance.

Flexor Withdrawal Response

Receptors: cutaneous.
Stimulus: nociceptive, a painful stimulus to the sole of the foot or the palm of the hand.
Response: withdrawal of the stimulated extremity. Repeated stimuli normally result in a diminishing response.
Area of integration: spinal cord.
Purpose: protection.
Age normally present: from birth throughout life.
Therapeutic use: developmental testing.

Galant Reflex (Trunk Incurvation Reaction)

Receptors: cutaneous.
Stimulus: a sharp touch from the 12th rib to the iliac crest.
Response: lateral trunk flexion toward the stimulated side.
Purpose: withdrawal.
Age normally present: 0 to 2 months.
Therapeutic use: developmental testing. Retention may interfere with development of symmetric stabilization of the trunk and with independent movement of the trunk and head. Avoid eliciting the reflex except for testing purposes.

*Compliments of Janet C. Lemke, Assistant Professor, Program in Physical Therapy, University of Wisconsin, Madison.

GLOSSARY OF REFLEXES AND REACTIONS *(Continued)*

True Grasp Reflex (Hand or Foot)

Receptors: cutaneous.
Stimulus: a moving tactile stimulus applied to the palm of the hand or the sole of the foot in a proximal to distal direction.
Response: flexion of metacarpo- or metatarsophalangeal and interphalangeal joints of the digits.
Area of integration: cerebral cortex.
Therapeutic use: developmental testing.

Instinctive Grasp Reflex

Receptors: visual.
Stimulus: the sight of an object to be grasped or stationary contact with the palm of the hand.
Response: reflex grasping with inability to release object.
Area of integration: motor cortex.
Purpose: to accommodate grasp to the size of an object.
Age normally present: at birth and then disappears.
Therapeutic use: developmental/neurologic testing. The reflex is often released in comatose patients.

Tonic Grasp Reflex (Not a True Grasp Reflex)

Receptors: proprioceptors of the flexor muscles of the hand and foot.
Stimulus: stretch of the finger or toe flexors, or moving pressure on the palm of the hand or the sole of the foot.
Response: fisting or curling of the fingers or toes.
Purpose: primitive posture for protection.
Age normally present: abnormal at any age.
Therapeutic use: developmental testing. Its presence implies hypertonicity, so it must be inhibited since it interferes with normal weight-bearing.

Hopping Reaction

Receptors: proprioceptors.
Stimulus: displacement of the body in a horizontal direction.
Response: movement of the legs so that the center of gravity remains over the base of support.
Area of integration: cerebral cortex.
Purpose: maintenance of upright posture.
Age of appearance: approximately 18 months.
Therapeutic use: developmental testing; used as a therapeutic procedure to improve balance.

Landau Reaction

Receptors: labyrinths.
Stimulus: hold infant horizontally in space with support under the thorax and abdomen.
Response: extension of the neck, trunk and hips.
Area of integration: midbrain.
Purpose: breaks up flexor dominance; develops extensor tone.
Age normally present: 4 months on.
Therapeutic use: developmental testing.

Marie-Foix Reflex

Receptors: proprioceptors of the extensors of the great toe.
Stimulus: forceful flexion of the great toe.
Response: sudden flexion of the knee, and flexion and abduction of the hip joint.
Area of integration: spinal cord.
Purpose: phylogenetic locomotion in prone.
Therapeutic use: this is a pathologic reflex; therefore, except for purposes of testing, it should not be elicited.

Moro Reflex

Receptors: joint receptors of the neck; proprioceptors of the neck muscles.
Stimulus: sudden extension of the head in relation to the trunk.
Response: flexion and abduction of the shoulder joints, extension of the elbow joints, extension of the fingers and abduction of the thumb, followed by extension and adduction of the shoulder joints with elbow joint flexion. A minimal response may consist of slight extension of the fingers.
Age normally present: 0 to 6 months
Therapeutic use: developmental testing. Retention of this reflex interferes with the development of sitting.

GLOSSARY OF REFLEXES AND REACTIONS *(Continued)*

Parachute Reactions (Protective Extension)

Receptors: semicircular canals.
Stimulus: quick displacement of the trunk in a downward, sideward or backward direction.
Response: arms (legs) extend to catch weight.
Purpose: prevention of damage to the head and/or trunk.
Age of onset: downward parachute–4 months.
sideward parachute–6 months.
forward parachute–7 months.
backward parachute–9 months.
Therapeutic use: developmental testing; used as a treatment procedure to increase protective reactions.

Placing Reaction

Receptors: cutaneous receptors on the dorsum of the foot or hand; proprioceptors of the wrist extensors or talotibial dorsiflexors; visual receptors.
Stimulus: contact of the dorsum of the foot or hand against the edge of a table.
Response: placing of the weight-bearing surface of the hand or foot upon the table.
Area of integration: cerebral cortex.
Age of appearance: 2 months, then gradually inhibited.
Therapeutic use: developmental testing.

Primary Standing Reaction

Receptors: proprioceptors of the muscles of the foot.
Stimulus: the trunk is supported in the upright position by the examiner. The stimulus is weight-bearing of the feet on a hard surface with the trunk inclined forward.
Response: righting of the body and acceptance of weight.
Area of integration: undetermined.
Purpose: primitive support.
Age of normal occurrence: 0 to 2 months.
Therapeutic use: developmental testing.

Primary Walking

Receptor: unknown.
Stimulus: elicit primary standing and then tilt the body forward slightly.
Response: reciprocal stepping motions in the lower extremities.
Area of integration: midbrain.
Purpose: primitive locomotion.
Age normally present: 0 to 2 months.
Therapeutic use: developmental testing.

Righting Reactions

Neck Righting Reaction

Receptors: proprioceptors in the neck muscles.
Stimulus: firm neck rotation, either active or passive.
Response: body follows in a logroll.
Area of integration: midbrain.
Purpose: rights body with respect to the head.
Age of onset: birth, and then gradually inhibited.
Therapeutic use: developmental testing; facilitation of rolling.

Labyrinthine Righting Reaction Acting on the Head

Receptors: otoliths.
Stimulus: tilt body.
Response: head realigns with the face vertical and the mouth horizontal.
Area of integration: midbrain.
Purpose: rights head with respect to gravity.
Age of onset: 1 month.
Therapeutic use: developmental testing; treatment procedure for developing better function of the labyrinths.

GLOSSARY OF REFLEXES AND REACTIONS (*Continued*)

Body Righting Reaction Acting on the Head

Receptors: pressure and cutaneous receptors on the body surface.
Stimulus: contact of the body with a solid surface.
Response: head righting with respect to gravity.
Area of integration: midbrain.
Age of onset: 4 to 6 months.
Purpose: rights head with respect to gravity; interacts with the labyrinthine righting reaction on the head to maintain the orientation of the head in space.
Therapeutic use: developmental testing.

Body Righting Reaction Acting on the Body (Body Derotative)

Receptors: cutaneous and/or pressure receptors.
Stimulus: rotation of the head or thorax.
Response: rolling over with rotation between the trunk and pelvis.
Area of integration: midbrain.
Age of onset: 6 to 8 months.
Purpose: develops trunk rotation.
Therapeutic use: developmental testing; treatment procedure for developing trunk rotation.

Optical Righting Reaction

Receptors: visual.
Stimulus: environmental relationships.
Response: head and body righting in relation to the environment.
Area of integration: midbrain.
Purpose: keeps the head and body oriented in space.
Age of onset: 1 month. As the child matures this reaction increases its dominance on the maintenance of posture. The other righting reactions become less important.
Therapeutic use: developmental testing; treatment procedure to develop interactions with other righting mechanisms.

Body Rotative

This is a chain reaction involving interaction of all the righting reactions. It results in the child's ability to roll over and then pull himself to a standing position.
Age of onset: 9 months.

Rooting

Receptors: cutaneous.
Stimulus: touch to the lateral perioral region.
Response: the tongue and face turn to the side of the stimulus.
Age normally present: birth to 2 months.
Purpose: exploratory; to find the source of food.
Therapeutic use: developmental testing.

Startle

Sometimes included with the Moro reflex but the stimulus is different.
Receptors: auditory.
Stimulus: loud noise.
Response: shoulder joint extension and abduction, extension at the elbow joint and fingers and abduction of the thumb, followed by shoulder joint flexion and adduction with total upper extremity flexion.
Age normally present: 0 to 6 months.
Therapeutic use: developmental testing. Retention of this reflex will interfere with development of sitting.

(*Note:* the startle reflex can also be elicited by any sudden stimulus such as light, noise, cold air or sudden movement. The child who is developing normally may initially respond to an unexpected stimulus, but will gradually habituate to it.)

Sucking

Receptors: cutaneous.
Stimulus: touch to the lips, tongue or palate.
Response: automatic sucking.
Area of integration: medulla.
Age normally present: 0 to 6 months.
Purpose: feeding reflex which is coordinated with swallowing and respiration.
Therapeutic use: developmental testing; used as a treatment procedure to facilitate swallowing and respiration.

GLOSSARY OF REFLEXES AND REACTIONS (*Continued*)

Swallowing

Receptors: cutaneous and/or pressure receptors of the tongue and palate.
Stimulus: food or liquid in the mouth.
Response: automatic swallowing.
Area of integration: medulla.
Age normally present: from birth throughout life.
Purpose: ingestion of food.
Therapeutic use: developmental testing; a treatment goal.

Tonic Labyrinthine Reflex

This is Magnus and de Kleijn's description.
Receptors: otoliths.
Stimulus and response:

1. extension of the neck, so that the cleft of the mouth is 45 degrees above the horizontal, results in maximum extension of all extremities.
2. flexion of the neck, so that the cleft of the mouth is 45 degrees below the horizontal, results in minimal extension of all extremities. (If hypertonicity exists, flexion of the extremities may be observed.)

Area of integration: medulla.
Age normally present: 0 to 4 months.

Tonic Labyrinthine Reflex

This is Tokizani's description.
Receptors: otoliths.
Stimulus: inversion of the head.
Response: head inverted to 180 degrees (downward) results in maximum extensor tone; head in the upright position results in minimal extensor tone.
Age normally present: throughout life.
Therapeutic use: facilitation of total body extension.

Tonic Lumbar Reflex

Receptors: joint and muscle proprioceptors in the lumbar area.
Stimuli and responses:

1. rotation of the trunk to one side results in flexion of the ipsilateral upper extremity and contralateral lower extremity; extension of the contralateral upper extremity and ipsilateral lower extremity.
2. lateral flexion of the trunk results in ipsilateral upper and lower extremity flexion.

Area of integration: midbrain.
Purpose: facilitates the development of trunk rotation and the respective limb adjustments.
Therapeutic use: treatment procedure to help develop trunk rotation.

EVALUATION OF THE OLDER CHILD AND ADULT

In general, the symptoms of CNS deficits may include:

1. *Sensory* deficits such as parasthesia (distortion of sensation) or anesthesia (total loss of sensation). These may be detected by observation, questioning the patient, and testing the sensation by pinprick, diffuse touch (as with a wisp of cotton) or vibration.
2. *Perceptual* deficits, which may include visual and/or auditory problems. For example, the patient with homonymous hemianopia may drift to one side while walking; those with auditory problems may have difficulty with localization of sound. Testing for perceptual deficits will be included with evaluation of the cranial nerves.
3. *Lack of conscious proprioception* (kinesthesia). This can be evaluated by moving the extremities while the patient's eyes are closed and asking him the position of the extremity. When administering such a test one must be careful not to give sensory clues that will aid the patient in determining how the part has been moved. For example, if one is examining by moving the great toe, the fingers of the examiner should be placed on the medial and lateral aspects of the toe rather than on the plantar and dorsal surfaces. Pressure on the plantar surface during extension and on the dorsal sur-

GLOSSARY OF REFLEXES AND REACTIONS *(Continued)*

Tonic Neck Reflexes

Asymmetric Tonic Neck Reflex

Receptors: proprioceptors of the cervical muscles; cervical joint receptors.
Stimulus: cervical intervertebral joint rotation with the neck in neutral flexion and extension.
Response: extension of the extremities on the side to which the face is turned; flexion of the extremities on the contralateral side. The response in the upper extremities is stronger than that in the lower extremities.
Area of integration: medulla.
Purpose: phylogenetic locomotion in prone.
Age normally present: 0 to 4 months. The normal response occurs inconsistently and is never strong.
Therapeutic use: developmental testing. Retention of this reflex interferes with development of symmetry and independent movements of the trunk and limbs; it may result in scoliosis.

Symmetric Tonic Neck Reflex

Receptors: proprioceptors of the cervical muscles; cervical joint receptors.
Stimuli and responses:

1. extension of the cervical intervertebral joints produces extension of the upper extremities and flexion of the lower extremities.
2. flexion of the cervical intervertebral joints produces flexion of the upper extremities and extension of the lower extremities.

Area of integration: medulla.
Purpose: breaks up the initial symmetry of upper and lower extremities.
Age normally present: 4 to 6 months.
Therapeutic use: developmental testing. Retention interferes with independent movement of the head and extremities.

Traction Response

Receptors: proprioceptors of the shoulder joint flexors and adductors and finger flexors.
Stimulus: stretch on shoulder joint flexors and adductors and finger flexors.
Response: upper extremity flexion and adduction with clenching of the fist.
Area of integration: undetermined.
Purpose: primitive posture for protection.
Age of onset: 5 months.
Therapeutic use: developmental testing.
(*Note:* the activity of PTS depends on the development of this reflex as well as the grasp reflex. The head will also right owing to the labyrinthine and optical righting reflex acting on it.)
PTS—Pull to sitting.

face during flexion will provide cutaneous clues regarding the direction of movement if tactile sensation is intact.

4. *Lack of motor control*. This can be evaluated by observation as well as a variety of tests. Motor deficits may manifest themselves in the form of tremor, a change in quality (spasticity, rigidity or hypotonicity), lack of control (chorea, athetosis, ballismus, etc.), or generalized or specific weaknesses in addition to decreased range of motion or abnormally increased mobility of the joints. Generalized and specific weaknesses may be determined by use of manual muscle testing, and range of motion may be measured by the use of a goniometer. In all cases a comparison of tone on one side of the body with that on the other may yield some valuable information. Manual muscle testing is not feasible in the presence of spasticity, rigidity or the dyskinesias. In these cases much can be learned about the correct treatment procedure from the reaction to cutaneous stimulation. For example, if a light, moving stimulus elicits a very hyperactive response it means that the patient is in a predominantly sympathetic state, and steps must be taken to calm him before proceeding with further treatment.
5. *Learning and behavioral disabilities*.

In connection with CNS deficits, it is extremely important for each health professional who works with a patient to have information about the integrity of the cranial nerves. Their dysfunction may explain some rather bizarre behavior. It takes only a few minutes to evaluate cranial nerve function and the results may produce rich dividends.

The first (olfactory) nerve may be tested by having small vials of liquids with characteristic odors available for the patient to smell.

The second (optic) nerve may be tested grossly by having the patient fix his gaze straight forward on an object. The test may be performed with both eyes open or with first one eye covered and then the other. The examiner, standing behind the patient, passes his hand from the periphery on one side to a point past the midline, and then repeats from the other side. The patient should indicate the point at which the examiner's hand is seen. If the patient is dys- or aphasic, have him raise a hand when he sees your hand. This is an easy way to detect homonymous hemianopia. Other types of hemianopia require more sophisticated examining techniques (see Patten, 1977).

Oculomotor (third) nerve dysfunction is very easy to detect. If the entire nerve is damaged the patient will present with ptosis (due to loss of function of the levator palpebrae superioris muscle), lateral deviation of the eye and lack of ability to look up (due to loss of function of all the extraocular muscles except the superior oblique and lateral rectus muscles), and loss of the pupillary light reflex on the ipsilateral side.

The trochlear (fourth) nerve innervates the superior oblique muscle, which rotates the eyeball downward and laterally. If the lateral and inferior rectus muscles and the inferior oblique muscle remain functioning, dysfunction of the superior oblique muscle is difficult to detect because the lateral rectus and inferior oblique muscles both pull the eyeball laterally and the inferior rectus muscle pulls the eyeball downward.

Although the interconnections of the trigeminal (fifth) nerve complex are very complicated, its function is not difficult to assess. Sensation in the distribution of the three divisions (ophthalmic, maxillary, mandibular) of the nerve may be tested in the same way that sensation is tested elsewhere on the body, i.e., touching with soft cotton, pinprick, etc. The function of the muscles of mastication (pterygoids, masseter and temporalis) may be observed and palpated bilaterally, and the strength of bite may be determined by having the patient bite down on a tongue depressor which the examiner then tries to pull from between the teeth. Never use the fingers to administer this test (for obvious reasons).

The abducens (sixth) nerve innervates the lateral rectus muscle. Therefore, if this nerve is damaged, the patient will be unable to obey the command to look in the direction of the side of the lesion. In fact he will have medial deviation on the side of the lesion with diplopia owing to the unopposed action of the medial rectus muscle.

Lesions of the facial (seventh) nerve are very obvious. If the nerve itself is damaged all the muscles of facial expression on the side of the damage will be weakened or nonfunctioning. Taste will be absent on the anterior two-thirds of the tongue on the side of the lesion, but this is not really disabling since taste is still present on the normal side and on the posterior part of the tongue, and in the area of the pharynx. The reader may remember that, if corticobulbar fibers which project to the facial nerve nucleus are damaged, there are regional differences in the distribution of weakness of the muscles of facial expression. The muscles of the lower two-thirds of the face on the side contralateral to the corticobulbar injury will be weakened or nonfunctioning, while those of the upper one-third of the face will retain their function.

Lesions of the vestibulocochlear (eighth) nerve are reflected by tinnitus and/or loss of hearing if the cochlear division is involved, and vertigo, nausea and vomiting if the vestibular division is involved. The two divisions of the nerve may be damaged selectively or collectively. Hearing losses usually are easily detected by the patient's behavior, and often by his subjective report that he cannot hear well. Damage to the vestibular division can be devastating to the patient as he may continually feel dizzy, which leads to nausea and vomiting. Those patients able to communicate do not hesitate to report their feelings to the health care personnel involved with their treatment. The function of the vestibular system can be tested in those who cannot communicate (especially brain-damaged children) by observation of their equilibrium reactions and vestibulo-ocular reflexes when they are tilted or spun.

Loss of function of the glossopharyngeal (ninth) nerve is not easy to test for without special diagnostic tools. If it is damaged bilaterally, which is rare, there will be loss of the gag reflex and loss of taste on the posterior one-third of the tongue.

If the vagus (tenth) nerve is damaged bilaterally, death occurs very rapidly. If it is damaged unilaterally, no special testing is required to detect the lesion. The patient will be hoarse because of weakness of the musculature of the larynx, and he may have a great deal of difficulty with swallowing (dysphagia) owing to weakness of the pharyngeal constrictors. Very often these patients must have a nasogastric tube in order to get adequate nutrition, and they often drool copiously because of inability to swallow their saliva.

Spinal accessory (11th) nerve lesions may be reflected by some hoarseness due to this nerve's contribution to the innervation of the muscles of the larynx, and by weakness of the sternocleidomastoideus and trapezius muscles. The sternocleidomastoideus functions in cervical intervertebral joint rotation to the opposite side, flexion and abduction. The trapezius functions primarily in shoulder girdle elevation, retraction and depression. Therefore, a lesion of the 11th nerve would produce some weakness in all of these movements.

The hypoglossal (12th) nerve is evaluated by having the patient protrude his tongue. If there is a unilateral 12th nerve lesion the tongue will deviate to the weak side owing to the unopposed action of the genioglossus muscle on the normal side (see Fig. 7–8).

It is not at all unusual to see several of the cranial nerves damaged concomitantly in conjunction with brain damage. Unfortunately, the author has seen as many as five of the cranial nerves dysfunctioning in one patient as a result of a cerebral vascular accident.

As part of the evaluation of a patient's over-all mental condition, the importance of determining the state of the autonomic nervous system cannot be overemphasized. The physician must ascertain whether the patient is functioning in the sympathetic or parasympathetic end of the spectrum, and other health care personnel can give important clues about this. For example, one patient may be in a constant state of lethargy, and another may be hyperactive and overreactive to stimuli. The former patient may be functioning too far in the parasympathetic, and the latter too far in the sympathetic end of the spectrum. Appropriate drug administration may or may not eliminate these extremes of behavior. When dealing with mentally retarded, developmentally disabled children or other patients who cannot communicate effectively, it is especially important to evaluate autonomic function at the beginning and during therapeutic rehabilitative procedures, because these individuals cannot provide verbal clues. If the patient is hyperactive on arrival for treatment, some time will be well spent in trying to calm him before meaningful treatment can be initiated. Means of accomplishing this include application of neutral warmth, slow stroking of the skin, a rocking motion, and so on. If the individual is in a hypoactive state, treatment may be prefaced by application of cold or heat, or more rapid forms of cutaneous stimulations, etc.

In addition to this type of work-up it is beneficial to practice the interpretation of lesions at different levels of the CNS. Ranson and Clark (1963) provide a number of case histories which are interesting and instructive to work through.

Generally, the higher in the CNS a relatively small lesion is located, the greater is the potential for retraining. For example, a patient with a cortical lesion has a relatively great potential for return of function because of the plasticity and redundancy in the CNS. New areas and pathways can be retrained to take over activities that formerly were functions of the damaged area. If the lesion is massive, however, the potential for retraining may not be too great, but it is worth working for. If the lesion is lower, e.g., in the spinal cord, there is not much chance of recovery of function below the level of the lesion, because the conduction pathways for the transmittal of information to and from the brain have been destroyed and will not regenerate. Of course, this is only true if the spinal cord has been completely transected. There may be partial return of function if the lesion is incomplete, and it is important to understand that often, upon initial evaluation, it will appear that the lesion is complete when in reality it is not. Therefore, it is important to proceed as if there is some potential for return of function below the level of the lesion until it has been definitely determined that there is not. The following case history emphasizes this point.

J. H., age 18, had sustained a neck injury

in an automobile accident. On admission to the hospital, x-ray examination revealed lateral displacement of the fifth cervical vertebra on the sixth so that the vertebral canal was completely interrupted at that point. The logical diagnosis was a complete severance of the spinal cord between C5 and C6, and this was entered in the patient's chart. He was placed in bed with cervical traction. Daily range of motion on the ward was ordered. Upon evaluation it was found that there was no sensation below the level innervated by C5, and no function of the muscles innervated by spinal segments below C5. Daily therapy consisted of complete range of motion exercises *and* complete muscle re-education techniques. Function and sensation gradually returned first in the upper extremities, then in the lower. Four months after admission the patient was discharged from the hospital walking with crutches and no braces. After an additional three months of outpatient treatment he was able to discard the crutches. His only difficulty is some slight spasticity in the lower extremities which only manifests itself when he attempts to run. The functional return in this case was remarkable, considering the original diagnosis, but it serves to emphasize that the diagnosis sometimes may be wrong, and this possibility should be borne in mind however infrequently such results may be attained.

This chapter has presented a few facts and evaluative procedures that may be utilized simply without any special diagnostic tools. For the interested reader there are several books which give more detailed accounts of the neurologic examination. Among these are *Neurological Differential Diagnosis (Patten, 1977)* and *Essentials of the Neurological Examination* (Alpers and Mancall, 1973).

REVIEW QUESTIONS

1. List the evaluative scales and procedures for neonates and infants discussed in this chapter. What are some of the advantages and disadvantages of each?
2. In general, what symptoms may be produced by CNS deficits? How does one go about determining the deficits?
3. Explain how to evaluate the function of each of the cranial nerves.
4. Why is the potential for retraining greater with relatively small lesions in higher CNS structures than in lower ones?

GLOSSARY

Acetylcholine A neurotransmitter, normally present in many parts of the body.

Acupuncture Puncture of specific peripheral nerves made with long, fine needles for diagnostic or therapeutic purposes, especially for the relief of pain.

Adiadokokinesia Inability to perform rapid, alternating movements, e.g., pronation and supination.

Adrenergic Relating to nerve fibers (usually sympathetic) that liberate epinephrine and norepinephrine.

Afferent Bringing to or into; e.g., afferent peripheral neurons bring information into the CNS.

Agnosia Absence of the ability to recognize the form and nature of persons and things, or of the perceptive faculty.

Agonist Denoting a muscle in a state of contraction, with reference to its opposing muscle, or antagonist.

Amygdaloid Resembling an almond; used to describe one of the nuclei of the brain.

Analgesia Loss of sensibility of pain.

Analgesic 1. Causing analgesia or freedom from pain; 2. a pain-stilling remedy.

Anastomosis A natural communication, direct or indirect, between two blood vessels or other tubular structures; also by extension, a passage of nerve fibers from one nerve to another.

Anencephaly Lack of development of the brain.

Anesthesia Loss of sensation.

Aneurysm A blood-containing sac or tumor connecting directly with the lumen of an artery or formed by a circumscribed enlargement of an artery.

Anorexia Loss of appetite for food.

Anoxia Oxygen lack, oxygen want, oxygen deficiency; more correctly, hypoxia.

Antagonist A muscle that opposes or resists the action of another muscle, its agonist.

Anterior primary divisions (also called ventral rami) The divisions of mixed spinal nerves that innervate the muscles and skin of the extremities and the anterolateral body wall. Anterior primary divisions contain all four functional components of spinal nerves.

Aphasia Speechlessness: the loss of the faculty of transmission of ideas by language in any of its forms — reading, writing, speaking or failure in the appreciation of the written, printed or spoken word — independent of disease of the vocal organs or the mind.

Apraxia 1. A disorder of voluntary movement, consisting of a more or less complete incapacity to execute purposeful movements, notwithstanding the preservation of muscle power, sensibility and coordination in general; 2. A psychomotor defect in which one is unable to apply to its proper use an object of which one can nevertheless give the name and describe the uses.

Arachnoid Resembling a cobweb; denoting specifically the arachnoid membrane, or middle layer of membrane that covers the brain and spinal cord.

Areflexia A condition in which the reflexes are abolished.

Arteriosclerosis (atherosclerosis) A fibrous overgrowth, mainly of the inner coat of an artery, associated with degenerative changes in the middle coat, causing thickening of the arterial wall with loss of elasticity and contractility.

Asphyxiation Unconsciousness due to suffocation or interference of any kind with oxygenation of the blood.

Association fibers Fibers that interconnect ipsilateral regions of the cerebral cortex.

Astrocyte Star-shaped cell — one of the CNS supportive glial cells of ectodermal origin.

Asynergia Incoordination; lack of ability of parts that normally act in unison to do so.

Ataxia Loss of muscular coordination.

Athetosis Without position or place — a condition in which there is a constant succession of slow, writhing involuntary movements, especially in the hands.

Atrophy A wasting of the tissues of a part or of the entire body.

Audiogenic Produced by sound.

Autogenic inhibition Inhibition of the muscle in which the stimulated sensory receptors (Golgi tendon organs) are located.

Autonomic Self-controlling; independent of outside influences; spontaneous — referring particularly to an involuntary portion of the nervous system concerned with visceral, vascular and other responses.

Avulsion A tearing away, e.g., the tearing of nerve roots from the spinal cord.

Axo-axonal synapse A synaptic contact between the axon of the presynaptic cell and that of the postsynaptic cell.

Axodendritic synapse A synaptic contact between the axon of the presynaptic cell and a dendrite of the postsynaptic cell.

Axon hillock A specialized part of the nerve cell body that serves as the usual point of origin of the axon.

Axoplasmic flow Movement of substances through the axon of the nerve cell.

Axosomatic synapse A synaptic contact between the axon of the presynaptic cell and the cell body (soma) of the postsynaptic cell.

B

Babinski reflex Extension instead of the normal flexion of the great toe, sometimes with flexion of the other toes, following stroking of the sole of the foot.

Ballismus Violent, forceful, flinging movements (ballistic), particularly involving muscles of the pelvis and proximal extremities, produced by damage of the subthalamic nucleus or its connections; if damage is unilateral the condition is called hemiballismus.

Bell's palsy A lower motor lesion of the facial nerve.

Bidextrous Having equal facility in the use of both hands.

Branchia The gills, or organs of respiration, in fishes; the analogue of the branchial arches in the human embryo.

Brown-Séquard's syndrome A right or left hemisection of the spinal cord.

Buccal Relating to the cheek.

Bulb Any globular or fusiform structure; the older literature referred to the brain stem as the bulb, hence the terminology corticobulbar fibers.

Bulbar Relating to a bulb, or a bulb shape; the bulbar region refers particularly to the brain stem.

C

Calcarine Spur-shaped; used in reference to one of the occipital lobe structures. The calcarine fissure is concerned with the cortical area which receives visual perception.

Caloric stimulation Stimulation by heat or cold.

Carotid Put to sleep; one of the two major arteries that supply the brain.

Catecholamines A specific class of neurotransmitters that includes epinephrine, norepinephrine and dopamine.

Cauda equina Horse's tail; specifically, the assemblage of spinal roots found in the dural sac of the lower one-third of the vertebral canal.

Caudal Relating to any anatomic structure that resembles a tail; inferior or, in the case of four-footed animals, posterior — i.e., toward the tail or coccygeal region.

Caudate Possessing a tail; name given to one of the basal ganglia of the brain.

Cephalic Relating to the head or direction toward the head.

Cerebellectomy Removal of the cerebellum.

Cerebellum Small brain; the part of the metencephalon that occupies the posterior cranial fossa posterior to the brain stem.

Cerebrum Brain.

Chiasm A decussation or crossing of two tracts — especially relating to the crossing of optic nerve fibers in the optic chiasm.

Cholinergic Relating to nerve fibers that cause effects similar to those induced by acetylcholine.

Chorea A disorder characterized by irregular, spasmodic, involuntary movements, in part graceful in character, of the limbs or facial muscles, especially of the distal limb musculature.

Choroid Like a membrane; particularly used in reference to the middle coat of the eyeball and to the plexuses in the cerebral ventricles that produce cerebrospinal fluid.

Chromatolysis The dissolution, dilution and dispersion of ribonucleic acid-containing structures (Nissl substance) in the cytoplasm of the nerve cell perikaryon, accompanied by peripheral displacement of the nucleus and swelling of the perikaryon.

Ciliary Relating to or resembling an eyelid or eyelash; refers to a muscle, ganglion and nerve in the eye; also refers to fine hair-like processes in a variety of cells.

Cingulate Girdle; to surround — cingulate gyrus — a band of association fibers in the medial portion of the cerebral hemispheres, passing from near the region of the anterior perforated substance over the superior surface of the corpus callosum. Some fibers then pass to the cuneus gyrus of the occipital lobe, others running inferior to the splenium of the corpus callosum and anteriorly as far as the uncus of the temporal lobe.

Clasped knife reflex Rigidity of the extensor muscles of a joint, which thus offer resistance to passive flexion up to a point when they give way rather suddenly, allowing the joint then to be easily flexed.

Clonus A sustained series of involuntary contractions and relaxations of a muscle that occur in rapid succession.

Cochlea Small shell — a cone-shaped cavity in the petrous portion of the temporal bone, forming one of the divisions of the labyrinth or internal ear; it consists of a spiral canal making 2½ turns around a central core of spongy bone, and containing the membranous cochlea in which is the organ of Corti, part of the terminal auditory apparatuses.

Coelom Belly, and relating to the abdominal cavity or hollow structure; also used in celiac artery, nerve and disease of the intestines.

Collateral Relating to the side — a secondary or accessory nerve accompanying the main stem.

Colliculus Small mound, hill or elevation, as seen in the midbrain (superior and inferior colliculi).

Commissural fibers Interconnected homotypic areas of the two hemispheres of the cerebral cortex.

Commissure A bundle of nerve fibers passing from one side to the other in the brain or spinal cord.

Congenital Born with, existing at birth; referring to certain mental or physical traits or peculiarities, diseases, etc., regardless of the cause.

Contralateral Relating to the opposite side of the body.

Contusion A bruise, a contused wound, an injury of the part without the skin being broken.

Corpus, corpora (pl.) Body, e.g., the corpus callosum.

Corpus callosum Hard body — the major commissural connections between the two cerebral hemispheres.

Cortex Bark, the outer layer of an organ or other structure of the body.

Craniectomy Excision of a portion of the skull.

Cribriform Sieve-like; containing many perforations, such as a portion of the ethmoid bone of the skull — the cribriform plate.

Crista A ridge, crest or elevated line projecting from a level or evenly rounded surface, e.g., those located in the semicircular canals; crista galli of the skull.

Crus Leg; refers to the ventral portion of the cerebral peduncles (crus cerebri).

Cuneate Wedge-shaped, as the cuneate gyrus of the occipital lobe.

Cytoarchitectonics The study of cell groupings in the central nervous system.

D

Decussation The point of crossing of two tracts, especially across the midline of the brain or spinal cord.

Dendro-dendritic synapse A synaptic contact between a dendrite of the presynaptic cell and one of the postsynaptic cell.

Dentate Notched, toothed, cogged; e.g., the dentate nucleus (one of the deep cerebellar nuclei).

Dermatome That cutaneous area which is supplied by a single dorsal root and its ganglion; also, the lateral portion of a mesodermal somite.

Diencephalon The interbrain — the posterior division of the prosencephalon from which are developed most of the third ventricle, thalami, hypothalamus, pineal body, and optic nerves and retinae.

Digastric Having two bellies, as does one of the suprahyoid muscles.

Diplopia Double vision.
Distal Farthest from the trunk.
Down's syndrome Mongolism.
Dura mater Hard mother; a tough, fibrous membrane that forms the outer sheath of the brain and spinal cord.
Dynamic polarization A state that allows unidirectional impulse transmission at chemical synapses.
Dysarthria Difficulty with articulation of words.
Dyskinesia Difficulty in performing voluntary movements.
Dysmetria Inability to gauge distances accurately together with inability to arrest a muscular movement at the desired point — either under- or overshooting of the target.
Dysphagia Difficulty with swallowing.
Dysphasia Difficulty in speaking caused by a brain lesion, but without any marked mental impairment.
Dyspraxia Impaired ability to perform an act previously well performed when voluntary movement, coordination, sensation and understanding are intact.

E

Ectoderm Outside skin; the outer layer of the three layers of cells formed from the inner cell mass in the blastocyst.
Efferent To bring out or to conduct outward, as an efferent nerve.
Emboliform Wedge-shaped; one of the deep cerebellar nuclei.
Embolism Sudden obstruction or occlusion of a vessel by a transported clot or vegetation, a mass of bacteria, or other foreign material.
Emetic Producing vomiting; an agent that produces vomiting.
Encephalopathy Any degenerative disease of the brain (encephalon).
Endocrine Denoting a gland that furnishes an internal secretion which is transported by blood or lymph and has a specific effect on another organ or part.
Endoderm The inner layer of the three layers of cells formed from the inner cell mass in the blastocyst.
Endolymph The fluid contained within the membranous labyrinth of the ear.
Endoneurial sheath An aggregation of collagen connective tissue fibers which ensheaths each axon and its surrounding Schwann cell in peripheral nerves.
Ependymal cells One of four types of glial cells of the central nervous system; these cells line the ventricles of the brain and the central canal of the spinal cord.
Epicritic To separate; judge — denoting a set or system of sensory nerve fibers that supply the skin and oral mucosa, by means of which one is enabled to appreciate the finer degrees of the sensations of pain, touch and temperature and to localize the same.
Epilepsy A chronic functional nervous system disorder, characterized by attacks of unconsciousness or convulsions or both, which may be associated with other mental disturbances.
Epineurial sheath A dense collagenous layer of connective tissue derived from the dura mater (a connective tissue covering of the brain) which ensheaths peripheral nerve trunks.
Etiology The causes of disease.
Euphoria A general state or feeling of well-being.
Exacerbation An increase in the severity of a disease or any of its symptoms.
Exteroceptors Sensory receptors located immediately under the skin or external mucous membranes.

Extrapyramidal systems Those descending nerve tracts that do not enter into the formation of the medullary pyramids.

F

Fascicle Small bundle.
Fastigial Sloping-roof nucleus in the white substance of the vermis of the cerebellum.
Fiber specific theory There are morphologically different sensory receptors for each quality of sensation.
Fissure A furrow, cleft or slit.
Flaccid Relaxed, flabby.
Flocculus A small flock of wool; a small lobe of the cerebellum at the posterior border of the middle cerebellar peduncle.
Foramen A natural aperture or perforation through a bone or a membranous structure.
Fornix Arch, vault; a bundle of nerve fibers that connect the hippocampus and the mamillary bodies.
Funiculus Small cord; column of the spinal cord. There are three spinal funiculi or columns: (1) anterior, between the anterior median fissure and the anterolateral sulcus; (2) lateral, between the anterior and posterior nerve roots; (3) posterior, between the posterior horn and the posterior median sulcus.

G

Gangliolysis Destruction of a ganglion.
Ganglion A collection of nerve cells usually located outside the CNS.
Gap junction A special type of cell — cell junction found at some synapses at which the extracellular space is almost completely obliterated by very close opposition of membranes of the two cells involved, with a resultant electrotonic coupling of the two cells.
Geniculate Pertaining to a knee (the geniculate nuclei of the thalamus; genu of the corpus callosum).
Genu Knee; used to designate any anatomic structure bent like a knee.
Glabrous Smooth; bald.
Glial cells Glue; the unexcitable tissues of the CNS of which there are four types: astrocytes; oligodendroglial cells; ependymal cells; and microglia.
Globose Resembling a globe.
Globose nucleus One of the deep cerebellar nuclei.
Globus pallidus Pale globe — one of the basal ganglia of the brain.
Glomerulus Small tuft or cluster, such as the complex of mossy fiber terminals, granule cell dendrites and Golgi cell axons within the cerebellum.
Gracilis Slight; slender.
Gustatory Relating to the sense of taste.
Gyrus Circle; convolution — one of the many prominent rounded elevations on the surface of the hemispheres of the brain that are separated by furrows called fissures or sulci.

H

Hematoma A blood cyst, a localized collection of blood; a tumor containing effused blood, usually due to a break in the wall of a blood vessel.

Hemiparesis Incomplete paralysis or weakness on one side of the body.
Hemiretina Half of one retina.
Hemorrhage Bleeding, a flow of blood, especially if very profuse.
Heteronymous motor neuron A motor neuron that projects to structures other than that in which the stimulated sensory receptors are located.
Hilton's law (partially stated) A joint is innervated by the nerves that supply the muscles that move (cross) that joint.
Hippocampus Sea horse; a gyrus of the brain.
Homologue Any part or organ of similar structure or composition to another one.
Homonymous hemianopia Loss of vision in a single peripheral visual field.
Homonymous motor neuron A motor neuron that projects back to the structure in which the stimulated sensory receptors are located.
Homunculus Little man.
Hydrocephalus Water head; a condition, usually congenital, marked by an excessive accumulation of fluid in the cerebral ventricles that dilates the ventricles, thins the brain and causes separation of the cranial bones; there may also be an accumulation of fluid in the subarachnoid space.
Hyperesthesia Abnormally increased sensation or increased sensitivity.
Hyperkinesia Excessive motility or motor activity.
Hyperneurotization Multiple innervation.
Hyperpolarization The membrane potential of a cell becomes more negative (moves further from the threshold for stimulation).
Hypertonicity Extreme tension; may refer to a hyperosmotic state or excess muscular tension.
Hypoesthesia Abnormally diminished sensation or decreased sensitivity.
Hypoglossal Beneath the tongue (the motor innervation to the tongue).
Hypokinesia Abnormally diminished power of movement, paresis.
Hypophysis The pituitary gland.
Hyporeflexia A condition in which the reflexes are weakened.
Hypothalamus Below the thalamus; a group of nuclei at the base of the brain in relation to the floor and walls of the third ventricle.
Hypotonia Reduced tension in any part — particularly used in reference to muscle tone; diminished resistance of muscles to passive movement.

I

Idiopathic Denoting a primary disease, one originating without apparent extrinsic cause.
Initial segment The part of a myelinated axon between the origin of the axon and the site where it becomes myelinated.
Insomnia Abnormal wakefulness; inability to sleep.
Insula Island of Reil, central lobe of the cerebrum, a cerebral lobe or group of convolutions in the depth of the fissure of Sylvius (lateral fissure).
Interoceptors Sensory receptors located within the walls of the respiratory, cardiovascular, genitourinary and gastrointestinal tracts.
Intractable Obstinate, resistant to treatment, difficult to control.
Intrinsic Inherent; belonging entirely to or situated entirely within a part.

Ipsilateral Situated on the same side.
Isometric contraction Contraction of muscle during which joint movement does not occur.

K

Kinesthesia Conscious position sense.

L

Labyrinth A maze or intricate system of intercommunicating passages; the internal ear, comprising the semicircular canals, vestibule and cochlea.
Lacrimal Pertaining to tears.
Lacuna A small depression, a gap or defect (venous lacunae associated with the superior sagittal sinuses).
Lamina A thin plate or flat layer, e.g., Rexed's laminar arrangement of the spinal cord, lamina terminalis.
Lemniscus A ribbon or band, or a bundle of nerve fibers in the CNS that subserve a particular function.
Lentiform Lens-shaped (term used for describing the shape of the putamen and globus pallidus).
Lesion A wound or injury; any pathologic or traumatic discontinuity of tissue or loss of function of a part.
Limbus Border; refers to the limbic system of the CNS.
Lingual Pertaining to the tongue, or tongue-shaped.
Lobectomy Excision of a lobe of any organ or gland.

M

Macula A spot; an oval area about 3 mm in length in the wall of both the saccule and utricle in the membranous labyrinth; each of these maculae consists of fusiform nucleated supporting cells, between which are nucleated flask cells that have a hair-like process projecting from the free extremity of each. On the surface of each macula is a collection of rhomboid calcium carbonate crystals called otoconia, statoconia or otoliths. The macula is in relation with the nerve fibers which terminate in arborizations around the hair cells. The macula is also that part of the retina concerned with most acute vision.
Mamillary Related to or shaped like a breast; related to the mamillary bodies of the hypothalamus.
Mandibular Related to the lower jaw.
Mastication Chewing food in preparation for swallowing and digestion.
Maxillary Pertaining to the upper jaw.
Meatus A passage or channel, especially the external opening of a canal, as in the auditory canal (external and internal acoustic meatus).
Medulla Marrow, a portion of the brain stem.
Meniere's disease An affection characterized clinically by vertigo, nausea, vomiting, tinnitus and progressive deafness, resulting from disease of the labyrinths.
Meninges Membranes, specifically the three membranes that envelop the brain and spinal cord: the dura mater, arachnoid and pia mater.

Meningocele A protrusion of the meninges through a defect in the vertebral column or skull.
Meningomyelocele A protrusion of the meninges and spinal cord through a defect in the vertebral column.
Mesencephalon Midbrain.
Mesenchyme An embryonic mesodermal tissue, consisting of cells forming a network, the meshes of which are filled by a homogeneous matrix; it gives origin to the connective tissues of the body as well as the blood and lymph vessels.
Mesentery Middle intestine; the fan-shaped fold of peritoneum that encircles the greater part of the small intestines and attaches to the posterior abdominal wall.
Mesoderm Middle skin; the middle of the three primary germ layers of the primitive embryo.
Metathalamus After thalamus; the portion of the thalamus that includes the two geniculate bodies.
Metencephalon After brain; the anterior of the two divisions of the rhombencephalon; from it are developed the pons and cerebellum and the pontine part of the fourth ventricle.
Microcephaly The condition of having a small head.
Microglial cells One of four types of glial cells in the CNS; they function as phagocytes.
Mitosis Thread splitting; indirect nuclear division, the usual process of cell division.
Monoplegia Paralysis of one limb.
Myelencephalon The posterior division of the rhombencephalon from which are developed the medulla oblongata and the medullary portion of the fourth ventricle.
Myelin A spirally disposed, discontinuous plasma membrane wrapping, produced by Schwann cells or oligodendroglial cells, that surrounds rapidly conducting axonal processes.
Myeloarchitectonics The organization of the nerve tracts in the spinal cord and brain stem, e.g., by staining with myelin stains.
Myotatic reflex Stretch reflex; a monosynaptic reflex.
Myotome Those striated somatic muscles which are derived from a single somite and therefore are innervated by the same spinal segment.

N

Necrosis Local death; the death of more or less extensive groups of cells with degenerative changes in the intercellular substance.
Neuralgia Pain of a severe, throbbing type in the course or distribution of a nerve.
Neuroblast An embryonic nerve cell that develops into a mature nerve cell.
Nociceptive Capable of appreciation or transmission of injurious influences.
Node of Ranvier A distinct gap between the myelin sheaths that coat some nerve cell axons; at these sites the myelin sheath is absent and the axon is enclosed only by Schwann cell processes.
Nodule Little knot; a small node in the vermis of the cerebellum which, together with the cerebellar flocculi, makes up the flocculonodular lobe.
Noxious Injurious, harmful.
Nucleus Little nut — 1. a mass of gray matter (aggregation of nerve cells) in any part of the brain or spinal cord; 2. a differentiated mass of protoplasm, the executive center of functional activity of the cell.

Nystagmus Rhythmic oscillations of the eyeballs, either horizontal, rotary, vertical or mixed, which occur rather slowly in one direction, then rapidly in the reverse direction; it is named for the direction in which the quick component occurs.

O

Obex Barrier; a small transverse medullary fold overhanging the opening from the fourth ventricle into the central canal of the spinal cord.
Occipital Relating to the back of the head and to a lobe of the brain.
Occlusion The act of closing or the state of being closed.
Olfactory Pertaining to the sense of smell.
Oligodendroglial cells One of four types of glial cells in the CNS; they are derived from the ectodermal cells and produce myelin in the CNS.
Ontogenesis The development of the individual, as distinguished from phylogenesis, or the evolutionary development of the species.
Ophthalmic Pertaining to the eye.
Orthodromic nerve conduction Depolarization of an axon in a direction from the nerve cell body toward the axon terminal.
Otolith Ear stone, also otoconia; calcium carbonate crystals present in a gelatinous membrane overlying the hair cells of the macula of the vestibular apparatus.

P

Palpebra Eyelid.
Paranoia A functional mental disorder marked by the presence of systematized delusions without other symptoms of insanity.
Paresthesia Abnormal sensation.
Parietal Relating to a wall — a lobe of the brain; one of the bones of the skull.
Parturition Childbirth, labor, giving birth to a child.
Peduncle Stalk or stem.
Percutaneous Performed through the skin.
Perikaryon That part of the cell that surrounds the nucleus (karyon); commonly used in reference to a nerve cell body.
Perineurial sheath A connective tissue sheath derived from the pia-arachnoid (two of the connective tissue coverings of the brain and spinal cord), which encloses groups of several axons.
Peristalsis The vermiform movement of the intestine or other tubular structure; a wave of alternate circular contraction and relaxation of the tube by which the contents are propelled onward.
Petrosal Stony; relating to the petrous portion of the temporal bone.
Petrous Resembling rock — of stony hardness; relating to the petrous portion of the temporal bone.
Phagocytosis The process of ingestion and digestion by the cells — most of the cells of the body concerned in nutrition or defense mechanisms possess this property; the substances ingested are other cells, bacteria, bits of necrosed tissue, foreign particles, etc.
Phylogenesis The complete history of evolutionary development of any plant or animal species; ancestral history of the individual, as opposed to ontogenesis, or the development of the individual.

Pia mater Tender mother; a delicate fibrous membrane that closely envelops the brain and spinal cord.

Piloerector Hair mover; relating to intrinsic skin muscles that raise the hair to a more erect position.

Piriform Pear-shaped; the piriform cortex is part of the olfactory system.

Pituitary Relating to a thick, nasal secretion; the pituitary gland was so named because it was formerly supposed to secrete the nasal mucus.

Plasticity The capability of being formed or molded, the quality of being plastic.

Plexus A braid; a network interjoining of nerves, veins or lymphatic vessels.

Pons Bridge; part of the brain stem located between the medulla and the midbrain.

Posterior primary divisions (also called dorsal rami) The divisions of mixed spinal nerves that innervate the muscles and skin of the back; posterior primary divisions contain all four functional components of spinal nerves.

Prognosis The foretelling of the probable course of a disease; a forecast of its outcome.

Projection fibers Nerve fibers that connect the cerebral cortex with other structures.

Prone Lying face downward.

Proprioception (conscious) Position sense represented by information from joint receptors by direct pathways to the cerebral cortex.

Proprioception (subconscious) Subconscious awareness of body position, muscle tension and movement represented in part by information from neuromuscular spindles and Golgi tendon organs by direct pathways to the cerebellum.

Proprioceptors Sensory receptors located in muscles, tendons and joints and labyrinths.

Prosencephalon Before brain; the anterior primitive cerebral vesicle, the forebrain, dividing secondarily into the telencephalon and diencephalon.

Protopathic Denoting a set or system of peripheral sensory nerve fibers that furnish a low degree of sensibility, enabling one to appreciate pain and temperature to a not very delicate extent, and not definitely localized.

Proximal Nearer to the trunk.

Pterygoid Wing-shaped.

Ptosis A falling; drooping, as of the upper eyelid, due to lack of function of m. levator palpebrae superioris.

Pulvinar A couch made from cushions; the posterior extremity of the thalamus which forms a cushion-like prominence that overhangs the superior colliculus.

Putamen Shell; one of a group of nuclei that comprise the basal ganglia; the larger and more lateral part of the lentiform nucleus.

Pyramidal system The corticospinal system which, in its descent, makes up the medullary pyramids.

Q

Quadrigemina Fourfold, denoting the corpora quadrigemina of the midbrain.

R

Radicular Pertaining to a nerve root.
Ramus Branch.
Redundant Exuberant, more than normal or necessary.
Reflex A reaction, an involuntary stereotyped movement or exercise of function in a part, excited in response to a stimulus applied to the periphery and transmitted to the CNS.
Remission A lessening in severity; a temporary abatement of the symptoms of a disease.
Reticular Resembling a little net.
Retina Net; the inner lining of the eye that is specialized for light reception.
Retrusion A backward thrust.
Rhombencephalon The hindbrain; it is derived from the posterior of the three primitive cerebral vesicles, dividing secondarily into the metencephalon and myelencephalon; it includes the pons, cerebellum and medulla oblongata.
Rigidity Abnormal stiffness or inflexibility.
Rostral Relating to any rostrum or anatomic structure resembling a beak. Common use — toward the beak, i.e., toward the front end of the neuraxis.
Rubro- Red.

S

Saccule Small sac; the smaller of the two membranous sacs in the vestibule of the labyrinth.
Sagittal Resembling an arrow; in the line of an arrow shot from a bow, i.e., a plane in an anteroposterior direction.
Sigmoid Resembling in outline the letter S or one of the forms of the Greek sigma, e.g., the sigmoid sinus formed by the dura mater of the brain.
Somatic Bodily; related to the body.
Somatodendritic synapse A synaptic contract between the cell body (soma) of the presynaptic cell and a dendrite of the postsynaptic cell.
Somatotopy Somatotopic organization; orderly representation of the body surface in the organization of an internal portion of the CNS.
Somite One of the pair of masses formed from the mesoderm between the digestive canal and the dorsal surface of the body in the embryo. Each somite consists of a myotome (contributes to somatic musculature), dermatome (contributes to subcutaneous structures) and a sclerotome (contributes to the vertebral column and related structures).
Spasticity A state of muscular rigidity and spasm with exaggeration of the deep tendon reflexes.
Sphincter A band or lace; an orbicular muscle which, when in a state of normal contraction, serves to close one of the orifices of the body.
Splanchnic Visceral.
Spongioblast A primitive neuroglial cell.
Stapedius A small muscle in the middle ear inserted into the neck of the stapes.
Stellate Star-shaped.
Stereognosis The appreciation of the form of an object by means of touch.

Strabismus Squinting; a constant lack of parallelism of the visual axes of the eyes.

Subclavian Below the clavicle, particularly the blood vessels that arise in this location.

Substantia gelatinosa A light-colored, glassy, semitranslucent substance, composed chiefly of neuroglia and small nerve cells, which forms most of the dorsal part of the posterior horn of the spinal cord.

Substantia nigra Black substance; a pigmented nucleus of the midbrain.

Sulcus A furrow or ditch, especially those on the surface of the brain.

Supine Lying on the back.

Synapse To clasp; the region where some part of one nerve cell contacts the perikaryon dendrite or axon of another nerve cell. Transmission of nervous activity from one cell to another occurs at these contact sites. The term may also include the neuromuscular junction.

Syndrome Running together; the aggregate of symptoms associated with any morbid process, and constituting together the picture of the disease.

Synergist A muscle that assists another in its action.

Syringomyelia The presence of abnormal cavities in the spinal cord (myelon).

T

Tectum Roof; a structure of the midbrain; the superior and inferior colliculi.

Tegmentum Cover; the dorsal portion of the pons and of the cerebral peduncle of the midbrain.

Telencephalon End brain; the anterior division of the prosencephalon from which are developed the cerebral hemispheres, the lateral ventricles, the anterior part of the third ventricle, the foramina of Monro and the olfactory nerves.

Temporal Relating to the temple, or temporal lobe of the brain.

Teratogenic Relating to agents that produce congenital abnormalities.

Thalamus Bedroom, inner chamber; a major nucleus of the diencephalon.

Thrombosis The formation of a clot; a plug more or less completely occluding a blood vessel or one of the cavities of the heart, formed by coagulation of the blood or a deposition of some of its formed elements.

Tic douloureux A form of trigeminal neuralgia due to degenerative changes in the nerve.

Tinnitus Subjective noises (ringing, whistling, booming) in the ears.

Tractotomy Operative section of any tract of the nervous system.

Transcutaneous Across the skin.

Trapezoid A four-legged table, hence a structure with four sides (trapezoid body of the auditory system), with two sides parallel and two diverging.

Trauma A wound; an injury inflicted, usually more or less suddenly, by some physical agent.

Trigeminal Triplet; pertaining to the fifth cranial nerve.

Trochlea Pulley; pertaining to the fourth cranial nerve.

U

Uncus Hook; any hook-shaped process or structure, specifically the hook-shaped anterior extremity of the hippocampal convolution.

Utricle A small sac; the larger of the two membranous sacs in the vestibule of the labyrinth.

V

Vagus Wandering; descriptive of the tenth cranial nerve.

Velum Any structure resembling a veil or curtain, e.g., portions of the roof of the fourth ventricle.

Ventricle A small cavity, e.g., the ventricles of the brain.

Vermis Worm; the narrow middle lobe or connecting mass between the two hemispheres of the cerebellum.

Vertigo The sense of feeling movement of oneself or of one's environment.

Vestibule An entrance court; a portion of the inner ear.

Villus Shaggy hair; a minute projection from the surface; used in reference to the arachnoid villi where cerebrospinal fluid is reabsorbed.

REFERENCES

This section is divided into two parts. Part I consists of those books and papers from which the author has obtained information for this book. It also includes additional sources, which the reader is invited to investigate to grow further in knowledge of the neurosciences. Part II lists some of the classics in the field of neuroscience for those who wish to learn more about the great investigators of an earlier time.

PART I

Alpers, B. J. and E. L. Mancall: Essentials of the Neurological Examination. F. A. Davis Co., Philadelphia, 1973.

Anderson, J.: Dynamic characteristics of Golgi tendon organs. Brain Res., *67*:531–537, 1974.

Andrews, C. L., L. Knowles and J. Hancock: Control of the tonic vibration reflex by the brain stem reticular formation in the cat. J. Neurol. Sci., *18*:217–226, 1973.

Angaut, P. and A. Brodal: The projection of the "vestibulocerebellum" onto the vestibular nuclei in the cat. Arch. Ital. Biol., *105*:441–479, 1967.

Angevine, J. B. and R. L. Sidman: Autoradiographic study of cell migration during histogenesis of the cerebral cortex in the mouse. Nature, *192*:766–768, 1961.

Arey, L. B.: Developmental Anatomy. W. B. Saunders Co., Philadelphia and London, 4th ed., 1974.

Asanuma, H. and I. Rosen: Functional role of afferent inputs to the monkey motor cortex. Brain Res., *40*:3–5, 1972.

Ayres, A. J.: Sensory Integration and Learning Disorders. Western Psychological Services, Los Angeles, 1977.

Barker, D.: The structure and distribution of muscle receptors. *In* Symposium on Muscle Receptors. D. Barker, Ed. Hong Kong University Press, 1962, pp. 49–57.

Barker, D., M. J. Stacey and M. N. Adal: Fusimotor innervation in the cat. Phil. Trans. R. Soc. Lond., Series B., Biol. Sci., *258*:315–346, 1970.

Baxendale, R. H. and J. R. Rosenberg: Crossed reflex actions of group I muscle afferents. J. Physiol., *251*:53, 1975.

Bessou, P. and Y. LaPorte: Responses from primary and secondary endings of the same neuromuscular spindle of the tenuissimus muscle of the cat. *In* Symposium on Muscle Receptors. D. Barker, Ed. Hong Kong University Press, 1962, pp. 105–119.

Birdsong, J. H. and A. S. McKinney: Long-range motor performance changes in levodopa-treated patients with Parkinson's disease. Neurology, *24*:107–115, 1974.

Bishop, B.: Vibratory stimulation. Phys. Ther., Part I,

54:1274–1282, 1974; Part II, 55:28–34, 1975; Part III, 55:139–143, 1975.

Bobath, B.: Very early treatment of cerebral palsy. Dev. Med. Child Neurol., 9:373–390, 1967.

Bobath, B.: Motor development, its effect on general development and application to the treatment of cerebral palsy. Physiotherapy, 57:526–532, 1971.

Bobath, K. and B. Bobath: The facilitation of normal posture reactions and movements in the treatment of cerebral palsy. Physiotherapy, 57:515–525, 1971.

Bowen, F. P., E. Brady and M. D. Yahr: Sensorimotor coordination in Parkinson's disease before and after levodopa therapy. Neurology, 23:1101–1106, 1973.

Bowsher, D.: Termination of the central pain pathway: the conscious appreciation of pain. Brain, 80:606–622, 1957.

Bowsher, D.: The termination of secondary somatosensory neurons within the thalamus of Macaca mulatta: an experimental degeneration study. J. Comp. Neurol., 177:213–227, 1961.

Boyd, I. A.: The structure and innervation of the nuclear bag muscle fibre system and the nuclear chain muscle fibre system in mammalian muscle spindles. Physiol. Trans. R. Soc. Lond., Series B, Biol. Sci., 245:81–136, 1962.

Boyd, I. A., C. Eyzaguirre, P. B. C. Matthews and G. Rushworth: The Role of the Gamma System in Movement and Posture. Association for the Aid of Crippled Children, New York, 1968.

Brain, R.: Speech Disorders, Aphasia, Apraxia and Agnosia. Butterworths, London, 1961.

Brazelton, T. B.: Neonatal behavioral assessment scale. Clin. Dev. Med., 50, 1973.

Brodal, A.: The Reticular Formation of the Brain Stem. Anatomical Aspects and Functional Correlations. Charles C Thomas, Springfield, Ill., 1957.

Brodal, A.: Neurological Anatomy (In Relation to Clinical Medicine). Oxford University Press, New York, London and Toronto, 1972.

Brodal, A. and B. Hoivik: Site and mode of termination of primary vestibulo-cerebellar fibres in the cat. Arch. Ital. Biol., 102:1–21, 1964.

Brodal, A., O. Pompeiano and F. Walberg: The Vestibular Nuclei and Their Connections, Anatomy and Functional Correlations. Charles C Thomas, Springfield, Ill., 1962.

Brown, I. and M. J. Meng: Fundamentals of Electrotherapy (Course Guide). American Printing and Publishing, Inc., Madison, WI, 1971.

Buchwald, J. S.: Proprioceptive reflexes and posture. Am. J. Phys. Med., 46:104–113, 1967.

Buchwald, J. S.: A functional concept of motor control. Am. J. Phys. Med., 46:141–150, 1967.

Bunge, R. P.: Glial cells and the central myelin sheath. Physiol. Rev., 48:197–251, 1968.

Burke, D., C. J. Andrews and J. W. Lance: Tonic vibration reflex in spasticity, Parkinson's disease and normal subjects. J. Neurol. Neurosurg. Psychiatry, 35:477–486, 1972.

Butzer, J. F., D. E. Silver and A. L. Sahs: Amantadine in Parkinson's disease. Neurology, 25:603–606, 1975.

Carpenter, M. B.: Human Neuroanatomy, 7th ed. Williams and Wilkins Co., Baltimore, 1976.

Carpenter, M. B.: Ventral tier thalamic nuclei. *In* Modern Trends in Neurology, Vol. 4. D. Williams, Ed. Butterworths, London, 1976.

Carpenter, M. B. and P. Peter: Nigrostriatal and nigrothalamic fibers in the Rhesus monkey. J. Comp. Neurol., 144:93–116, 1972.

Carpenter, M. B., B. M. Stein and B. Peter: Primary vestibulocerebellar fibers in the monkey: distribution of fibers arising from distinctive cell groups of the vestibular ganglia. Am. J. Anat., *135*:221–250, 1972.

Casey, K. L.: The neurophysiological basis of pain. Postgrad. Med., *53*:58–63, 1973.

Cauna, N.: Fine structure of the receptor organs and its probable functional significance. *In* Touch, Heat and Pain. A. V. S. de Rueck and J. Knight, Eds. Ciba Foundation Symposium, Little, Brown and Co., Boston, 1966, pp. 117–127.

Chase, T. N., E. M. Holden and J. A. Brody: Levodopa-induced dyskinesias. Arch. Neurol., *29*:328–330, 1973.

Clark, D. L., J. R. Kreutzberg and F. K. W. Chee: Vestibular stimulation influence on motor development in infants. Science, *196*:1228–1229, 1976.

Cogan, D. G.: Neurology of the Ocular Muscles, 2nd ed. Charles C Thomas, Springfield, Ill., 1975.

Colonnier, M.: The fine structural arrangement of the cortex. Arch. Neurol., *16*:651–657, 1967.

Copenhaver, W. M., D. E. Kelly and R. L. Wood: Bailey's Textbook of Histology, 17th ed. Williams and Wilkins Co., Baltimore, 1978.

Cunningham's Textbook of Anatomy, 11th ed. G. J. Romanes, Ed. Oxford University Press, 1972.

Darian-Smith, I. and G. Mayday: Somatotopic organization within the brain stem trigeminal complex of the cat. Exp. Neurol., *2*:290–309, 1960.

Denny-Brown, D.: Motor mechanisms — Introduction: the general principles of motor integration. *In* Handbook of Physiology, Sect. 1, Vol. II. J. Field, Ed. American Physiological Society, Washington, D. C., 1960.

DeRobertis, E. D. P., F. A. Saez and E. M. F. DeRobertis, Jr.: Cell Biology, 6th ed. W. B. Saunders Co., Philadelphia, 1975.

Dietrichson, P., J. Presthus and R. Holmsen: Treatment of Parkinsonism with L-dopa and a decarboxylase inhibitor. Eur. Neurol., *13*:339–349, 1975.

Doudlah, A. M.: A Motor Developmental Checklist. Perceptual — Motor Research Section, Central Wisconsin Colony and Training School, 317 Knutson Drive, Madison, WI 53704. Copyright 1976, State of Wisconsin, Department of Health and Social Services.

Eccles, J. C.: The Physiology of Synapses. Springer-Verlag, Berlin, Gottingen, Heidelberg, 1964.

Eccles, J. C.: Functional organization of the cerebellum in relation to its role in motor control. *In* Muscular Afferents and Motor Control. R. Granit, Ed. Almquist and Wiksell, Stockholm, 1966.

Eccles, J. C., R. Llinas and K. Sasaki: The excitatory synaptic action of climbing fibers on the Purkinje cells of the cerebellum. J. Physiol., *182*: 268–296, 1966.

Eccles, J. C., R. Llinas and K. Sasaki: The inhibitory interneurones within the cerebellar cortex. Exp. Brain Res., *1*:1–16, 1966.

Eccles, J. C., R. Llinas and K. Sasaki: Parallel fibre stimulation and responses induced thereby in the Purkinje cells of the cerebellum. Exp. Brain Res., *1*:17–39, 1966.

Eccles, J. C., R. Llinas and K. Sasaki: The mossy fibre-granule cell relay of the cerebellum and its inhibitory control by Golgi cells. Exp. Brain Res., *1*:82–101, 1966.

Eldred, E.: The dual sensory role of muscle spindles. *In* The Child with Central Nervous System Deficit. U.S. Dept. of Health, Education and Welfare, 1965, pp. 8–31.

Eldred, E. and B. Fujimori: Relations of the reticular formation to muscle spindle activation. *In* Reticular Formation of the Brain. H. H. Jaspers, Ed. Little, Brown and Co., Boston, 1958.

Eldred, E., R. Granit and P. A. Merton: Supraspinal control

of the muscle spindles and its significance. J. Physiol., *122*: 498–523, 1953.

Endo, K., T. Araki and N. Yagi: The distribution and pattern of axon branching of pyramidal tract cells. Brain Res., *57*:484–491, 1973.

Englander, R. N., M. G. Netsky and L. S. Adelman: Location of human pyramidal tract in the internal capsule: anatomic evidence. Neurology, *25*: 823–826, 1975.

Engle, C. A. and B. H. Schofield: A review of the central response to peripheral nerve injury and its significance in nerve regeneration. J. Neurosurg., *37*:195–203, 1972.

Epstein, F., G. Hochwald and J. Ransohoff: A volume control system for the treatment of hydrocephalus: laboratory and clinical experience. J. Neurosurg., *38*:282–287, 1973.

Faull, R. L. M. and J. B. Carman: Ascending projections of the substantia nigra in the rat. J. Comp. Neurol., *132*:73–92, 1968.

Felix, D. and M. Weisendanger: Pyramidal and non-pyramidal motor cortical effects on distal forelimb muscles of monkeys. Exp. Brain Res., *12*:81–91, 1971.

Feringa, E. R., R. D. Johnson and J. S. Wendt: Spinal cord regeneration in rats after immunosuppressive treatment. Arch. Neurol., *32*:676–683, 1975.

Fitzgerald, M. J. T.: The innervation of the epidermis. *In* The Skin Senses. D. R. Kenshalo, Ed. Charles C Thomas, Springfield, Ill., 1968, pp. 61–83.

Fox, C. A., D. E. Hillman, K. A. Siegesmund and C. R. Dutta: The primate cerebellar cortex: a Golgi and electron microscope study. *In* The Cerebellum, Progress in Brain Research, Vol. 25. C. A. Fox and R. S. Snider, Eds. Elsevier Publishing Co., Amsterdam, 1967.

Frankenburg, W. K., and J. B. Dodds: Denver Developmental Screening Test. University of Colorado Medical Center, 1969.

Freeman, W. and J. W. Watts: Psychosurgery, Intelligence, Emotion and Social Behavior Following Prefrontal Lobotomy for Mental Disorders, 2nd ed. Charles C Thomas, Springfield, Ill., 1949.

Fry, W. J., R. Krumins, F. J. Fry, G. Thomas, S. Borbely and H. Ades: Origins and distribution of some efferent pathways from the mammillary nuclei of the cat. J. Comp. Neurol., *120*:195–258, 1963.

Gardner, F.: The nerve supply of muscles, joints and other deep structures. Bull. Hosp. Joint Dis., *21*:153–161, 1960.

Gauthier, G., O. Juge and A. Birchler: Parkinsonian syndromes. Treatment by association of L-dopa plus decarboxylase inhibitor. Eur. Neurol., *11*:133–157, 1974.

Gaze, R. M. and M. J. Keating, Eds.: Development and regeneration in the nervous system. Br. Med. Bull., *30*, 1974.

Gazzaniga, M. S.: The Bisected Brain. Appleton-Century-Crofts, New York, 1970.

Gazzaniga, M. S., J. E. Bogen and R. W. Sperry: Observations on visual perception after disconnexion of the cerebral hemispheres in man. Brain, *88*:221–236, 1965.

Gernandt, B. E., M. Iranyi and R. B. Livingston: Vestibular influences on spinal mechanisms. Exp. Neurol., *1*:248–273, 1959.

Gesell, A. and C. S. Amatruda: Developmental Diagnosis. Normal and Abnormal Child Development. Hoeber Division, Harper and Row, New York Evanston and London, 1969.

Gildenberg, P. L.: Stereotaxic lower cervical cordotomy for the treatment of intractable pain. Confin. Neurol., *34*:275–278, 1972.

Granit, R.: Receptors and Sensory Perception. Yale University Press, New Haven, 1975.

Granit, R. and R. Burke: The

control of movement and posture. Brain Res., *53*:1–28, 1973.

Grant, G.: Projection of the external cuneate nucleus onto the cerebellum in the cat: an experimental study using silver methods. Exp. Neurol., *5*:179–195, 1962.

Grant, G.: Spinal course and somatotopically localized termination of the spinocerebellar tracts. An experimental study in the cat. Acta Physiol. Scand., *56*: Suppl. 193:1–45, 1962.

Grant, G. and O. Oscarsson: Mass discharges evoked in the olivocerebellar tract on stimulation of muscle and skin nerves. Exp. Brain Res., *1*:329–337, 1966.

Gray, E. G.: Electron microscopy of presynaptic organelles of the spinal cord. J. Anat., Lond., *97*:101–106, 1963.

Gray, E. G. and R. W. Guillery: Synaptic morphology in the normal and degenerating nervous system. Int. Rev. Cytol., *19*:111–182, 1966.

Gray, H.: Anatomy of the Human Body, 29th ed. Lea and Febiger, Philadelphia, 1975.

Guillery, R. W.: Degeneration in the posterior commissural fornix and the mammillary peduncle of the rat. J. Anat., *90*:350–370, 1956.

Guillery, R. W.: A light and electron microscope study of neurofibrils and neurofilaments at neuro-neuronal junctions in the lateral geniculate nucleus of the cat. Am. J. Anat., *120*:583–604, 1976.

Guth, L. and C. D. Clemente, Eds.: Growth and regeneration in the central nervous system. Exp. Neurol., *48*, 1975.

Guyton, A. C.: Textbook of Medical Physiology, 3rd ed. W. B. Saunders Co., Philadelphia, 1976.

Hakim, S., F. D. de la Roche and J. D. Burton: A critical analysis of valve shunts used in the treatment of hydrocephalus. Dev. Med. Child Neurol., *15*:230–255, 1973.

Hamori, J. and J. Szentagothai: Identification under the electron microscope of climbing fibers and their synaptic contacts. Exp. Brain Res., *1*:65–81, 1966.

Harris, G. W. and R. George: Neurohumeral control of the adenohypophysis and regulation of the secretion of TSH, ACTH and growth hormone. *In* The Hypothalamus. W. Haymaker et al, Eds. Charles C Thomas, Springfield, Ill. 1969.

Hepp-Reymond, M. C. and M. Weisendanger: Unilateral pyramidotomy in monkeys: effect on force and speed of a conditioned precision grip. Brain Res., *36*:117–131, 1972.

Herman, R. and S. A. Mecomber: Vibration-elicited reflexes in normal and spastic muscle in man. Am. J. Phys. Med., *50*:169–183, 1971.

Homma, S., K. Ishikawa and S. Watanabe: Optimal frequency of muscle vibration for motoneuron firing. J. Chiba Med. Soc., *43*:190–196, 1967.

Hongo, T., E. Jankowska and A. Lundberg: The rubrospinal tract. I. Effects on alpha motoneurons innervating hindlimb muscles in cats. Exp. Brain Res., *7*:344–364, 1969.

Hongo, T., N. Kudo and R. Tanaka: Effects from the vestibulospinal tract on the contralateral hindlimb motoneurones in the cat. Brain Res., *31*:220–223, 1971.

Houk, J. C. and E. Henneman: Responses of Golgi tendon organs to active contractions of the soleus muscle of the cat. J. Neurophys., *30*:466–481, 1967.

Houk, J. C. and W. Simon: Responses of Golgi tendon organs to forces applied to muscle tendon. J. Neurophysiol., *30*:1466–1481, 1967.

Houk, J. C., J. J. Singer and E. Henneman: Adequate stimulus for tendon organs with observations on mechanics of ankle joint. J. Neurophys., *34*:1051–1065, 1971.

Hultborn, H. and A. Lundberg: Reciprocal inhibition during

the stretch reflex. Acta Physiol. Scand., *85*:136–138, 1972.

Humison, G. L.: Animal Tissue Techniques. W. H. Freeman and Co., San Francisco, 1972.

Hyden, H.: The neuron. *In* The Cell: Biochemistry, Physiology, Morphology, Vol. 4. J. Brachet and A. I. Mirsky, Eds. Academic Press, New York, 1960.

Iggo, A.: Electrophysiological and histological studies of cutaneous mechanoreceptors. *In* The Skin Senses. D. R. Kenshalo, Ed. Charles C. Thomas, Springfield, Ill., 1968.

Indeck, W. and A Printy: Skin application of electrical impulses for relief of pain (in chronic orthopedic conditions). Minn. Med., *58*:305–309, 1975.

Janetta, P. J.: Microsurgical approach to the trigeminal nerve for tic douloureux. Progr. Neurol. Surg., *7*:180–200, 1975.

Jones, E. G. and R. Y. Leavitt: Retrograde axonal transport and the demonstration of non-specific projections to the cerebral cortex and striatum from thalamic intralaminar nuclei in the cat, rat and monkey. J. Comp. Neurol., *54*:349–378, 1974.

Jones, E. G. and T. P. S. Powell: Connexions of the somatic sensory cortex of the Rhesus monkey. I. Ipsilateral cortical connexions. Brain, *92*:477–502, 1969.

Jones, E. G. and T. P. S. Powell: Connexions of the somatic sensory cortex of the Rhesus monkey. II. Contralateral cortical connexions. Brain, *92*:717–730, 1969.

Jones, E. G. and T. P. S. Powell: Connexions of the somatic sensory cortex of the Rhesus monkey. III. Thalamic connexions. Brain, *93*:37–56, 1970.

Josif, G., O. Pompeiano, P. Strata and U. Thoden: The effect of stimulation of spindle receptors and Golgi tendon organs on the cerebellar anterior lobe. Arch. Ital. Biol., I & II., *110*:476–542, 1972.

Kantner, R. M., D. L. Clark, L. C. Allen and M. F. Chase: Effects of vestibular stimulation on nystagmus response and motor performance in the developmentally delayed infant. Phys. Ther., *56*:414–421. 1976.

Katz, B.: Nerve, Muscle and Synapse. McGraw-Hill Book Co., New York, 1966.

Katz, B.: The Release of Neural Transmitter Substances Charles C Thomas, Springfield, Ill., 1969.

Keller, J. H. and P. J. Hand: Dorsal root projections to nucleus cuneatus of the cat. Brain Res., *20*:1–17, 1970.

Kemp, J. M. and T. P. S. Powell: The corticostriate projection in the monkey. Brain, *93*:525–546, 1970.

Kennedy, W. R.: Innervation of normal human muscle spindles. Neurology, *20*:463–475, 1970.

Kennedy, W. R., H. deF. Webster and K. S. Yoon: Human muscle spindles: fine structure of the primary sensory ending. J. Neurocytol., *4*:675–695, 1975.

Kerr, F. W. L., L. L. Kruger, H. O. Schwassman and R. Stern: Somatotopic organization of mechanoreceptor units in the trigeminal nuclear complex of the monkey. J. Comp. Neurol., *134*:127–144, 1968.

Knott, M., and D. E. Voss: Proprioceptive Neuromuscular Facilitation, 2nd ed. Harper and Row, Inc., Hagerstown, Md., 1968.

Krayenbuhl, H. and J. Siegfried: Dentatotomies or thalamotomies in the treatment of hyperkinesia. Confin. Neurol., *34*:29–33, 1972.

Kuypers, H. G. J. M. and D. G. Lawrence: Cortical projections to the red nucleus and the brain stem in the Rhesus monkey. Brain Res., *4*:151–188, 1967.

Landgren, S. and H. Silfvenius: Projection to cerebral cortex of group I muscle afferents from the cat's hindlimb. J. Physiol. Lond., *200*:353–372, 1969.

Larsell, O. and J. Jansen: The Comparative Anatomy and Histology of the Cerebellum. The Human Cerebellum, Cerebellar Connections and Cerebellar Cortex. University of Minnesota Press, Minneapolis, 1972.

Lawrence, D. G. and D. A. Hopkins: Developmental aspects of pyramidal motor control in the Rhesus monkey. Brain Res., *40*:117–118, 1972.

Lawrence, D. G. and H. G. J. M. Kuypers. The functional organization of the motor system in the monkey. I. The effects of bilateral pyramidal lesions. Brain, *91*:1–14, 1968.

Leksell, L., B. A. Meyerson and D. M. Forster: Radiosurgical thalamotomy for intractable pain. Confin. Neurol., *34*:264, 1972.

Lemire, R. J., J. D. Loeser, R. W. Leech and C. A. Ellsworth, Jr.: Normal and Abnormal Development of the Human Nervous System, Harper and Row, Inc., Hagerstown, Md., 1975.

Lieberman, A. N.: Parkinson's disease: a clinical review. Am. J. Med. Sci., *267*:66–80, 1974.

Liu, C. N. and W. W. Chambers: An experimental study of the corticospinal system in the monkey (Macaca mulatta). The spinal pathways and preterminal distribution of degenerating fibers following discrete lesions of the pre- and postcentral gyri and bulbar pyramid. J. Comp. Neurol., *123*:257–284, 1964.

Liu, H. M.: Schwann cell properties. 1. Origin of Schwann cells during peripheral nerve regeneration. J. Neuropathol. Exp. Neurol., *32*:458–473, 1973.

Livingston, R. B.: Mechanics of cerebrospinal fluid. *In* Physiology and Biophysics. T. C. Ruch and H. D. Patton, Eds. W. B. Saunders Co., Philadelphia, 1965.

Loeser, J. D.: The management of tic douloureux. Pain, *3*:155–162, 1977.

Loeser, J. D., R. G. Black and A. Christman: Relief of pain by transcutaneous stimulation. J. Neurosurg., *42*:308–314, 1975.

Loewy, A. D., J. C. Araugo and F. W. L. Kerr: Pupillodilator pathways in the brainstem of the cat; anatomical and electrophysiological identification of a central autonomic pathway. Brain Res. *60*:65–91, 1973.

Mann, M. D.: Axons of dorsal spinocerebellar tract which respond to activity in cutaneous receptors. J. Neurophysiol., *6*:1035–1050, 1971.

Mann, M. D.: Clarke's column and the dorsal spinocerebellar tract. A review. Brain Behav. Evol., *7*:34–83, 1973.

Mars, H.: Levodopa, carbidopa and pyridoxine in Parkinson disease. Arch. Neurol., *30*:444–447, 1974.

Martin, W. E., R. B. Loewenson, J. A. Resch and A. B. Baker: Parkinson's disease (clinical analysis of 100 patients). Neurology, *23*:783–790, 1973.

Marx, J. L.: Analgesia: how the body inhibits pain perception. Science, *195*:471–473, 1977.

Massion, J.: The mammalian red nucleus. Physiol. Rev., *47*:383–436, 1967.

Matthews, P. B. C.: Muscle spindles and their motor control. Physiol. Rev., *44*:219–287, 1964.

McGraw, M. B.: The Neuromuscular Maturation of the Human Infant. Hafner Publishing Co., New York and London, 1966.

McIntyre, A. K.: Central projection of impulses from receptors activated by muscle stretch. *In* Symposium on Muscle Receptors. D. Barker, Ed. Hong Kong University Press, 1962, pp. 19–29.

Melzack, R. and P. D. Wall: Pain mechanisms: a new theory. Science, *150*:971–979, 1965.

Meyers, R. E.: Function of corpus callosum in interocular transfer. Brain, *79*:358–363, 1956.

Milani-Comparetti, A. and E. A. Gidoni: Pattern analysis of motor development and its disorders. Dev. Med. Child Neurol., *9*:625–630, 1967.

Milani-Comparetti A. and E. A. Gidoni: Routine developmental examination in normal and retarded children. Dev. Med. Child Neurol., *9*:631–638, 1967.

Miller, S. and D. Oscarsson: Termination and functional organization of spino-olivocerebellar paths. *In* The Cerebellum in Health and Disease. W. S. Fields and W. D. Willis, Eds. Warren H. Green, Inc., St. Louis, 1970.

Mones, R. J.: Parkinson's disease treated with L-dopa. N.Y. State J. Med., *72*:2749–2750, 1972.

Moore, R. Y., R. K. Bhatnagar and A. Heller: Anatomical and chemical studies of a nigro-neostriatal projection in the cat. Brain Res., *30*:119–135, 1971.

Mountcastle, V. B.: Medical Physiology, Vol. II, 13th ed. C. V. Mosby Co., St. Louis, 1974.

Munger, B. L., L. M., Pubols and B. H. Pubols: The Merkel rete papilla — a slowly adapting sensory receptor in mammalian glabrous skin. Brain. *29*:47–61, 1971.

Murphy, J. T. and N. H. Sabah: Cerebellar Purkinje cell responses to afferent inputs. II. Mossy fiber activation. Brain Res., *25*:469–482, 1970.

Nathaniel, E. J. H. and D. R. Nathaniel: The ultrastructural features of the synapses in the posterior horn of the spinal cord in the rat. J. Ultrastr. Res., *14*:540–555, 1966.

Nauta, W. J. H.: The central visceromotor system: a general survey. *In* Limbic System Mechanisms and Autonomic Function. C. H. Hockman, Ed. Charles C Thomas, Springfield, Ill., 1972.

Nauta, W. J. H. and H. G. J. M. Kuypers: Some ascending pathways in the brain stem reticular formation. *In* Reticular Formation of the Brain. H. H. Jasper et al., Eds. Henry Ford Hospital International Symposium, Little, Brown and Co., Boston, 1958.

Noback, C. R. and L. K. Laemle: Structural and functional aspects of the visual pathways of primates. *In* The Primate Brain, Advances in Primatology, Vol. I. C. R. Noback and W. Montague, Eds. Appleton-Century-Crofts, New York, 1970.

Nyberg-Hansen, R.: Origin and termination of fibers from the vestibular nuclei descending in the medial longitudinal fasciculus. An experimental study with silver impregnation methods in the cat. J. Comp. Neurol., *122*:255–268, 1964.

Nyberg-Hansen, R.: Anatomic demonstration of gamma motoneurons in the cat's spinal cord. Exp. Neurol., *13*:71–81, 1965.

Nyberg-Hansen, R.: Sites and mode of termination of reticulospinal fibers in the cat. An experimental study with silver impregnation methods. J. Comp. Neurol., *124*:71–99, 1965.

Orbach, J. and K. L. Chow: Differential effects of resection of somatic areas I and II in monkeys. J. Neurophysiol., *22*: 195–203, 1959.

Oscarsson, O.: Functional organization of the spino- and cuneocerebellar tracts. Physiol. Rev., *45*:495–522, 1965.

Oscarsson, O.: Termination and functional organization of a dorsal spino-olivocerebellar path. Brain Res., *5*:531–534, 1967.

Oscarsson, O.: Functional significance of information channels from the spinal cord to the cerebellum. *In* Neurophysiological Basis of Normal and Abnormal Activities. M. D. Yahr and D. P. Purpura, Eds. Raven Press, New York, 1967.

Palay, S. L. and V. Chan-Palay:

Cerebellar Cortex. Cytology and Organization. Springer Verlag, Berlin, 1973.

Patten, J.: Neurological Differential Diagnosis. Harold Starke, Ltd., Springer Verlag, New York, Heidelberg, Berlin, 1977.

Peele, T. L.: The Neuroanatomical Basis for Clinical Neurology. McGraw Hill Book Co., New York, 1976.

Penfield, W. and H. H. Jasper: Epilepsy and the Functional Anatomy of the Human Brain. Little, Brown and Co., Boston, 1954.

Penfield, W. and T. Rasmussen: The Cerebral Cortex of Man. A Clinical Study of Localization of Function. Macmillan Co., New York, 1950.

Peters, A., S. L. Palay and H. DeF. Webster: The Fine Structure of the Nervous System. W. B. Saunders Co., Philadelphia, 1976.

Pickford, M.: Neurohypophysis-antidiuretic (vasopressor) and oxytocic hormones. *In* The Hypothalamus, W. Haymaker et al., Eds. Charles C Thomas, Springfield, Illinois, 1969.

Pinder, R. M.: The pharmacology of Parkinsonism. *In* Progress in Medicinal Chemistry, Vol. 9. G. P. Ellis and G. B. West, Eds. Butterworths, London, 1973.

Poggio, G. F. and V. B. Mountcastle: A study of the functional contributions of the lemniscal and spinothalamic systems to somatic sensibility. Bull. Johns Hopkins Hosp., *106*:266–316, 1960.

Pompeiano, O. and A. Brodal: Spinovestibular fibers in the cat. An experimental study. J. Comp. Neurol., *108*:353–382, 1957.

Powell, T. P. S., W. M. Cowan and G. Raisman: The central olfactory connexions. J. Anat., *99*:791–813, 1965.

Powell, T. P. S. and V. B. Mountcastle: Some aspects of the functional organization of the cortex of the postcentral gyrus of the monkey: a correlation of findings obtained in a single unit analysis with cytoarchitecture. Bull. Johns Hopkins Hosp., *105*:133–162, 1959.

Proske, U. and D. M. Lewis: The effects of muscle stretch and vibration on fusimotor activity in the lightly anaesthetised cat. Brain Res., *46*:55–69, 1972.

Raisman, G.: Neural connexions of hypothalamus. Br. M. Bull., *22*:197–201, 1966.

Raisman, G.: The connexions of the septum. Brain, *89*:317–348, 1966.

Raisman, G., W. M. Cowan and T. P. S. Powell: The extrinsic afferent, commissural and association fibres of the hippocampus. Brain, *88*:963–996, 1965.

Ralston, H. J., III: The synaptic organization in the dorsal horn of the spinal cord and in the ventrobasal thalamus in the cat. *In* Oral-Facial Sensory and Motor Mechanisms. R. Dubner and Y. Kawamura, Eds. Appleton-Century-Crofts, New York, 1971.

Rexed, B.: Some aspects of the cytoarchitectonics and synaptology of the spinal cord. *In* Organization of the Spinal Cord, Progress in Brain Research, Vol. 2. J. C. Eccles and J. P. Schade, Eds. Elsevier Publishing Co., Amsterdam, 1964.

Rhoton, A. L., J. L. O'Leary and J. P. Ferguson: The trigeminal, facial, vagal and glossopharyngeal nerves in the monkey. Arch. Neurol., *14*:530–540, 1966.

Richter, C. P. and L. N. Bartemeier: Decerebrate rigidity of the sloth. Brain, *49*:207–225, 1926.

Rivera-Dominguez, M., F. A., Mettler and C. R. Noback: Origins of cerebellar climbing fibers in the Rhesus monkey. J. Comp. Neurol., *155*:331–342, 1974.

Robers, W. J.: Tendon organ function. Brain Res., *28*:345–350, 1971.

Rood, M. S.: Neurophysiological mechanisms utilized in

the treatment of neuromuscular dysfunction. Am. J. Occup. Ther., *10*:220–225, 1956.

Rose, J. E.: Organization of frequency sensitive neurons in the cochlear complex of the cat. *In* Neural Mechanisms of the Auditory and Vestibular Systems. G. L. Rasmussen and W. E. Windle, Eds. Charles C Thomas, Springfield, Ill., 1960.

Rose, J. E., R. Galambos and J. R. Hughes: Microelectrode studies of the cochlear nuclei of the cat. Bull. Johns Hopkins Hosp., *104*:211–251, 1959.

Rosenberg, J. R. and K. W. Lindsay: Asymmetric tonic labyrinthine reflexes. Brain Res., *63*:347–350, 1973.

Rosenbluth, J.: Functions of glial cells. *In* The Central Nervous System. O. T. Bailey and D. E. Smith, Eds. Williams and Wilkins Co., Baltimore, 1968.

Rothman, K. J. and R. R. Monson: Survival in trigeminal neuralgia. J. Chronic Dis., *26*:303–309, 1973.

Salmon, G. and G. Lazorthes: Atlas of the Arteries of the Human Brain. Sandoz Co., Paris, 1971.

Saper, C. B., A. L. Loewy, L. W. Swanson and W. M. Cowan: Direct hypothalamo-autonomic connections. Brain Res., *117*:305–312, 1976.

Saper, C. B., N. D. Yamodis and A. D. Loewy: Edinger-Westphal nucleus: projections to medulla and spinal cord. Abstr., Soc. Neurosci., *III*, 1977.

Sasaki, K., S. Kawaguchi, Y. Matsuda and N. Mizuno: Electrophysiological studies on cerebello-cerebral projections in the cat. Exp. Brain Res., *16*:75–88, 1972.

Scalzi, H. A. and H. M. Price: The arrangement and sensory innervation of the intrafusal fibers in the feline muscle spindle. J. Ultrastr. Res., *36*:375–390, 1971.

Scarff, J. E.: Unilateral prefrontal lobotomy for relief of intractable pain and termination of narcotic addiction. Surg. Gynecol. Obstet., *89*:385–392, 1949.

Schaltenbrand, G. and C. N. Woolsey, Eds.: Cerebral localization and organization. *In* Proceedings, Symposium, World Federation of Neurology, Lisbon, Portugal, 1960.

Scheibel, M. E. and A. B. Scheibel: Structural organization of nonspecific nuclei and their projection toward the cortex. Brain Res., *6*:60–94, 1967.

Schwartz, D. W. F., L. Deecke and J. M. Frederickson: Cortical projection of group I muscle afferents to areas 2, 3a and the vestibular field in the Rhesus monkey. Exp. Brain Res., *17*:516–526, 1973.

Shapovalov, A. I. and N. R. Gurevitch: Monosynaptic and disynaptic reticulospinal actions on lumbar motoneurons of the rat. Brain Res., *21*:249–263, 1970.

Skoglund, S.: Muscle afferents and motor control in the kitten. *In* Nobel Symposium on Muscle Control and Reflex Afferents. R. Granit, Ed. 1967.

Stauffer, E. K. and J. A. Stephens: The tendon organs of cat soleus: static sensitivity to active force. Exp. Brain Res., *23*:279–291, 1975.

Strominger, N. L. and A. I. Strominger: Ascending brain stem projections of the anteroventral cochlear nucleus in the Rhesus monkey. J. Comp. Neurol., *143*:217–242, 1971.

Stuart, D. G., C. G. Mosher, R. L. Gerlach and R. M. Reinking: Mechanical arrangement and transducing properties of Golti tendon organs. Exp. Brain Res., *14*:274–292, 1972.

Sugita, K., N. Mutsuga, Y. Takaoka and T. Doi: Results of stereotaxic thalamotomy for pain. Confin. Neurol., *34*:265–274, 1972.

Swanson, L. W.: Immunohistochemical evidence for a neurophysin-containing autonomic pathway arising in the paraventricular nucleus of the hypothalamus. Brain Res., *128*:346–353, 1977.

Swash, M. and K. P. Fox: Muscle spindle innervation in man. J. Anat., *112*:61–80, 1972.

Szabo, J.: Projections from the body of the caudate nucleus in the Rhesus monkey. Exp. Neurol., *27*:1–15, 1970.

Torvik, A.: Phagocytosis of nerve cells during retrograde degeneration. An electron microscope study. J. Neuropathol. Exp. Neurol., *31*:132–145, 1972.

Travis, A. M.: Neurological deficiencies after ablation of the precentral motor area in Macaca mulatta. Brain, *78*:155–173, 1955.

Travis, A. M.: Neurological deficiencies following supplementary motor area lesions in Macaca mulatta. Brain, *78*: 174–198, 1955.

Travis, A. M. and C. N. Woolsey: Motor performance of monkeys after bilateral, partial and total cerebral decortications. Am. J. Phys. Med., *35*:273–310, 1956.

Van Buren, J. M. and R. C. Borke: Variations and Connections of the Human Thalamus. Springer-Verlag, New York, 1972.

VanGilder, J. C. and J. L. O'Leary: Topical projection of the olivocerebellar system in the cat: an electrophysiological study. J. Comp. Neurol., *140*:69–80, 1970.

Volpe, E. P.: Human Heredity and Birth Defects. Bobbs-Merrill, New York, 1971.

Walberg, F.: Cerebellovestibular relations: anatomy. Progr. Brain Res., *37*:361–376, 1972.

Walberg, F.: Descending connections from the mesencephalon to the inferior olive: an experimental study in the cat. Exp. Brain Res., *21*:145–156, 1974.

Walker, A. E.: Internal structure and afferent-efferent relations of the thalamus. *In* The Thalamus. D. P. Purpura and M. D. Yahr, Eds. Columbia University Press, New York, 1966.

Williams P. and R. Warwick: Functional Neuroanatomy of Man (from Gray's Anatomy, 35th British Ed.) W. B. Saunders Co., Philadelphia, 1975.

Woolsey, C. N.: Patterns of sensory representation in the cerebral cortex. Fed. Proc., *6*:437–441, 1947.

Woolsey, C. N.: Organization of somatic sensory and motor areas of the cerebral cortex. *In* Biological and Biochemical Bases of Behavior. H. F. Harlow and C. N. Woolsey, Eds. University of Wisconsin Press, Madison, 1958.

Woolsey, C. N. and D. Fairman: Contralateral, ipsilateral and bilateral representation of cutaneous receptors in somatic areas I and II of the cerebral cortex of pigs, sheep and other mammals. Surgery, *19*:684–702, 1946.

Woolsey, C. N., P. H. Settlage, D. R. Meyer, W. Spencer, T. P. Hamuy and A. M. Travis: Patterns of localization in precentral and "supplementary" motor areas and their relation to the concept of a premotor area. A. Res. Nerv. Ment. Dis. Proc., *30*:238–264, 1951.

Woolsey, C. N. and G. H. Wang: Somatic areas I and II of the cerebral cortex of the rabbit. Fed. Proc., 4:79, 1945.

PART II

Brodmann, K.: Vergleichende Localisationlehre der Grosshirnrinde in ihren Prinzipien Dargestellt auf Grund des Zellenbaues. J. A. Barth, Leipsig, 1909.

Cajal, S. Ramón Y.: Histologie du Système Nerveux de L'homme et des Vertebrates, 2 Vols. Norbert Maloine, Paris, 1909, 1911.

Cajal, S. Ramón Y.: Degeneration and Regeneration of the Nervous System, Vol. I. Translated by R. M. May, Oxford University Press, London, 1928.

Langley, J. N.: The Autonomic Nervous System, Vol. 1. W. Heffner and Sons, Cambridge, 1921.

Sherrington, C. S.: The Integrative Action of the Nervous System. Yale University Press, New Haven, 1906.

Waldeyer, W.: Ueber einege neuere Forschungen und Gebiete der Anatomie des Centralnervensystems. Dtsch. Med. Wochenschr., *17*:1891.

INDEX

Page numbers in *italic* type refer to illustrations.
Page numbers followed by (t) refer to tables.